S

NUMBER 47

THE HISTORY OF MEDICINE SERIES

ISSUED UNDER THE AUSPICES OF
THE LIBRARY OF
THE NEW YORK ACADEMY OF MEDICINE

ESSAYS ON THE HISTORY OF MEDICINE

Selected from the Bulletin of the New York Academy of Medicine

Edited by

SAUL JARCHO, M.D.

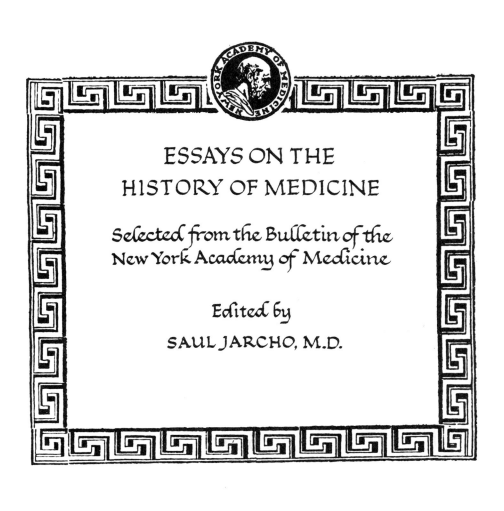

Published by
Science History Publications/USA
a division of
Neale Watson Academic Publications, Inc.
156 Fifth Avenue, New York, N.Y. 10010

Library of Congress Cataloging in Publication Data
Main entry under title:

Essays and notes on the history of medicine.

Bibliography: p.
Includes index.
1. Medicine--History--Addresses, essays, lectures.
I. Jarcho, Saul. II. New York Academy of Medicine.
Bulletin. [DNLM: 1. History of medicine--Collected
works. WZ5 5E78]
R131.E78 610'.9 76-11770
ISBN 0-88202-066-8

Designed and manufactured in the U.S.A.

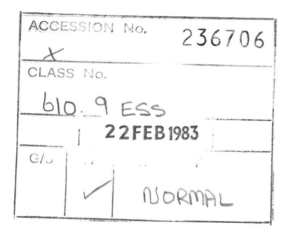

Contents

Medicine in New York

Paleopathology

Medical Numismatic Notes

PREFACE

At a meeting held on January 13, 1976 under the chairmanship of Dr. William Ober the Library Publications Committee of the New York Academy of Medicine resolved to publish a selection of historical articles and notes that had appeared in the Academy's *Bulletin.* In these writings, contributed by Fellows of the Academy and non-Fellows, by physicians and non-physicians, and by professional historians, amateur historians, and by scholars in many disciplines, history had been interpreted broadly and included not only medical history as ordinarily presented but also ancillary subjects such as paleopathology, medical geography and cartography, and medical numismatics. Some of these subjects are almost totally without other representation in contemporary medical journalism, especially in clinical periodicals. The papers of Fielding H. Garrison, published in 1966 under the Committee's auspices, had proved successful by customary criteria and offered both precedent and encouragement for the present eclectic enterprise.

From the plethora of available papers only a relatively small number could be chosen. The choices were designed to reflect the modern broad interpretation of the history of medicine. With this as a general principle an effort was made to provide representation of major chronologic periods, of various continents and countries, and of men, books, ideas, and ideals. At the same time it was recognized that the diversity of the choices would reveal anew the broad scope which the *Bulletin* has attempted to maintain as a medical journal that sets before the world an attractive combination of technical, sociological, and humanistic writings.

This being said, it was necessary to make the familiar choice between a chronological and topical arrangement. It was found that without undue violence the majority of the papers could be put into approximate chronological order from antiquity to modern times. Four additional papers form a separate group on medicine in New York. Two other essays exemplify aspects of paleopathology. The two last papers represent the *Bulletin's* special series on medical numismatics.

Should the present assemblage gain approval, the Committee will consider the publication of collected articles on clinical, technical, and social aspects of medicine. Materials of this character necessarily form the bulk of the *Bulletin's* content.

The selections contained in this book lead naturally to considerations of scope. How far can the present collection be deemed representative of present-day research and writing in the history of medicine?

Let us consider first the temporal aspect of this question. It did not prove difficult for the present editor to assemble a series of contributions which represent Greco-Roman antiquity, the Middle Ages, the Renaissance, and each century of more recent times. Among articles published in the *Bulletin* writings on medicine in the Middle Ages proved to be scarce, especially in comparison with the relative abundance of articles on ancient medicine—most especially Greek. That the Greeks outnumber the Romans in our indices will astonish no one: Nowadays a few physicians read Hippocrates but, so far as can be ascertained, very few read Celsus and rarely does anyone have the hardihood to cull the medical passages out of Pliny. Among Greek writers nearly all the attention goes to Hippocrates and Galen; the Byzantine clinicians apparently are unread.

The geographical scope of the *Bulletin's* medico-historical articles, represented by the present selection, also deserves attention. The history of medicine as herein represented proves to be the history of medicine in the United States and in parts of western Europe—chiefly Great Britain, France, Germany, Austria, Italy, and Greece. An exceptional essay in our series deals with Brazil, another with Australia. Assuredly historical studies are made in other countries and about other countries, but few have reached us. There has been no representation of Africa or Asia.

A different consideration is that of subject matter. A reader courageous enough to study tables of contents—whether the tables in the present book or those in successive volumes of the *Bulletin of the New York Academy of Medicine* or those in American periodicals devoted specially to the history of medicine—soon recognizes that the various parts of clinical medicine receive unequal attention from students of medical history. Infectious diseases—from the plague of Athens to poliomyelitis and beyond—have long been favored. Much has been written also about the history of nutritional disease and about diseases of the heart, lungs, kidneys, and other useful organs. In general these subjects come within the history of what to-day are called internal medicine and public health. Much has been written also about therapeutics, pediatrics, pathology, surgery, and anesthesiology. Much has been written about the history of psychiatry.

Nowadays the number, volume, and verbosity of writings in the history of psychiatry contrast with the scarcity of writings on the history of neurology; indeed, the contrast may tell us something about the relative influence of these two subjects in American life.

The other medical specialties contribute little to recent medico-historical periodical writing. There are few articles on the history of ophthalmology, obstetrics, urology, proctology, plastic surgery, dermatology, physiotherapy, and radiology.

These inequalities are difficult to explain. They probably depend in part on differences in temperament; some prefer the pen, others the scalpel. In part the differences depend also on differences in education. Another factor is simply that of number. It is obvious that the specialties least represented in medico-historical bibliographies are the specialties that have the smallest number of practitioners. Some specialist physicians prefer to publish their occasional historical efforts in the periodical journals of their own specialty.

This leads us to a difficult question, more or less unanswerable. To what extent should clinical periodicals publish articles on the history of medicine? In actual practice the determining factors appear to be the tastes or wishes of the reader and of the editors. Surveys being troublesome, unreliable, and expensive, editors of medical periodicals rarely engage in them but prefer to rely on their own opinions or the opinions of consultants. The occasional unsolicited letter or oral comment from a reader may be welcomed if it is encouraging or shrugged off if it is adverse, but can scarcely be a guide to policy.

In actual practice most clinical journals publish no more than occasional historical papers. The annual historical and literary issues of the *Journal of the American Medical Association* will be remembered long and favorably as bright exceptions. Some specialty journals publish historical articles regularly or frequently. As the economic condition of American clinical periodicals glides from dubious to precarious, articles on history may be viewed as an expensive intrusion which competes with technical subject matter.

It must also be noted that unwise policy has permitted or forced a catastrophic reduction of standards at all stages of American education—elementary, secondary, collegiate, and postgraduate. As a result, the American is more and more likely to be a technician who has been trained by technicians, rather than an educated man educated by scholars. Because of these processes, dominant for several decades, humanistic interests and humanistic research and writing are on the defensive in contemporary American medicine. This is true despite the recent upsurge of aggressive humanitarianism; enthusiasts, indeed, confuse the two terms and the two attitudes.

It appears impossible to foretell whether the remaining decades of the present century will improve the American intellectual climate and will secure a more favorable reception of the history of medicine. Prognosis being the weakest part of medicine, it may be best to avoid prediction and to rely on hope.

For assistance of many different kinds thanks are due to Sylvan Levey, Franklin Furness, Phylis Furth, June Beasley Fairclough, Barbara Sonnier, Francoise Duvivier, and Neale Watson.

For the Committee:

SAUL JARCHO, M. D.,
Editor-in-Chief
Bulletin of the New York Academy of Medicine
March, 1976

THE ORIGINS OF MODERN SCIENTIFIC THINKING

GREGORY I. ALTSCHULLER

Consultant in Medicine
The Roosevelt Hospital
New York, N. Y.

MEDICINE always has had and always will have two aspects: one scientific and the other clinical, in the broadest sense of the words. In different periods of history one or the other has dominated the mind of the medical man but both aspects have always been present.

Speaking of the origins of modern scientific thinking implies, therefore, also discussing the origins of scientific medicine. Some of the great natural philosophers of ancient Greece, as well as some of the outstanding scientists of modern times, have been physicians who contributed greatly both to physical sciences and to medicine. However, specific problems of medicine, important as they are and however closely they are connected with the development of scientific thinking, will be discussed only briefly in this essay.

Richard Mead, M.D. (1673-1754), physician to Sir Isaac Newton and physician-in-ordinary to King George II of England, was one of the most prominent and successful physicians in London, widely known for his professional skill and his literary reputation and respected for his kindness and generosity. He was a protégé of Dr. John Ratcliff, who presented him with his famous gold-headed cane as a token of respect and friendship.[1]

Dr. Mead lived at the time when somewhat primitive iatrochemical and iatrophysical theories impressed the minds of many leading medical men. He belonged to a small group of English physicians who at the very beginning of the 18th century attempted to apply the methods and principles of mathematics and of physical science to medicine. He acquired knowledge of these methods and became an ardent adept of the iatrophysical school while studying medicine in Padua and Leyden.[2] However, he avoided the most extreme theories of his teacher, John Pitcairn, representative of the iatromathematical school in England, although in his paper on "Mechanical Account of Poisons" (1702)

Dr. Mead tried to explain the action of poisons as the effect on the stomach of "small knives and daggers" he had observed under his microscope. In his later works he attempted to explain the influence of celestial bodies on the course of various diseases by gravitational attraction, by variations in the atmospheric pressure, and by similar factors. His ideas about the importance of quantitative mathematical methods as applied to medicine are best expressed in the following passage:

> . . . It is very evident that all other Methods of improving Medicine have been found ineffectual by the Stand It has been at these Three or Four thousand years, and since late Mathematicians have set themselves to the study of It, Men do already begin to talk so Intelligibly and Comprehensively even about abstruse Matters that it may be hoped in a short time, if Those who are designed for this Profession, are early, while their Minds and Bodies are Patient of Labour and Toil, initiated in the Knowledge of Numbers and Geometry, that Mathematical Learning will be the Distinguishing Mark of a Physician from a Quack, and He, who wants this necessary Qualification will be as ridiculous as One without Greek or Latin.[3]

Even if this enthusiastic prediction has not come true in the past 200 odd years, ours is the age of computers, and we are coming rather close to the ideas of Dr. Mead.

What are the characteristics of modern science? Without making any attempt at an accurate definition, we might summarize them as follows. Modern science is characterized by a desire to discover the laws of nature. These laws must be of general order and few, the tacit assumption being, as in ancient Greece, that there exists in nature an *order* and that nature loves simplicity ("*natura simplicitatem amat*"). All laws of nature must be expressed in mathematical language, and qualities must be replaced by quantities. Numbers and measurements are the basic tools of modern science, and deduction is combined with induction.[4]

Newton's universal law of gravitation is of such a general order. Since the time of Newton two important forces have been added to the force of gravity: the *electromagnetic force*, known since the time of Michael Faraday, and the *intra-atomic, nuclear force*, which became known in the 20th century. James C. Maxwell's field theory, first described in his paper "A Dynamical Theory of the Electromagnetic Field" (1865),[5] gradually replaced the older Newtonian concept of force and became one of the most important discoveries of modern physics. It led to Albert Einstein's theory of relativity and to his concept of a four-dimension continuum that forms the world of events.[6] In its final development matter and field became only two forms of energy which differ quantitatively but not qualitatively.[7]

Modern physicists accept the force of attraction that holds things together, such as the force of gravity and a centrifugal force which causes the expansion of the universe or the repulsion of particles with an opposite electrical charge.

Of great importance is the use of models and experiments instead of the simple observation of nature. Niels Bohr's model of the atom and the double helix as the model of DNA described by James D. Watson and Francis H. C. Crick are examples of the use of models in modern science. Experiments are the most important tools in modern scientific research, whether the laws of nature are discovered on the basis of experiments, as in Newtonian theory or, as in the epistemological approach of Einstein and other modern scientists, an experiment proves or disproves theoretical concepts deduced by the scientist from certain a priori assumptions.

The results of his theoretical investigations are applied by the modern scientist to problems of practical importance. This last point is the one which makes such a great difference between the work of ancient natural philosophers and of modern scientists.

In ancient Egypt, as well as in Babylon and Assyria, there was a highly developed technology but no science in the proper sense of the word. Pyramids were built, and also temples, an elaborate system of roads, mines on the Sinai Peninsula, and endless canals on which the very life of Egypt depended. In medicine hundreds of detailed prescriptions—some empirical, others rather magical—were recorded in papyri. A perfectly organized hierarchy of physicians existed that would gladden the heart of the 18th century professor Johann Peter Frank, famous author of the *System einer vollständiger medicinischer Polizey*. There was a Chief of the Secrets of Health, the Guardian of the Imperial Anus, and a whole network of inspectors, supervisors, and superintendents of various ranks who controlled the activities of thousands of physician-specialists; each took care of only one part of the body. In addition to these there were ordinary physician-magicians.[8]

But behind this imposing structure there was very little knowledge of pathology, very little rational theory. Physiology begins when man enters into speculations about the significance of three basic substances essential to life: air and food, both coming from the outside world, and blood within the body itself. The only rational pathology created by ancient Egypt was the theory of *WeHeDuW*, or *perittoma* in its later Greek version, related to the universal observation of the decay of all organic matter. It was probably based on the observation that the decomposition of a corpse starts in the large intestine. The decay of organic matter produces heat and odor. In the body of a sick man this decay or the process of putrefaction produces a pyogenic principle *WeHeDuW* which can pass into the bloodstream and cause fever and rapid pulse. Thus a state of pyemia is created which, if not treated properly, endangers health and life. Before the poisonous residues are absorbed into the bloodstream, they must be removed by enemas or purges or, later, by bloodletting. The Egyptian idea of putrefaction of the ingested food in the intestine as the major etiological principle of most illnesses was taken over by the Cnidians, still later elaborated by Galen,[9-11] and became the logical basis for bloodletting, which dominated therapeutics for centuries, until the beginning of the 19th century. The wide use of enemas and purges known to the Egyptians and to many African tribes since time immemorial could also be rationalized by physicians on the basis of the theory of *WeHeDuW* or *perittoma*. It is interesting to note that the absorption of poisonous matter from the intestines with advancing age was believed to be an inescapable process, which led eventually to the destruction of the body.[12, 13]

The theory of *WeHeDuW* seems to be the only rational pathological idea created by the Egyptian physicians. The Egyptians and Babylonians knew much more about astronomy through millennia of observation of the movements of celestial bodies. They knew, for instance, the difference between the calendar year and the solar year. They had a very cumbersome system of mathematics based on the decimal system but with separate symbols for the numbers 1, 10, 100, 1000, and so on. All this had been all-important for the practical pragmatic minds of the Egyptians. But there was very little theoretical basis for this knowledge.

In ancient Greece science had existed as a rational system from the time of the Milesians, but technology was completely neglected. The reason for this basic difference between the two cultures is complex and probably can be best understood as a result of the difference between the pragmatic mind of the Egyptian and the philosophical, contemplative mind of the Greek. The ancient Greek wanted to understand the world and the laws of nature but saw no need for any change or improvement which required manual work unworthy of a man of intelligence. In the words of Aristotle: ". . . It is owing to their wonder that men both now begin and at first began to philosophize. . . . They wondered originally at the obvious difficulties, then advanced little by little and stated difficulties about the greater matters and the phenomena of the sun and of the stars and about the genesis of the universe. And the man who is puzzled and wonders thinks himself ignorant. . . . Therefore, since they philosophized in order to escape from ignorance, evidently they were *pursuing science in order to know*, and not for any *utilitarian end*. . . ."[14]

It was left to man of the late Renaissance and of the 17th century—adventurous, daring, free from the chains of scholasticism—to try to understand the laws of nature in order to tame nature, to exploit and to conquer it. Scientific, rational thinking was then first applied to day-to-day problems of practical importance, and out of this new-found union of science and technology was born the enormous progress of both modern scientific thinking and of modern technology.

But long before this union occurred the great minds of ancient Greece had laid down the foundations of rational scientific thinking and, for the first time in the history of mankind, they tried to replace *mythos* by *logos*. They tried to discover the general laws of nature and they tried to explain the discrepancy between the unity of the cosmos and the plurality of sense-observed phenomena, between the eternal orderly movements of celestial bodies and the chaotic movements of sense-objects on earth.

Deduction was their main tool in analyzing observed phenomena, and only gradually did the quantitative approach to nature replace the old qualitative approach. But the endeavor to exploit nature, to apply the new discoveries to practical problems, to apply science to technology, was alien to them.

These limitations of ancient science are important. But without the cosmologists of Miletus, without the atomists and Anaxagoras, there would have been no foundation on which to build modern science.

Science and the Evolution of Language

Replacing quality by quantity, replacing poetical descriptions of events by mathematical formulas had been a great step forward. It gave man a powerful tool for understanding nature and the laws of nature. But it required the growth of rational logical thinking instead of the mythical explanation of observed facts. The truth of logical thought can and must be investigated, and it can and must be accepted by all once proved right. Mythical truth is always *revealed* as such and must be accepted without any proof or argumentation.

It is obvious that the development of rational ideas requires a certain degree of linguistic development. The appearance of new scientific concepts and terms is the result of the evolution of language. It took almost five centuries, from the time of Homer to Plato and Aristotle, before the basic concepts of science and philosophy and abstract terms and concepts such as infinity, space, velocity, continuum, matter, force, and time evolved gradually in ancient Greece. It is a very long way from *the* horse of the hero of Homer to a concept of *a* horse, an abstract term. Words change their meaning. The "psyche" of Homer meant only a vital force which leaves the body when a man dies. The psyche as soul, as a thinking and feeling principle, appeared much later. The "aether" meant to Empedocles the most rarified substance, the fill of the universe. It was the Fifth Substance for Aristotle, identical to *pneuma* for the Stoics, and again something quite different to Galen, to René Descartes, to Newton, to the scientists of the 19th century or to Einstein and his followers.[15-18]

The same is true of mathematical thinking. It is a long way from natural and rational numbers or even from the irrational numbers of the Pythagoreans to the invention of analytical geometry by Descartes or of calculus by Leibnitz. The Romans simplified the cumbersome system of the Egyptians by using fewer symbols (X, C, D, M) and, to a very limited degree, the place-value property. But only with the Indo-Arabian system in the second half of the first millennium A.D., when the integer zero was introduced with the full use of the place-value property, did a real development of mathematics become possible.

The ancient Greeks had a fully developed system of logical thinking and of philosophical concepts but their mathematics remained rather primitive.

Science and the Rise of the Individual

Homer lived in the ninth century B.C., about two generations before the time of King David and King Solomon of Biblical tradition. The world of Homer was that of heroes dominated by deities. Homer sang to the courts of Achaean princes, and the heroes of Homer's epics had all the characteristics of an ideal warrior: courage, magnanimity in victory, dignity in defeat. The hero was fearless and strong, an ideal of a man close to the image of the Homeric gods. But his knowledge of things was deceptive, and his fate was in the hands of gods who had the complete knowledge of things. And both men and gods had to obey the forces of time and fate.[19]

The attitude of men toward the acquisition of knowledge gradually changed. Xenophanes (ca. 540 B.C.) taught that man could acquire knowledge, though incomplete, not as a gift of gods but by his own industry and perseverance. He denied the existence of anthropomorphic gods. For him there was only one God, "who sees all over, thinks all over and hears all over" and who had a real knowledge of things. The knowledge of man would always be partial, but whatever knowledge he could acquire, he would gain only by a long seeking.[20-22]

Alcmeon (500 B.C.), the greatest of the pre-Hippocratic physicians, belonged to the same philosophical school of Croton in southern Italy that is connected with the names of Xenophanes and Pythagoras. He was probably the first known to practice anatomical dissections and to make experiments on animals. He was the first to state that the brain and not the heart is the seat of the senses and of the intellect. He described the optic nerves and their crossing and he assumed that the optic nerves conduct the perception of light into the brain. The function of the brain, Alcmeon thought, is to transmit the sense of perception, to recollect, and thus to lead to the acquisition of knowledge. Only conjecture based on facts born out of perception may lead, according to Alcmeon, to some knowledge of invisible reality. Thus he introduced the concept of induction as a way to acquire knowledge.[23, 24]

In his medical teachings Alcmeon was very close to the basic ideas of Pythagoras, and to Alcmeon we owe the fundamental principles of humoral pathology. Health, he believed, is a state of perfect harmony, disease is a disturbance of this harmony, and cure is the return to the original state of harmony. Many of the ideas of the Hippocratic school can be traced to this great physician of Croton.

Man slowly asserted his right to be independent from the whims of anthropomorphic gods. Archilochus was born about 650 B.C. at Paros, son of a nobleman and a slave girl. He moved from Paros to Phasos and there took part in the wars against the Greek invaders from the mainland. He fought in many wars and belonged to the type of mercenary soldiers who served in the armies of Pharaoh Psammetichus I and who helped him to liberate Egypt from the Assyrians. Archilochus was a soldier and a poet. He saw war without any illusions; he saw in it not only heroic deeds but also blood, suffering, and cruelty. Instead of the glorification of heroes he sang about the naked realities of war. Not the gods but man was the center of his attention.[25]

And then came Sappho of Lesbos and Anacreon, who asserted themselves in their lyrics as human beings and emphasized the reality of human passions, of love and hate. The beautiful monodic songs of Sappho are the revolt of individualism against the chains of hesiodic theogony. Man wanted to think for himself and to know and to feel reality.[26, 27]

About 700 years before the birth of Sappho, in the middle of the 14th century B. C., a spiritual revolution took place in Egypt at a time when the country was ruled by the young Pharaoh Ikhnaton, a dreamer and philosopher, "the world's first idealist and the world's first individual." It was a revolt of a dreamer against the powerful priesthood and against centuries-old tradition. Ikhnaton introduced the worship of a new supreme god, Aton, that was a new name for the old sun-god Re. Temples were built and new rituals and symbols were created. Hymns were written which resemble closely the psalms of King David. Ikhnaton insisted on "living in truth," and in the religion, the art, and in the poetry of his time one observes the passionate desire to see and understand the realities of life instead of an idealization of the world of the dead.[28] Beautiful love songs appeared; they are preserved in the papyri and many of them are surprisingly similar to the Song of Songs of the Bible. They were recently recreated from learned translations of egyptologists by outstanding American and Russian poets.[29, 30]

But Ikhnaton, philosopher and spiritual reformer, could not defend his kingdom against the forces of external and internal enemies. After his death (1358 B.C.) the short-lived Egyptian spiritual revolution came to an end, the new temples were destroyed, and the old traditions and the old way of life were restored by the combined forces of the priesthood and powerful courtiers. A decline of the empire followed and only after years of stagnation in art and economics was the orderly organization that Egypt had once enjoyed gradually brought back.[31]

The spiritual revolution in Egypt ended with the death of Ikhnaton. The outburst of individualism in Greece in the seventh century B.C., which had been the result of a centuries-long process of evolution of language and thought helped to clear the way for the rational approach to nature. The revolt of the individualism that had been spearheaded by the Greek lyrics of the seventh century B.C. seems to have much in common with a similar movement that took place in Western Europe at the end of the 16th and the beginning of the 17th centuries. The Elizabethan poets and musicians (Thomas Morley, John Wilbye) began to write madrigals in which they used not only translations of the sonnets of Petrarch and Tasso but folk songs and love songs known to the man in the street, somewhat like the rock songs of our time. At the same time a group of young musicians and poets (the Camerata) gathered in a back room of a palace in Florence and discussed passionately the new creative art later called by the traditionalists "baroque," a derogatory term meaning ugly, irregular. The operas of Claudio Monteverdi were written then. In them the man on the stage was not submerged in the majestic polyphony of the early Renaissance but spoke and sang about his sorrows and passions and joys. The same revolt spread all over Europe. About 20 years later John Milton, long before writing his *Paradise Lost*, published his tracts on divorce and the famous *Areopagitica* in defense of freedom of the press. The teleologically oriented philosophy of the Middle Ages changed gradually and gave way to a new philosophy and a new science. Copernicus in the early 16th century proved by mathematical reasoning that the earth is not the center of the universe; the immensity of the universe was soon proved, contrary to medieval religious and philosophical teachings. And then, in 1687, the young Isaac Newton wrote his brilliant *Principia* in which he proved that the same laws of nature govern the movements of the stars, the sun, the moon, and sense objects on earth.

The revolt of individualism in Europe, once started, continued to grow and can be traced in the birth of the English novel and in the creation of sonata-form with its conflict of human passions brought to perfection by Haydn, Mozart, and Beethoven; it dominated music until our time. The baroque movement in art and science led the way to Cartesian philosophy and to the mathematization of science by Galileo Galilei, Newton, and Leibnitz. The development of modern science began in the 17th century and never stopped.

The Early Milesians

The birth of rational philosophy in Greece took place in the city of Miletus, founded by Ionian settlers soon after the Dorian invasion of the Greek mainland.[32] Miletus very early became the center of a lively trade with its eastern neighbors and with Egypt. In the course of time these commercial ties brought cultural influences. And two medical schools, the cradles of Hippocratic and Asclepiadic medicine, were founded on the tiny islands Cos and Cnidos off the shores of Miletus.[33]

The three great Milesians—Thales, Anaximenes, and Anaximander—all tried to solve the basic problem which is still puzzling the theoretical physicist today: What is the nature of matter? For the first time in the history of mankind they attempted to solve the problem by rational methods outside the realm of religion, myth, and magic. How is one to explain the unity of the universe and the plurality of the sense-perceived world? What is real and what is only an illusion? In our time Pierre Teilhard de Chardin, the late theologian, philosopher, and scientist, devoted the first chapter of his book *The Phenomenon of Man* to this problem of unity and plurality.[34] The explanation given by the Milesian philosophers might seem naive to us; primordial matter was water for Thales, air for Anaximenes, and *arche* for Anaximander, substance without limits, ageless and eternal. But the approach of these thinkers was radically different from that of Homer or Hesiod. Ocean for Homer was a mythical unity—the origin of men and gods. To Thales water was the water we see and drink, which becomes ice and vapor. If for Homer the rainbow was a bridge walked by the messengers of the gods, for Anaximenes it was a result of "the beams of the sun falling on the thick, condensed air." This was not yet a scientific discovery but a first attempt at a rational explanation of an observed natural phenomenon. And the statement of Anaximenes that the plurality of sense-objects was caused "by the virtue of rarefication and condensation of air in different substances" was a first attempt to substitute quantity for quality.[35]

Anaximander, another Milesian, wrote that all life comes from the sea and that the present forms of animals including man are the result of their evolving through a process of adaptation to the environment: "Living creatures arose from moist element as it was evaporated by the sun. . . . Man was like another animal, namely as a fish in the beginning, he was born from animals of another species. . . . While other animals quickly found food for themselves, man alone requires lengthy period of suckling. Hence had he been originally as he is now, he would never have survived."[36]

Anaximander was not a precursor of Charles Darwin, but nevertheless his was the stroke of intuition of a genius. He was the first to use models and drawings while explaining the movements of the stars to his pupils.

What fascinated these first natural philosophers was the striking discrepancy between the majestic order and constancy of the movements of celestial bodies and the chaotic changes observed daily in the sense-perceived world.

This discrepancy led Parmenides, the great philosopher of Elea, to whom Plato owed so much, to speak of all observed changes as pure illusion and to accept as real only the unchangeable, motionless eternal Being: "What is—is uncreated and indestructible for it is complete, immovable and without end. . . . Nor was it ever, nor will it be, for now it is, all at once, a continuous one. . . ."[37] This discrepancy led Leucippus to state that nothing occurs by chance but there is a reason and necessity for everything.[38] The idea of order in nature and of causality had been the basis of the philosophical quest of the first Milesians and still is an assumption accepted a priori by every scientist: "Without the belief that it is possible to grasp the reality with our theoretical constructions, without the belief in the inner harmony in our world, there could be no science. This belief is and always will be the fundamental motive for all scientific creation."[39]

Empedocles and the Pythagoreans

Thales, Anaximenes, and Anaximander taught the monistic theory of the universe. Primordial eternal matter had been for them either water, air, or an "eternal Being." It was Empedocles of Akragas who first broke with this monistic tradition. For him the eternal elements, unchangeable and indivisible, are four, not one, and the plurality of sense-objects results from the endless variety of combinations of those four primordial elements: "For all of these (fire and water and earth and air) are equal and alike in age . . . and nothing comes into being besides these, nor do they pass away. . . . For out of these spring all things that were and are and shall be—trees and men and women, beasts and birds and the fishes that dwell in the waters, yea and the gods that live long lives and are exalted in honors. For there are these alone, but running through one another, they take different shapes—so much does mixture change them. . . ."[40]

These four "roots" of all things were identified with the cold, the hot, the moist, and the dry. And the four elements of Empedocles remained the basis of scientific medicine and of humoral pathology for the next two thousand years. To Hippocrates they became black bile, yellow bile, blood, and phlegm, and they can be traced in one form or another in the writings of Galen and Avicenna and in the writings of all great medical men to the end of the 17th century. The four elements of Empedocles were eternal and equal parts of primordial matter. The same four elements in Plato's *Timaeus* became not substances but geometrical forms which become matter only when put together.[41] Much later, with the acceptance of Aristotelian metaphysics, they became not equal but different in their dignity and value, and the lighter elements, air and fire, were considered *nobler* than earth and water.

This number 4 had been borrowed by Empedocles and Alcmeon from Pythagoras and his school. The Pythagoreans formed a secret society with a complicated ritual, strict rules of behavior, and a belief in the transmigration of the soul and in reincarnation.[42] Aside from the mystical elements in their teachings, the essence of the cosmos to the Pythagoreans was numbers. Numbers were for them spatial concepts; the number 1 represented a point; 2, a line; 3, a plane, and 4, a solid. All things are numbers and can be properly expressed only in numbers. The quality of musical pitch corresponds to a measurable length of a string and therefore can be replaced and explained by a mathematical formula. Thus the harmony of the sounds depends on a proper choice of numerical values, and the harmony of the spheres depends on the eternal harmony of the heavens.[43]

To the pythagoreans the number 4 and all even numbers were unlimited and all odd numbers were limited. A whole allegorico-metaphysical philosophy developed later on the basis of this theory of numbers. Numbers became symbols. The number 3 represented a man, and 2 a woman, so that marriage could logically be said to be represented by number 5. Great minds of the 16th century were preoccupied with this mystery of numbers. In England in 1570 John Dee maintained in his address *To the Unfained Lovers of Truthe* that the universe consisted of "Numbrings."[44] Galileo wrote once in terms almost Platonic that ". . . philosophy is written in that vast book which stands forever open before our eyes, I mean the Universe, but it cannot be read until we have learned the language and become familiar with the characters in which it is written. It is written in mathematical language and the letters are triangles, circles and other geometrical figures without which means it is humanly impossible to comprehend a single word. . . ."[45]

Pythagoras knew irrational numbers too, such as the square root of 2; his pupils called them "devoid of logos." They knew that irrational numbers are squeezed between the integers and that this confinement can be narrowed indefinitely and that *reality can be approached only through approximation.* The pythagoreans kept this knowledge secret for about 200 years, until their society declined completely. Archimedes in the third century B.C. used this principle in calculating the famous "pi," the ratio of the circumference of a circle to its diameter, by inscribing and circumscribing regular polygons with ever-increasing numbers of sides. Pythagoras applied numbers to the sensory world and to the cosmos in general; he replaced qualities by quantities as does modern science.[46]

Plato divorced numbers from all sense-perceived objects and applied them to the world of ideas or forms. His authority made impossible any real progress in the quantitative analysis of the sensory world for nearly 2,000 years. Similarly the authority of Aristotle, who firmly believed in the immobility of the earth, made it impossible for the scientists of many generations to accept the heliocentric theory of earth movements taught by Aristarchus of Samos as early as 270 B.C.[47]

It seems, however, that in the 20th century we are again approaching the platonic teachings of the relation between the world of ideas and the sensory world. The elementary particles of Plato's *Timaeus* were in the final analysis not substances but mathematical forms. The only mathematical forms available at that time were such geometrical forms as regular solids and triangles. In modern quantum theory there can be no doubt that the elementary particles will also be mathematical forms but of much more complicated nature.[48] Matter and energy are expressed by the modern theoretical physicist in the form of mathematical abstractions, and the network of these abstractions becomes the only reality, not unlike the platonic world of ideas in contrast to which the sense-perceived world becomes a pure illusion.

Empedocles introduced not only the four fundamental elements as the building blocks of nature but he was the first to introduce the concept of force as the cause of the movements of matter. He recognized two forces, which he called Love and Strife. In using these poetical terms he wanted to indicate that one force brings things together, whereas the other pulls them apart: "At one time it grew to be only one out of many; at another, it divided up to be many instead of one. . . . And these things never cease continually changing places, at one time all uniting in one through *Love*, at another each borne in different directions by the repulsion of *Strife*."[49] We might replace his terms by concepts more familiar to us: attraction and repulsion. The centrifugal force of Huygens and the force of attraction which became the starting point that led to the discovery of the great law of gravitation by Newton are quite similar to the two forces of Empedocles, who in the fifth century B.C. came so close to the ideas of the great men of the 17th century A.D.

Some other statements of Empedocles show the greatness of his intuition. He stated that light as it propagates through space requires time to reach the observer. One of the late commentators, Philoponus, described his opinion as follows: "Empedocles said that light is a streaming substance which, emitted from the source of light, first reaches the region between earth and sky and from there comes to us; but we are not conscious of this movement, because of the speed." Thus for the first time the idea of the velocity of light had been clearly expressed.[50, 51]

More than 2,000 years later Galileo in his *Dialogues Concerning Two New Sciences*, first published in 1637, expressed the opinion that . . . "the familiar bit of experience is that sound, in reaching our ear, travels more slowly than light; it does not inform me whether the coming of the light is instantaneous or whether, although extremely rapid, it still occupies time. . . . The fact that the speed of sound is as high as it is, assures us that the motion of light cannot fail to be extraordinary swift. . . ." And Galileo proceeds to devise a method by which one might accurately ascertain whether ". . . The propagation of light is really not instantaneous."[52] His method, while logically correct, could not be properly applied with the primitive experimental techniques of his time. However, about 50 years later Olaus Roemer, the Danish astronomer, proved in 1675 that the velocity of light is finite. He used astronomical observations to calculate the speed of light, contrary to the terrestial method suggested by Galileo. By observing the revolutions of the first satellite of Jupiter at the different positions of the earth on its orbit around the sun, Roemer calculated the velocity of light to be 308,000 kilometers per second, or very close to what we know it to be.

His calculations were checked and found to be correct by the greatest authority of the time, Huygens.[53] Much later, with the refinement of the experimental technique, Armand H. L. Fizeau confirmed his result by terrestial experiments as did Albert A. Michelson in the 20th century.[54]

Empedocles taught that air has the properties of a body or matter; this was an entirely new concept.[55] But much more important for the further development of science and medicine was his theory of the "shedding of particles" by all objects. Those particles or "effluences flow from all things that have come into being." The infinitesimal indivisible particles enter our sense organs and are the true basis of sensation, vision, and smell. Perception is due to the meeting of an element in us with the same element outside. This takes place when the pores of the organ of sense are neither too large nor too small for the "effluences" which all things are constantly emitting. However, Empedocles believed that hearing is produced when the air moved by the voice sounds inside the ear.[56]

The idea of the emission of particles had been fully developed by the atomists, especially by Democritus, whose "atoms" were really "effluences." To Democritus the only reality consisted of atoms and the void; this led him to distinguish between the real or primary qualities and the secondary qualities. Galen quotes Democritus as saying ". . . all the qualities of the things perceived by us result from collision of the atoms. In reality there no white, no black, no yellow, or red, or bitter or sweet. . . . Colors exist by convention, sweet by convention, bitter by convention, in truth nothing exists but the atoms and the void." And in another fragment: ". . . Senses give us no information about the reality but only the interplay of atoms."[57]

Johannes Kepler, who lived at the time of the revival of pythagorean and neoplatonic ideas and of platonic geometrical atomism, but long before the atomism of Democritus and Epicurus became common knowledge, thought ". . . that knowledge offered the mind by the senses is obscure, contradictory and untrustworthy. The real world is a world of quantitative characteristics only, the differences are differences of numbers alone."[58] Somewhat later Galileo, who even more than Kepler believed in the mathematical foundation of nature, insisted, contrary to the vague theories of the Pythagoreans, that exact mathematical methods must be applied to studies of nature. The reality of the universe is geometrical; the ultimate characteristic of nature, the primary qualities, are those of which certain mathematical knowledge is possible: number, figure, position, magnitude, motion. All other qualities are subjective. ". . . I think that these tastes, odors, colors . . . on the side of the object in which they seem to exist are nothing else but mere names, but hold their residence solely in the sensitive body. . . ."[59]

This and similar opinions which are so close to the statements of Democritus led, a few decades later, to the Cartesian dualism. Still later, at the very end of the 17th century they were fully developed by John Locke. Locke, the first of the English empiricists, famous author of *An Essay concerning Human Understanding*, philosopher, and physician, was a close friend of Dr. Thomas Sydenham and a contemporary of Dr. Richard Mead. Locke also accepted fully the Newtonian concept of nature as essentially mechanical in its dynamics and corpuscular in its structure. He believed that all our knowledge is based on perception and that ". . . perception is the first operation of our intellectual faculties and the inlet of all knowledge in our minds." The objective cause of perception is direct or indirect contact with the object, and Locke distingushed between the real or primary qualities such as solidity, extension, figure, and motility and the secondary qualities which are "in truth nothing in the objects themselves but powers to produce various sensations in us by their primary qualities. . . . For it being manifest that there are bodies and good store of bodies each whereof are so small that we cannot by any of our senses discover either their bulk, figure, or motion . . . and that the different motions and figures, bulk and number of such . . . insensible particles of matter . . .

affecting the several organs of our senses, produce in us the different sensations which we have from the smells and the colors of the bodies. . . ."[60]

The materialistic philosophy of Locke was fought violently by his younger contemporary, George Berkeley, who for philosophical and religious reasons denied the very existence of the external world. However, Locke's theory of the working of the human mind, opposed in England by Berkeley and later by David Hume,[61] had been further developed in France by the French sensualists and by Etienne B. de Condillac, whose famous expression "penser c'est toujours sentir" defines best the views of that school.

The ideas of Condillac (1715-1780) were systematized about 20 years after his death by a group of outstanding medical men: M. F. X. Bichat, Pierre J. G. Cabanis, Philippe Pinel, and François Magendie—all well known in the history of medicine. Radical analytical empiricism characterized the methods of these thinkers, who later became known as the Ideologues and whose strictly materialistic philosophy in many aspects resembled the philosophy of Locke.[62]

The Shedding of Particles and the Miasmatic Pathogenesis of Diseases

Another aspect of the theory of the empedoclean shedding of particles and of the democritean emission of atoms was the miasmatic theory of the pathogenesis of infectious diseases. The word miasma had been used as a medical term since the time of Hippocrates but in the course of centuries it changed its meaning many times. To Hippocrates "miasma" meant some vaguely defined contamination of the air; when air spoiled by miasma is inhaled "men turn sick." Galen, who wrote extensively about miasmas, connected them with the concept of putrefaction and spoke of "putrid miasmas" that flow in the air and are the cause of fever and disease in those who are susceptible.[63] The authority of Galen kept the concept of putrid miasmatic effluvia alive for centuries long after the existence of an invisible *contagium animatum vivum* was postulated as a cause of disease in human beings, animals, and even plants by Girolamo Fracastoro, who wrote in 1546 that "the contagium of putrefaction goes from one body to another whether adjacent or distant," and that "these seeds *(seminaria prima)* have the faculty of multiplying and propagating rapidly." Girolamo

Fracastoro, one of the greatest scientists of the 16th century, expressed ideas very close to the theories of modern pathology and epidemiology.[64] However, a miasmatic etiology of major epidemic diseases—of cholera, typhus, yellow fever, and plague—in its more modern version had been accepted and passionately defended up to the second half of the 19th century by the majority of the most prominent European physicians.[65] Austin Flint, in the fifth edition of his *Treatise on Principles and Practice of Medicine*, written in conjunction with William H. Welch and published in 1881, i.e., on the very threshold of the new bacteriological era, wrote, "that infectious diseases may or may not be communicable by means of contagium. If communicable—it is a communicable infectious disease. If not communicable, it is an infectious, miasmatic disease."[66] The ancient concept of miasmatic propagation of diseases, which originated in the works of ancient Greek scientists, disappeared forever from the pages of the medical textbooks in the bacteriological era. But in 1888 Dr. Louis Smith, clinical professor of children's diseases at Bellevue Hospital Medical College in New York City, still believed that most children "developed diphtheria by inhaling infectious sewer gas."[67]

The Atoms and the Void

The rational scientific thinking of the Greek natural philosophers reached its heights in the two opposite schools of thought represented on one side by the atomists and on the other side by Anaxagoras and later by the stoics. The ideas of both schools are of great significance and are closely related to the development of modern scientific concepts of matter, space, and force.

The atomists, whose main representative was Democritus, one of greatest geniuses of the ancient world (460-370 B.C.), also included Leucippus (ca. 460 B.C.), Epicurus and his school (341-270 B.C.) and, finally, the Roman poet T. Lucretius Carus (d. 55 B.C.).

The world of the atomists, with a few differences between the teaching of Democritus and of the epicureans, consisted of an infinite number of invisible and indivisible atoms of various sizes and shapes which moved constantly in a void or vacuum. The matter of which the atoms are made is uniform or, as stated by Aristotle: "the nature of them all is, they say, the same, just as if each one separately were a piece of gold. Matter is eternal . . . nothing can be created out of nothing nor can it be destroyed and returned into nothingness."[68-70] This is a sort of law of conservation of matter, and it was first postulated by Parmenides of Elea, who was born at the end of the sixth century B.C. and was still alive in 449 B.C. when he conversed with the young Socrates in Athens.[71] He wrote: "What is, is uncreated and indestructible; for it is complete, immovable and without end. . . . Nor was it ever nor will it be; for now it is, all at once and continuous one. . . ."[72]

The atoms of Leucippus and Democritus move perpetually in the infinite void, overtake each other and collide; ". . . some of them rebound in random directions, while others interlock because of the symmetry of their sizes, shapes, positions, and arrangements, and remain together. This was how compound bodies were begun."[73] However, the atomists never explained what force causes the movements of the atoms. They accepted it as a fact as they postulated the existence of atoms.

Epicurus modified slightly the teachings of Leucippus and Democritus by introducing the concept of the weight of atoms, which according to Democritus differed only in their shape and size. However, both agreed on the existence of a void ". . . because unless there is a void . . . there can not be *many*, since there is nothing to keep them apart. . . ." The atoms of Epicurus move through the void with equal speed "nothing colliding with them. For neither will the heavy move more quickly than the small and light . . . nor again the small more quickly than the great having their whole course uniform when nothing collides with them either." This conclusion based on pure deduction is very close to the famous law of inertia of Galileo, who wrote that an "undisturbed body continues to move uniformly in a straight line or remains at rest." Galileo also discovered terrestrial acceleration and thus cleared the way for Newton's law of gravitation and for the newtonian concept of mass as different from weight. Galileo was first to make motion the object of exact mathematical study.[74]

Mathematical analysis was unknown to the ancients. The absolute determinism of Democritus did not explain the creation of the world. Epicurus admitted spontaneous deviation of the atoms from their predetermined course in the void and by this act of the "free will" of the atoms explained the possibility of their collision as the starting point of the creation of matter.[75]

If we replace the size and the shape of the atoms by their atomic weight and allow the absolute void of Democritus to be filled with an extremely rarefied matter (the ancients called it ether; for the Stoics it was *pneuma*),[76, 77] we arrive at the theory of matter and the universe that was valid and was taught in physics and chemistry to the very end of the 19th century.

Democritus stated emphatically that the atoms, the fundamentals of nature, are not perceptible to the senses. The senses give us only the interplay of atoms. It is impossible to know how each thing is in reality.

All sensation depends on the contact of atoms of various shapes with our organs of sense. However, perception varies with the state of the body of the perceiver: "For this reason one kind of atom sometimes produces the opposite sensation while the opposite produces the original one."

Epicurus modified this complete negation of the values of our sensations. Three hundred years later Lucretius summed up the opinion of Epicurus in the following sentence: "You will find that the concept of truth was originated by the senses and that the senses cannot be rebutted. . . . If they are not true, then reason in its entirety is equally false."[78]

For the atomists all qualities were replaced by quantities. How can one explain the infinite variety of sense-perceived objects? Democritus, as quoted by Aristotle, gave a brilliant analogy as an explanation of the plurality of the sensory world: atoms are like letters of the alphabet, per se they are devoid of quality or meaning. But letter-atoms acquire meaning when combined into syllables and words. Change one letter in a word and its meaning is changed. Change one atom in a combination of atoms and the properties of the matter are changed. What is true for the letters is also true for the atoms. "Tragedy and comedy are both composed of the same letters."[79-81]

Pythagoreanism, Atomism, and the Birth of Modern Science

Atomism in all its various forms, as the geometrical atomism of Plato's *Timaeus* or as that of Democritus, Epicurus, or the Roman poet Lucretius, together with the revival of pythagoreanism, became the most important major link between the ancient Greek philosophers and the great minds of the 16th and 17th centuries, who created the foundations of modern science and technology. Plato's *Timaeus* attracted attention and fascinated the medieval thinkers as early as the 11th century, when Aristotle was still known only as the author of books on logic. Toward the end of the Middle Ages Aristotelian philosophy and metaphysics with its teleology, its strict homocentrism and geocentrism, and its attitude to nature as mainly qualitative, with logic and not mathematics as the real key to knowledge, united in the minds of medieval men with the Christian theology. However, the platonic ideas of the world as fundamentally geometrical, simple, and harmonious—together with the pythagorean theory of the importance of numbers—remained a powerful counterpart of the dominant Christian and Aristotelian philosophy. All or almost all of the medieval thinkers were deeply religious. But once the world is accepted as essentially geometrical and quantitative in the platonic and pythagorean sense, a mathematical approach to knowledge is legitimate and is not in conflict with the basic teachings of religion.

At the very end of the Middle Ages Nicholas of Cusa (1401-1464), a theologian, a cardinal since 1448, a man deeply interested in platonic philosophy as well as in mathematics and in physical science, wrote that "number is the first model of things in the mind of the Creator" and that "knowledge is always measurement." He insisted on quantitative measurements of time and weight, with the use of a balance for physical, physiological, and even mathematical investigations. His book on philosophy bears a curious title *De Docta Ignorantia* (the learned ignorance); in it he wrote about the relativity and imperfection of human knowledge.[82, 83] Nicolaus Copernicus, who was born 10 years after the death of Nicholas of Cusa, lived in a time of great cultural, economic, and social upheaval when many conflicting, strange, and radical ideas had to be faced by intelligent men in Western Europe. Copernicus studied mathematics and astronomy at the University of Cracow and early accepted the pythagorean doctrine of numbers and the geometrical atomism of Plato. He spent several years in Italy and, while studying mathematics under Domenico Maria de Novara, professor of astronomy in Bologna, became dissatisfied with the orthodox, ptolemaic theory of the movements of celestial bodies. In Padua he studied medicine with Girolamo Fracastoro. In 1504 he returned to Germany. The revolutionary idea that dominated his thinking all his life matured slowly but by now he was certain that he could offer a better, simpler, and more harmonious explanation of the movements of the earth and the planets than did the followers of Ptolemy. He postulated the diurnal rotation of the earth around its axis and annual motion of the earth around the sun. By doing so he was concerned only with giving a more accurate and simpler explanation of the observed facts by replacing the 80 ptolemaic epicycles by his 34. However, by placing the sun in the center of the universe instead of the earth and by reviving the heliocentric theory of Aristarchus of Samos that was familiar to him, Copernicus met intense opposition both on theological and scientific grounds. He worked on his great book *De Revolutionibus* all his life, and it was published in 1541, two years before his death.[84] Copernicus was helped in writing it by a young mathematician, Rhaeticus, who stayed with him as a devoted student and admirer. One may doubt whether the great book of Copernicus would have been written if this young and talented mathematician and devoted disciple had not stayed with the aging genius and helped him to accomplish his work.

The heliocentric theory of Copernicus had been understood and accepted in his time by few but was bitterly criticized by many. Melanchthon wrote about this "Sarmatian (Slavic) astronomer who moves the earth and fixes the sun." And Martin Luther spoke with disdain of "the fool who will overturn the whole art of astronomy." Aristotelian philosophy dominated the minds of a majority of intelligent people of his time to whom daily experience proved beyond any doubt the immobility of the solid, massive, and stable earth.[85]

However, about 50 years later the great revolutionary idea of Copernicus was seized and fully developed by a young genius, Johannes Kepler (1571-1630).

As a young man Kepler had been impressed by the importance of the sun in the heliocentric system of Copernicus. In 1593, while still a student in Tübingen, he wrote that "the sun alone by virtue of its dignity and power is suited for this motive duty and worthy to become the home of God himself not to say the first mover."[86] For the rest of his life Kepler was involved in the mystical implications of the neoplatonic and pythagorean theories of numbers and in the allegorical symbolism of celestial bodies. To the platonics the universe was fundamentally geometrical, and Kepler accepted fully the geometrical atomism of Plato's *Timaeus:* God created the world in accordance with the principles of perfect harmony;[87] real knowledge is mathematical; and knowledge acquired through the senses is deceptive and unreliable. However, Kepler above all else was a brilliant mathematician, and within the framework of the neoplatonic and pythagorean philosophy of numbers he searched constantly for new harmonies of the universe, primarily for the mathematical harmonies of the movements of celestial bodies. Kepler endeavored to verify the harmonious simplicity of the world of Copernicus by exact mathematics, never disregarding as irrelevant the deviations between the observed facts and the results of pure deduction.

Very important and fortunate for the great discoveries of Kepler were those of one of the greatest astronomers of his time, Tycho Brahe; irritable, arrogant, and full of prejudices, he despised and distrusted all the calculations and conclusions of Copernicus. Yet he admitted young Kepler, an admirer of Copernicus and his heliocentrism, as an assistant to his observatory and his workshop near Prague, where he lived in semiexile.[88]

There, for a year and a half, until the death of Brahe, Kepler was able to obtain full knowledge of Brahe's methods and observations; after the death of his master, he was able to use the enormous factual material collected by Brahe during almost 40 years of patient and precise astronomical observation.

Kepler, after years of incessant work, found new mathematical harmonies in his three famous laws of planetary motion. But pythagorean mysticism dominated his mind, as did platonic geometric atomism. As late as 1619 in his book *Harmonices Mundi*, while describing his third law of planetary motion which he called the "harmonic law," Kepler discussed in great detail the "music of the spheres" and made a serious attempt to express it in the form of musical notation.[89-92]

A deeply religious man, Kepler nevertheless firmly defended the right of the philosopher or scientist to seek the truth about the real nature of the world. "In theology," wrote he, "to be sure, the force of authorities is to be weighed; in philosophy, however, that of causes. . . . Worthy of sainthood is the dutiful performance of moderns who, admitting the meagreness of the earth, yet deny its motion. But truth is more saintly for me, who demonstrate by philosophy, without violating my due respect for the doctors of the church, that the earth is both round and inhabited at the antipodes and of most despicable size and finally is moved among the stars."[93]

Kepler's great and voluminous book, *Astronomia Nova*, remained unnoticed and was read by only a few scientists, partly because of its poor latinity and unclear style. However, it was accepted enthusiastically by Galileo, then a young professor of mathematics in Padua.

Galileo was born in 1564 and was a contemporary of Kepler, with whom he maintained a lively correspondence for many years. His philosophy, like that of Kepler, was essentially pythagorean and platonic, and geometric atomism was the basis of his theory of matter. However, the mysticism of pythagoreanism had much less importance for him than for Kepler. Even long before the atomism of Democritus and Epicurus became well known through the writings of Pierre Gassendi, Galileo adopted some of the concepts of the atomic theory of matter. Nature to him was geometrical and mathematical because God was a geometrician in his labors, and "matter consists of infinite number of small indivisible units (atoms)." In his search for an explanation of the events of nature, Galileo asked "How?" instead of "Why?" and he patiently applied exact mathematics and experiments in his studies of motion. The philosophical and theological problems of the "ultimate cause" or of the creation of the world were all-important to him,[94] but he wrote cautiously that "considerations of this kind belong to a higher science than ours. We must be satisfied to belong to that class of less worthy workmen who procure from the quarry the marble out of which, later, the gifted sculptor produces those masterpieces which lay hidden in this rough and shapeless exterior."[95] He had boundless admiration for his predecessors, for Aristarchus and Copernicus, but he turned his attention from the movements of celestial bodies to the motions of the objects on earth, which became the object of exact mathematical studies and painstaking experiments. The problems of terrestrial dynamism led him to the discovery of the law of inertia, to the concept of acceleration, and to the refutation of the Aristotelian theory of motion. However, mass to Galileo was still equivalent to weight; it was Newton who first expressed mass in terms of force, and force in terms of mass, in his law of gravitation.

By the middle of the 17th century pythagoreanism had lost the influence it had had in the preceding century. With great progress in new branches of mathematics the geometrical platonic approach to nature gave place to algebraic analysis. But atomism as taught by Democritus and particularly by Epicurus became familiar as never before to the philosophers and scientists through the work of Gassendi, whose *Syntagma Philosophicum* appeared in 1649. One of the chapters of this fruit of his life-long studies was titled *De Atomis* and subtitled *Quid dicatur atomus et qui illius assertores* ("what is the atom and who are those who accept it").

Gassendi devoted his attention almost exclusively to the atomism of Epicurus and Lucretius. Unlike Kepler and Galileo, he did not apply atomism—whether geometrical or that of Epicurus—to new discoveries. His was an erudite, not a creative mind, and he oscillated all his life between the teachings of the atomists and the tenets of Christian theology. A stubborn defender of atomism, he characteristically stated that the heliocentric theory of Copernicus would be the best if it did not contradict the teachings of the Church.

Whatever his limitations, Gassendi was the first in modern times to defend atomism openly and to make the atomism of Epicurus known and popular.[96]

Newton's corpuscular atomistic theory of matter was the last in the long line of revivals of the theory of matter of Democritus by the founders of modern science. Newtonian theories had a very great impact on the development of science in general and of physics in particular for about 200 years. Not until the very end of the 19th century had Newtonian classical physics been gradually replaced by new theories based on new ideas and confirmed by new experiments. The ideas of atoms and the void were replaced by the concept of the continuum.[97]

Anaxagoras and the Stoics

Anaxagoras was born about 488 B.C. and died in 428 B.C., the year Plato was born. He was one of the founders of the continuum theory of matter. In many respects his ideas were a logical development of the pluralistic theory of Empedocles, as opposed to the monism of the first Milesians. But, contrary to Empedocles and the atomists, he postulated an absolute continuum of matter. To Anaxagoras matter consisted of an infinite number of infinitesimal, invisible, and indivisible particles, real and eternal—each particle containing something of everything, unlike the atoms of Democritus. Any finite object is made up of an infinite number of these infinitely small particles (Anaxagoras called them "seeds"), and the stream of these invisible building blocks of matter makes the continuum the substrate of all objects and also the "fill of the universe." Our sense perception is too weak to allow us to know the truth, "visible existences are only the sight of the unseen," but sensations prove the existence of physical reality.

The continuum of Anaxagoras was a dynamic and active concept, not the immovable unchangeable eternal *one* of Parmenides. And the infinite variety of sense objects was to him the result of endless combinations of an infinite number of particles and not of combinations of a finite number of atoms which differ from one another only by their shapes and sizes.

Of even greater importance than his theory of matter was Anaxagoras' concept of *force* which causes the movements of everything, a concept of a dynamic organic force which he called "mind" (*nous*). This force differs from matter because it is incorporeal, it cannot be perceived, and it can be known only by the effect it exerts on matter.

This "cosmic mind" of Anaxagoras permeates everything: it is the source of changes in the universe, of all motion as well as of static order. There is a complete analogy between the mind of the individual, be it man, animal, or even a plant, which as an organizing principle controls the functioning of the living organism, and the cosmic mind which controls the whole universe, as it is the embodiment of the idea of natural law which governs the ordered behavior of physical reality. This cosmic mind of Anaxagoras is not unlike the dynamic force of modern physics which we call energy. It seems that in his concept of matter and of the unifying dynamic cosmic force Anaxagoras was much closer than the atomists to the 20th century theories of modern physicists.[98, 99]

Many years after the death of Anaxagoras his rational materialistic approach to natural philosophy was severely criticized by Plato in the *Laws*. In the 10th book of his *Laws* Plato wrote: ". . . when you and I argue that there are Gods and produce the sun, moon and stars as Gods or divine beings, if we would listen to the aforesaid philosophers we should say that they are earth and stones only which can have no care at all of human affairs. . . ."[100] And in another statement: "All that moves in the heaven appears to them to be full of stones and earth and other soulless bodies which dispense the causes of the whole cosmos."

Anaxagoras was the first scientist who tried to apply the same approach to the explanation of terrestrial and celestial phenomena. His attempt was naive and primitive. Two thousand years later Newton's universal law of gravitation proved in exact mathematical terms the identity of the laws which govern the movements of objects both on earth and in the heavens.

Anaxagoras had been accused of atheism and sentenced to life imprisonment. Pericles, his pupil and friend, saved him from prison, and Anaxagoras was exiled to a small island on the eastern shores of the Mediterranean. He died there at the age of 70, respected and beloved by many.

The theory of the continuum and the denial of the existence of the void was also the basic concept of the physics of the Stoics. Their main representatives were Zeno (332-262 B.C.), Chrysippus (280-207 B.C.), and Poseidonius (135-51 B.C.). To the Stoics the cosmos was a single harmonious organism governed and united by *pneuma*, the "spirit" which makes the whole world a single unit. The Stoics postulated the existence of *pneuma* as a kind of primordial matter very similar to the soul, which fills the universe, both objects and the space between objects. In the words of a late commentator, "Chrysippus . . . supposes that the whole of nature is united by the pneuma which permeates it and by which the world is kept together and is made coherent and interconnected."[101]

The denial of the void and the assumption of a continuum led the Stoics to the wave theory of the propagation of physical phenomena contrary to the theory of the atomists: "The air is not composed ot particles, but it is a continuum which contains no empty spaces. If it is struck by an impulse it rises in circular waves proceeding in straight sequence to infinity, until all the surrounding air is stirred, just as a pool is stirred by a stone which strikes it. But whereas in this latter case the movement is circular, the air moves spherically." And in another statement quoted by a late commentator: "We hear because the air between the voice and the hearer is struck and expands in spherical waves which reach our ears. . . ."[102]

Newton, in the English edition of his *Opiticks*, published in 1704, about 2,000 years after Anaxagoras and the Stoics, accepted the main principles of the ancient atomists, i.e., the existence of the atoms and of the void. He also accepted, with certain reservations, the existence of ether as "a most subtle spirit which pervades and lies hid in all gross bodies." This subtle substance which, according to Newton, might be of various degrees of rarity and density, fills the universe; it is inside matter and outside it. Newton's theory of light was atomistic and corpuscular. To him the rays of light were very small particles emitted from luminous objects which hit other objects. In other words, matter hits matter.[103, 104]

Robert Hooke, one of the founders of the Royal Society of London, and soon after him Huygens, one of the greatest mathematicians of his time, taught that light consists of spherical waves which hit the particles of ether and cause thus an infinite number of secondary waves: "Light takes time for its passage . . . it spreads, as sound does, by spherical surfaces and waves, for I call them waves from their resemblance to those which are seen to be formed in water when a stone is thrown in it. . . ." (quoted by Einstein).[105] This is a theory of a continuum that denies the existence of the void accepted by the atomists and Newton. And thus Newton, the atomist, and Huygens, the teacher of the continuum, repeated in the 17th century the controversy that existed in 500 B.C. between the atomism of Democritus and the theories of Anaxagoras and the Stoics.

It seems that today there are still two accepted ways of explaining the nature and the propagation of light: one corpuscular, in the form of the photons of the quanta theory, and the other based on the wave theory of light.

The evolution of scientific thought is a part of the general evolution of culture. In any period of history man's search for an explanation of observed natural phenomena depends on the interrelation of the fundamental theological and philosophical assumptions and on the degree and refinement of the experimental technique which exists at this particular time. The short-lived spiritual revolution in Egypt in the 15th century B.C. created new ideas and new attitudes toward nature and art; even after it came to a sudden end, it continued to influence generations of medical men. The pythagoreans and their theory of numbers as well as the atomism of ancient Greece had enormous influence on the development of modern science in the 16th and 17th centuries and played a major role in replacing the medieval scholastic, Aristotelian philosophy of man's relation to the universe by cartesian and newtonian rationalism and the mathematization of science and nature.

Fundamental religious and philosophical assumptions and postulates are always the background of the search for scientific truth, and they define the direction this search will follow. The concept of the four basic elements of Empedocles which replaced the monistic theory of the early Milesians had been in turn denied by the atomists, who on the basis of pure deduction postulated the existence of invisible and indivisible atoms and of the void. The atomistic theory of matter and newtonian classical physics dominated scientific thinking until the end of the 19th century, but then new philosophical assumptions, a new dynamic concept of space and time, gradually destroyed the very foundation of newtonian physics, and the growth of technology and the refinement of experimental techniques broke down the indivisible atom and led to the search for subatomic particles as ever-elusive elementary building blocks of matter, and finally to the dissolution of the very concept of matter into a continuum of fields and energy.

The philosophical and scientific revolution of our time is just another step in the never-ending search for truth which started thousands of years ago in ancient Greece.

REFERENCES

1. MacMichael, W.: *The Gold-Headed Cane,* 5th ed. London, Kimpton, 1923, pp. 39-110.
2. MacMichael, W. and Hawkins, F.: *Lives of British Physicians.* London, Murray, 1830, pp. 155-167.
3. Rotblat, J., ed.: *Aspects of Medical Physics. The First International Conference on Medical Physics,* Harrogate, 1965. London, Taylor & Francis, 1966, pp. 4-5.
4. Carnap, R.: *Philosophical Foundations of Physics.* New York, Basic Books, 1966. pp. 105-114.
5. Bork, A. M.: Maxwell and the vector potential. *Isis 58*:210, 1967.
6. Holton, G.: Einstein, Michelson and the crucial experiment. *Isis 60*:160-167, 1969.
7. Einstein, A. and Infeld, L.: *The Evolution of Physics.* New York, Simon & Schuster, 1950, pp. 255-260.
8. Sigerist, H.: *A History of Medicine,* vol. 1: *Primitive and Archaic Medicine.* New York, Oxford Univ. Press, 1951, pp. 320-324.
9. Galen: *De Methodo medendi.* Liber XI, cap. 8, Kühn, C. G., ed., 10. Leipzig, Cnobloch, 1823-1831, p. 753.
10. Galen: *De Sanitate tuenda.* In: Op. cit., Liber 1, cap. 3. Kühn, 6, p. 8.
11. Galen: Op. cit., cap. 12. Kühn, C. G., ed. 6 pp. 63-64 ff.
12. Steuer, O. and Saunders, J. B. de C. M.: *Ancient Egyptian and Cnidian Medicine.* Berkeley, Univ. Calif. Press. 1959, pp. 21-30.
13. Saunders, J. B. de C. M.: *The Transisition from Ancient Egyptian to Greek Medicine.* Lawrence, Kansas, Univ. Kansas Press, 1963, pp. 20-30.
14. Aristotle: Metaphysics, In: *The Basic Books of Aristotle,* McKeon, R. ed. New York, Random, 1941, book 1, chap. 2, 982-b, p. 692.
15. Galen: *De Plenitudine Liber,* cap. 3. Kühn 7, p. 522-525.
16. Wilson, L. G.: Erasistratus, Galen and the Pneuma. *Bull History Med. 33*: 293, 1959.
17. Snell, B.: *The Discovery of the Mind.* New York, Harper, 1960, pp. 228-245.
18. Einstein, A. and Infeld, L.: Op. cit., pp. 183-185.
19. Auden, W. H.: In: *The Portable Greek Reader.* New York, Viking,

1948, pp. 17-24.
20. Burnet, J.: *Early Greek Philosophy,* 4th ed. London, Black, 1930, p. 119.
21. Snell, B.: Op. cit., pp. 139-143.
22. Copleston, F. S. J.: *A History of Philosophy.* New York, Doubleday, 1962, vol. 1, part 1, p. 65.
23. Castiglioni, A.: *A History of Medicine.* New York, Knopf, 1941, pp. 135-137.
24. Snell, B.: Op. cit., pp. 146-147.
25. Snell, B.: Op. cit., pp. 46-54.
26. *The Portable Greek Reader,* op. cit., pp. 499-501.
27. Snell, B.: Op. cit., pp. 55-57.
28. Seton, L.: *The Art of the Ancient Near East.* New York, Praeger, 1961, pp. 175-185.
29. Pound, E. and Stock, N., transls.: *Love Poems of Ancient Egypt.* New York, New Directions, 1962.
30. Akhmatova, A. transl.: *Lirika Drevnego Egypta.* Moscow, Khudozhestvennaia Literatura, 1966.
31. Breasted, J. H.: *A History of Egypt.* New York, Bantam, 1964, pp. 297-319.
32. Bury, J. B.: *A History of Greece.* New York, Modern Library, pp. 56 ff.
33. Sudhoff, K.: *Kos and Knidos.* Muenchen, Verlag der Muenchner Drucke, 1927, pp. 285-300.
34. de Chardin, T.: *The Phenomenon of Man.* New York, Harper, 1965, pp. 39-44.
35. Burnet, J.: Op. cit., pp. 73-77.
36. Burnet, J.: Op. cit., pp. 70-71.
37. Burnet, J.: Op. cit., pp. 174-175.
38. Burnet, J.: Op. cit., p. 340.
39. Einstein, A. and Infeld, L.: Op. cit., p. 313.
40. Burnet, J.: Op. cit., p. 209.
41. Plato: *Timaeus.* Lee, H. D. P., transl. New York, Penguin, 1964, pp. 31, 67-68.
42. De Vogel, C. J.: *Pythagoras and Early Pythagoreanism.* Assen, Netherlands, Van Gorcum, 1966 chaps. 2 and 3, pp. 20-51.
43. Helm, E. E.: The vibrating string of the pythagoreans. *Scientific American 217*:92-104, 1967.
44. Patrides, C. A.: The numerological approach to cosmic order during the English renaissance. *Isis 49*:394.
45. Burtt, E. A.: *The Metaphysical Foundations of Modern Physical Science,* rev. ed. London, Routledge & Kegan Paul, 1932, p. 64.
46. Sambursky, S.: *The Physical World of the Greeks.* London, Routledge & Kegan Paul, 1960, pp. 26-46.
47. Sambursky, S.: Op. cit., pp. 70-71 and 207-208.
48. Heisenberg, Werner. *Physics and Philosophy.* New York, Harper, 1962, pp. 71-72.
49. Burnet, J.: Op. cit., pp. 207-208.
50. Burnet, J.: Op. cit., p. 239.
51. Sambursky, S.: Op. cit., p. 20.
52. Galileo, G.: *Dialogues Concerning Two New Sciences,* Crew, H. and de Salvo, A., transls. New York, Dover, 1954, pp. 42-43.
53. Sagnac, P. and de Saint-Leger, A.: *Peuples et Civilisations.* La Preponderance Française, 2d ed. Paris, Presses Univ. France, 1944, pp. 286-287.
54. Einstein, A. and Infeld, L.: Op. cit., p. 96.
55. Burent, J.: Op. cit., p. 229.
56. Burnet, J.: Op. cit., pp. 247-249.
57. Galen, C.: *De Elementis ex Hippocrate,* Liber 1, cap. 2. Kühn, 1, p. 415-419.
58. Burtt, E. A.: Op. cit., pp. 56-57.
59. Galileo, G.: *Discoveries and Opinions of Galileo. The Assayer.* St. Drake, S., transl. New York, Doubleday, 1957, p. 274.
60. Locke, J.: An Essay Concerning Human Understanding. In: *The Empiricists.* New York, Doubleday, 1961, pp. 26-33.
61. Berkeley, G.: *The Principles of Human Knowledge.* New York, Meridian, 1963, pp. 81-96.
62. Rosen, G.: The Philosophy of Ideology and the Emergence of Modern Medicine in France. *Bull. Hist. Med. 20:* 328, 1946.
63. Galen: *De Differentiis Febrium.* Liber 1, cap. 6. Kuhn, 7, pp. 289-290.
64. Castiglioni: Op. cit., pp. 455-459.
65. Ackerknecht, E.: Anti-contagionism between 1821 and 1867. *Bull. Hist. Med. 22*:562-593, 1948.
66. Flint, A.: *A Treatise on the Principles and Practice of Medicine,* 5th

ed. Henry Lee's Sons, 1881, p. 98.
67. Rosen, G.: *A History of Public Health.* New York, M.D. Publications, 1958, pp. 287-90.
68. Aristotle: *De Caelo.* Bk. 1, chap. 7, 276a, op. cit., p. 412.
69. Aristotle: *De Generatione et Corruption,* bk. 1, chap. 1, 314a and bk. 1, chap. 7, 325a. Op. cit., pp. 470 and 497.
70. Sambursky, S.: Op. cit., pp. 111-113.
71. Copleston, F. S. J.: Op. cit., p. 65.
72. Burnet, J.: Op. cit., pp. 174-175.
73. Sambursky, S.: Op. cit., p. 113.
74. Sambursky, S.: Op. cit., 162-163.
75. Lucretius: *On the Nature of Things,* chap. 2. Munro, H. A. J. transl. New York, Doubleday, 1960, pp. 37 ff.
76. Galen: *De Plenitudine Liber,* cap. 3. Op. cit., p. 525.
77. Sambursky, S.: Op. cit., p. 134 ff.
78. Lucretius: Op. cit., pp. 104-05.
79. Aristotle: *De Generatione et corruption,* bk. 1, chap. 1, 315b. Op. cit., p. 473.
80. Aristotle: *Metaphysics,* bk. 1, chap. 4, 985b. Op. cit., p. 697.
81. Burnet, J.: Op. cit., p. 336, footnote 4.
82. Burtt, E. A.: Op. cit., p. 43.
83. Sarton, George: *Six Wings. Men of Science in the Renaissance.* Indiana Univ. Press, 1957, pp. 77-78.
84. Burtt, E. A.: Op. cit., pp. 24-39.
85. Sarton, G.: Op. cit., pp. 55-62.
86. Burtt, E. A.: Op. cit., pp. 48 ff.
87. Kepler, J.: *Harmonices Mundi,* liber. 5, cap. 3, pp. 299, 308. In: *Gesammelte Werke,* Casper, M., ed. Muenchen, Beck'sche, 1940, vol. 6.
88. Sarton, G.: Op. cit., pp. 66-67.
89. Helm, E. E.: Op. cit., pp. 97-98.
90. Kepler, J.: *Harmonices Mundi,* liber. 5, cap. 4. In: op. cit., 316.
91. Burtt, E. A.: Op. cit., p. 58 and footnote 45.
92. Kepler, J.: Concerning the more certain fundamentals in astrology. Meywald, E., transl. *Amer. Astrol.* July, pp. 7-12: August, pp. 17-23, 1941.
93. Kepler, J.: *Astronomia Nova.* In: *Gesammelte Werke,* op. cit., vol. 3, pp. 33-34.
94. Burtt, E. A.: Op. cit, pp. 87 ff.
95. Galileo, G.: *Two New Sciences,* op. cit., p. 194.
96. Rochot, B.: *Les Travaux de Gassendi (1592-1655) sur l'Epicure et sur l'Atomisme.* Paris, Librairie Philosophique J. Vrin, 1944, pp. 168.
97. Heisenberg, W.: Op. cit., pp. 59-70.
98. Sambursky, S.: Op. cit., pp. 190-91.
99. Gershenson, D. E. and Greenberg, D. A.: *Anaxagoras and the Birth of Scientific Method.* New York, Blaisdell, 1964, pp. 5-26.
100. Plato: In: *The Works of Plato. The Laws.* Jowett, B. transl. New York, Tudor, 1948, p. 454.
101. Sambursky, S.: Op. cit., pp. 134 ff.
102. Sambursky, S.: Op. cit., p. 138.
103. Newton, I.: *Opticks.* London, Smith & Walford, 1704, Definition 1 and pp. 138 ff.
104. Newton, I.: *Philosophiae Naturalis Principia Mathematica,* Liber 3, edi. ultima. Amsterdam, 1714, pp. 484 ff.
105. Einstein A. and Infeld, L.: Op. cit., pp. 110-111.

THE STRUCTURE OF GALEN'S DIAGNOSTIC REASONING*

WALTHER RIESE

Emeritus Associate Professor of
Neurology, Psychiatry, and the History of Medicine
Medical College of Virginia
Richmond, Va.

THE major epistemological problem raised by diagnosis is implied in the constituents of this mental procedure and their interrelations. The names of diseases, their diagnoses, and classifications are correlative terms. The constituents of diagnosis recur as the criteria of subdivisions in our classificatory schemes. We reach a diagnosis by identifying a given disease, and we identify a disease by relating it to its *genus* of which the disease is a *species*, and the lowest, i.e., the final, division of our classificatory scheme. The variants or subgroups of a given disease result from differences in etiology, in the sites, and in the natures of lesions. Which of the constituents should be given the highest rank in the hierarchy? The physician trying to reach a diagnosis must realize that it is quite arbitrary to give preference to the anatomical, or the pathological, or any other element of his diagnosis or principle of classification.

An example may illustrate the diagnostic rules here offered. The diagnostician would begin with the statement that in a given case one of the basic functions of animal or human life, e.g., voluntary movement, is disordered. He would then proceed to localize the level of the nervous system involved in the type and scope of the paralysis encountered; next would come the tentative impression of the pathological nature of the lesion and, finally, the presumable etiology. I submit that the mental procedure here outlined is more fitting for the dignity and greatness of human intelligence than any diagnosis ready-made by automatic routine, though the latter too may serve purposes of its own.

In a chapter of his *De Locis Affectis*,[1] in which Galen gives rules for diagnosis, he states that one must study above all the *function* disturbed.

*This work was supported in part by Public Health Service Research Grant RO 3-MH-12975 from the National Institute of Mental Health, Bethesda, Md.

The disorder of the specific function of an organ is designated as its specific or pathognomonic system. This, he continues, is the only indispensable constituent of disease with which those symptoms resulting from variations in type and intensity of the lesions cannot compete.[2] Referring to Asclepiades in his treatise *On Medical Experience*, Galen distinguished "prognostic" symptoms, which precede the disease; diagnostic ones, which appear along with it; and therapeutic symptoms, which follow the disease. In his book *On the Best Sect* Galen analyzed the symptoms from the standpoint of their therapeutic implications. He pointed out that there are no two cases in which symptoms are identical as to type, number, intensity, and chronological order. Since the days of Hippocrates, prognosis was the main concern of the ancient physician; the thesis of the chronological significance of symptoms is illustrated in *On Medical Experience* by the different prognostic values of symptoms, identical in nature but different in chronological order.

Galen taught that treatment is a kind of symptom-formation; that the effect of a given therapeutic procedure that preceded certain occupations and manipulations was different from the effect of the same procedure when it succeeded them. Thus he expressed by the term consistency the chronological place of symptoms as the ultimate criterion of disease. What finally emerges is a most rational doctrine of diseases —since the decisive criterion, namely the order of symptoms or the moment of their appearance, remain purely formal determinants devoid of any perceptive qualities.

Next in diagnosis comes the examination of the part involved. This may be called the *regional* constituent of diagnosis. In the history of medicine the founders of morbid anatomy, Morgagni, Bichat, Virchow, and others are credited with the introduction and elaboration of the anatomical conception of disease which, we are told, could not come into existence before the rise of anatomy during the Renaissance. This certainly holds true for the more substantial contributions made by these eminent physicians to local diagnosis. But in principle the regional constituent, so powerful in our modern conception of disease, was enunciated by Galen, and it remains unintelligible that in this respect the Roman physician was denied the credit he deserved, though the title alone of his work *De Locis Affectis* should have aroused the historian's alertness and sense of justice. It remains true, however, that

Galen's anatomy was, for centuries, the standard. But in many ways it was inaccurate; this occurred not only because of technical imperfections and inexactitudes, but because it was based upon dissection of animals only. Neuburger reports that Galen only twice obtained, through accident, possession of a human skeleton—once in the case of a corpse washed out of its grave by a river in flood, the second body being that of an executed robber.[3] Permission to dissect the bodies of enemies killed in battle was of very little value to science, since the technically ill-equipped surgeons attached to the Roman army were not in a position to derive much advantage from this source. Galen dissected chiefly the anthropoid apes, bears, swine, ungulates, ruminants, an elephant, birds, fishes, and snakes.

The third constituent of Galen's conception of disease, which is at the same time the next step in diagnosis, is the examination of the type of the lesion in the part involved. In this matter neither Galen's thought nor his terminology is clear beyond doubt. In some instances the lesions seem almost indistinguishable from the functional disturbances. For example, Galen includes in the category of lesions the two great "communities" established by the sect of the methodists, namely, the laxum and the strictum. In other instances, as in tumor, inflammations, tumefaction, stone, or foreign body,[4] the lesions definitely assume the anatomico-pathological meaning of modern terminology. It was indeed morbid anatomy which, in the course of medical history, gave the final shape to this constituent of our concept of disease. What is not subject to doubt is that lesions occupy the second rank in the hierarchy of the constituents of the Galenic conception of disease. You should by all means first detect the organ whose function is impaired, he said, and then determine the type of the lesion.[5] That Galen believed in anatomico-pathological entities is probably not too daring an assumption. Once the borders of health and temperament are crossed and disease is established, he said, the latter no longer changes its nature. He qualified this by citing inflammation as a well-defined species regardless of its site; to the modern physician inflammation is often a chapter of neuropathology. The character of a species of diseases is conceived by Galen along the lines of *structural* organization. In fact, diseases are interpreted as analogous with "homoiomeres," i.e., things composed of similar parts. Once formed, a disease has a type of its own from the very beginning; the intensity and extent (of the lesions) alone are subject to variation. The same idea was expressed many centuries later by Bichat in his *Anatomie Générale.*

"I always try," Galen said, "to discover the region affected primarily or secondarily and responsible for the disordered function. As soon as I feel certain," he concluded, "to have found this region, I try to discover the nature of the disorder *(diathesis);* I derive my indication from both these concepts, considering not only the type of the remedy and its dosage but also the age of the patient, his constitution, the season, place, and all of the Hippocratic criteria." These diagnostic rules are to be found in the tenth chapter of the second book of Galen's *De Optima Secta,* dedicated to Thrasybulos.

The source from which Galen derived his diagnostic signs are identical with the various constituents of the structure of diagnosis, i.e., the region involved, the symptoms and, third, the causes of diseases, not to mention the specific dispositions of each individual. Galen considered pain a diagnostic sign of utmost importance; he believed it to assume a specific character in accordance with the site of its origin.

Galen strongly defended the causal nature of disease, though, of course, he could not as yet outline a true doctrine of causes. But his idea of a special diathesis persisting after elimination of its cause *(cessante causa non cessat morbus),** is an anticipation of a doctrine of causes. His use of the term is not unequivocal. He assigns the term to dyscrasias or to humoral disturbances as well as to foreign agents and influences. The latter are closer to the Hippocratic tradition. In medical thought *causal thought* emerges as an organizing principle of memory and history. The empiricist's neglect of the investigation of causes, his tendency to consider all phenomena on the same level indiscriminately, deprives him of the advantage of distinguishing between essential and accidental ones–i.e., between salient causes and simple concomitants.

The search for causes in illness due to moral factors is much more difficult than in those due to physical factors. It is true that the method of this search is still the same: namely the method of analogy. But since in morals, a field of individual experiences, the previous experiences that serve as analogies for present experiences are alive and usable only to the extent that a sincere investigator has experienced them himself, the investigator is involved more particularly and more per-

*The cause may cease, but the disease lingers on.

sonally than in the search for physical causes. Every informed physician knows the difficulties which so often make it almost impossible for him to distinguish the so-called organic origin of a given symptom from its so-called "psychogenic" origin. This is because the search for causes is almost never a search for present, perceptible phenomena, but for past phenomena, which must be reconstructed in thought. To this difficulty, which is fundamental, is added one arising from the fact that the symptom itself includes no differentiating element that reveals the dynamics of its origin, even when fraudulent or simulated. The richness of the structural and functional design, that is to say, the potentiality of the organism to adapt itself to multitudinous conditions, is notably counterbalanced by the limited number of reactions. So it is that, despite their individual stamp, the number and nature of symptoms are limited. *Illnesses due to moral causes have no symptomatology of their own,** a conclusion that supports the argument that there are no specific causes.

Finally, the Galenic conception of disease implies a genetic constituent, namely the history of disease. Galen committed himself to the rule that in each case one must investigate not only the present but also the past symptoms, using the patient and also the relatives as his informants. Galen might have been influenced by Rufus of Ephesus. Centuries earlier, Hippocrates had laid down the principles and the terms of a study of the natural history of disease. Up to modern times, the generations succeeding the Greeks had nothing basically new to add to the historical view of disease presented for the first time in its definite shape in the writings of the *corpus hippocraticum.*

The history of medicine can be written in terms of the history of disease concepts. Each school of thought developed its own conception of disease. All conceptions of disease can be reduced to one of the constituents of the conception of disease, and each conception of disease is only an accentuation of one of the Galenic constituents.

---

*This statement is only a specific expression of the general fact that no symptom, as such, reveals its origin. Several factors can give rise to the same symptom. The observation of paralysis still does not tell us that its cause and *etiology* is not the same as symptomatology. However, the organism is exposed at all times to innumerable influences; it seems to be distinguished by the poverty rather than the abundance of its types of reaction. No classification, hence no diagnosis, would be possible if the number of symptoms were unlimited. Man seems to be better equipped to receive the messages of the world in which he is destined to live than to act upon this world. The experience that a given symptom lends itself to the most diverse causal interpretations comes under the rule that all objective behavior, even when normal, can be explained by different causes. The action of man does not necessarily reveal his thought. We thus catch a true picture of the limitations and delusions of the art of interpreting symbolic actions, gestures, facial expressions and, therefore, of the sources of the inevitable misunderstandings in interhuman relations. The famous unity of soul and body, which certain enthusiastic spirits preach to us, still defies observational and experimental proof.

The modern physician trying to reach a diagnosis, proceeds in the same way and uses the same intellectual avenues as his Roman forerunner. The perfection which the contemporary physician reaches as compared to his predecessor is a perfection in technique, but not in thought.

Symptoms have always been considered the most significant criteria of disease. Symptoms are related to functions as to their rational roots. But functions must be conceived as first and direct manifestations of life; they no more, and also no less, facilitate and enhance conditions of life in action. Long before their relations to the organs involved and to the lesions encountered (i.e., to their regional and pathological sources) were studied and known, diseases were identified and classified according to their symptomatology, which represents the oldest chapter of clinical medicine and the oldest constituent of diagnosis. In fact, in the history of medical thought, symptomatology even preceded diagnosis; the case histories embodied in the *corpus hippocraticum* carry a minute descriptive and chronological analysis of symptoms, though they carry no diagnosis. *The latter is the most significant contribution of modern medicine as opposed to ancient medicine.* But as long as the symptom is interpreted as no more than a disturbed function *(functio laesa)* it is devoid of any dynamic character. Only too obviously, the concepts of loss or disturbance implied in the Galenic definition of the symptom as *functio laesa* do not in themselves imply any positive constituent such as force or power. Johann Georg Zimmermann, the 18th century Swiss medical philosopher, added to this type of symptom that of *epigennema.*

That Zimmermann thus introduced the "natural forces of the body" as opposing forces (as so many effects of the combat which takes place between nature and disease) was undoubtedly a dynamic conception of the symptom which seems to merge into another ancient idea, i.e., that of the *vis medicatrix naturae,* the dynamic nature of which is revealed by its very name *(vis).*

But it was Galen himself who wrote a treatise *On The Natural Faculties,* one of his most popular works and one of the very few that have been rendered into English. The term faculty is almost synonymous with the term force or power, and Galen introduced a special force for each physiological phenomenon—a force of growth, a force of preservation, a force of retention. None of these faculties or forces, however, appears in his diagnostic reasoning. The reason for this strange omission remains undisclosed. Did he anticipate the danger of an ontological interpretation?

It is true that in the course of the history of medical thought and philosophy in general, the faculties finally assumed the character of self-sufficient entities; the term implied this meaning up to the 19th century, more specifically in the writings of Gall,[6-8] whose influence on medicine and anthropology can hardly be overstated. It must be said, perhaps for the first time, that Galen was not responsible for this ontology. Just as it may be said of any other cause, he said that a given faculty exists only in relation to its own effect. One would be mistaken in conceiving a faculty as something concrete or perceptible, residing in a substance as we reside in our houses. To say that a faculty exists only in thought, I submit, would be the logical though somewhat generous conclusion of Galen's thesis. Not knowing the nature of the acting cause, he also said, one calls it a faculty. It would be difficult to reconcile this agnosticism with any ontology. Finally, Galen requested that a systematic investigation of the number and nature of the faculties should always start with the acts and not with the powers themselves. In fact, there are as many faculties as there are real acts, which a modern reader would be tempted to call life processes. Again, the rule implies an anti-ontological approach, since it is precisely the criterion of ontology to make the hypothetical entity (faculty) and not the concrete phenomenon the starting point of the whole investigation. In his enlightening note Daremberg[9] referred to a similar passage in Aristotle,[10] ". . . In the order of investigation the question of what an agent does precedes the question, what enables it to do what it does." The whole problem is of far greater than academic proportions. Galen's authority was uncontested in medical thought for more than 1,500 years. The analysis here submitted shows that he was not responsible for any dogmatic ontology or dogmatic vitalism that arose in his name at any period of medical history.

Galen's division and classification of the faculties certainly contributed to their dogmatic use and to the ontology initiated by that use. This is most obvious in his interpretation of nutrition. In this process numerous faculties are believed to be involved, namely an alterative or assimilative faculty that, however, presupposes an attractive or epispastic one. Assimilation in its turn was thought to be preceded by adhesion, and this, again, by presentation. Finally, the retentive faculty ensured a prolonged stay of the present juice at the part.[11, 11a] Here, then, was a most rational, most sober, and most admirable interpretation of nutrition though made by analytic thought alone.

According to Sarton, it was Galen's gratuitous postulation of special forces for each need, even more than his teleology, that risked stopping, and did stop, scientific investigations.[12]

The moment one arrives at the idea of the healing power of nature and, above all, at the concept of *organ* which it comprises, one has adopted the Aristotelian doctrine of final causes. This brings us back at once to the idea of the usefulness of the parts of the human body, an idea to which Galen devoted one of his most significant and important treatises (*De usu partium*). According to Daremberg, Galen is here concerned less with showing the functions of the parts than with demonstrating the relation between their organization and the functions which they have to fulfil. And the eminent French medical historian goes on to conclude that we are dealing not so much with a work of physiology as with an anatomical treatise composed according to the doctrine of final causes. Indeed, Galen contrasts function with usefulness of the parts. Thus he defines function as an active and efficacious movement, while usefulness is nothing more than what is popularly called "convenience."

In another passage Daremberg maintains that Galen in the treatise on the usefulness of the parts is concerned neither with anatomy nor physiology proper: he is not inquiring into how a thing is and how an act is performed, but into why a disposition exists and in what way this disposition may contribute efficaciously to action. Analogously, Galen distinguishes between the usefulness of the parts and "natural problems," which comprise questions of organization, of structure and the explanation of physiological action, but not what concerns the usefulness of the parts.

Adopting the Aristotelian thesis that the body is the instrument of the soul, Galen reaches the conclusion that the same parts are very dissimilar in different animals because the souls themselves differ. Thus he allows himself to be drawn into a veritable symbolism of bodily structure which, he believes, is adapted to the habits and faculties of the soul. This idea is hardly compatible with the Cartesian thesis of an absolute difference and a strict separation between the *res extensa* and the *res cogitans,* a thesis that originated, it is true, more than 1,500 years after Galen. But the study of the usefulness of the parts constitutes for Galen "the principle of a perfect theology," which he believed to be "a greater and far more important work than the whole of medicine." Galen's symbolism of the bodily structure is especially apparent when he speaks of cerebral structures, which he designates as psychical organs. This designation is assuredly precarious in attributing to tissues qualities, such as psychical qualities, which are foreign to them and which belong rather to the faculties and functions. In the physical organs the function is innate, while in the psychical organs it springs from the principle of feeling and of movement.

This is why muscles, which have no innate principle of feeling and of movement, are always in need of nerves to supply them as the sun sheds light upon all the beings upon which it shines.* This distinction between the two orders of organs brings Galen back once more to the problems of diagnosis. However, the observation that "this is why it occurs only in the case of organs endowed with feeling and movement that sometimes without being in any way injured they nevertheless lose their function" demands today a stricter, more technical, broader interpretation. Indeed, it demands complete mastery of the problem and the results of the doctrine of cerebral localization, which arose, it is true, almost 2,000 years after Galen.** But this gap, which an informed contemporary reader cannot fail to discover in Galen's thought, takes nothing away from his diagnostic advice "to examine and determine first of all what activities occur in the organs considered as psychical or as physical; as physical, for example, the change resulting from contact with adjacent objects; as psychical, the feeling arising from this change."

Let us conclude this chapter on the principle of usefulness by citing Galen's view that knowledge of usefulness is no less indispensable for the diagnosis of the affections of a part than knowledge of functions. ("If walking is prevented because a nerve or muscle of the leg is injured, it is likewise prevented when a bone is broken or dislocated

*This metaphor appears again in the *Essai de Psychologie Physiologique* by C. Chardel (Paris, Bureau d'Encyclopédie Portative, 1831), who considers it to be a demonstrated truth that life is a fluid analogous to an electromagnetic fluid, and that it likewise owes its origin to solar emanations (*op. cit.,* p. 129). He also says that "the cerebral gland in animals seizes the solar rays which the arterial blood brings to it and composes from them a fluid almost as subtle as light. . . ." (*op. cit.,* pp. 124-25).

**In my *History of Neurology*[13] I conceded (p. 80) that Galen made observational, experimental, and clinical contributions to cerebral localization, and that these contributions mark the truly modern elements in Galenism. Other modern elements are to be found in his first attempt to use unmasking psychology as instrumental in the treatment and cure of nervous disorders.

from its socket": this is an example of the fortunate application drawn from the treatise on the usefulness of the parts to the diagnosis of affected parts hidden in the depths of the body.) Still speaking in Galenic terms, function is an active movement, but those movements which take place in certain parts when other parts move are designated as passive or sympathetic movements. It is precisely in this analysis of movements that Galen arrives at a conclusion of the greatest significance, namely, the definition of an organ. In relation to the prime mover, which is the principle of the soul, muscles must be considered as an organ. The concept of an organ is, therefore, linked with that of the soul or, better still, with that of life. An organ is more than just a part.

In the 19th century Hughlings Jackson, a most eminent clinician and interpreter of nervous function and nervous disease, divided all symptoms into negative and positive, the former covering loss of function or functional deficiencies resulting from the disease process, such as paralysis and speechlessness; the positive symptoms being the activities and overactivities of the healthy parts, now left to themselves, such as tremor and hallucinations.

In this view, the positive symptoms represent new modes of functioning and behavior thrown into action as best suited to cope with the tasks with which a damaged nervous system still has to cope. Symptoms thus conceived emerge as true organs, provocative as the term may appear when separated from its anatomical attribute. This interpretation can be traced back to Galen and, in the final analysis, to Aristotle. It conveys a strong teleological element which many a physician might be reluctant to accept today, though the rule still stands that one must treat the person rather than attack his symptoms immediately and indiscriminately. The person must be understood to be more than a compound of functioning units, and display direction and purposeful action. The interpretation also brings home to the contemporary physician the spontaneous recovering and healing tendencies embodied in positive symptoms and their corollaries, the compensatory satisfactions. In using the latter term we have crossed the border of physiology to invade psychology.* Galen's little known and hardly practiced talent as a diagnostician of the human soul enabled him to

*Ilza Veith, in a short and thoughtful paper, explored Galen's psychology for the first time, and in terms of modern psychology.[21]

identify the roots, the nature, and the manifestations of human passions.[13-20, 27] He finally emerges as a moral philosopher on equal footing with his inalienable merits and rights as a philosopher of science and medicine.

In diagnosis, medical thought seeks to grasp a body of vital manifestations and to assign it a place in the terminology of diseases. It is a labor of assemblage, of synthesis, and of classification of human knowledge. No relation of man to man seems to be implied. Thus at first approach we really see no moral problem raised by diagnosis. However, the origin of diseases or their etiology is included in their very nature and therefore in diagnosis. Now the idea of sin as a cause of disease appears in primitive medicine. With Paracelsus, in the 16th century, this idea reappears in its Christian form; it reaches its peak with Heinroth in the early 19th century. Among recent authors, C. von Monakow upholds the thesis that disease may result from a betrayal of the interests both of the community and of humanity. In all ages man has incriminated his passions as causes of disease, and insofar as these passions are included in ethics, a definitely moral problem is raised by the diagnosis of diseases caused by passions. We need not be surprised to see the passions occupy a prominent place among etiological factors admitted by a school of thought which favors the "moral" treatment of insanity, e.g., in the writings of Philippe Pinel and Jean E. D. Esquirol. But other factors figure in the etiology of diseases and reflect even more eloquently the relations of man to man and hence, of their moral nature. La Rochefoucauld, in a brief chapter, "On the Origin of Disease" in his *Reflexions Diverses,* has drawn up a list: just so many vices, just so many causes of disease;* and Rousseau states that the miseries and diseases of civilized man must be attributed to a ceaseless search for satisfactions exceeding his natural needs and a boundless avidity. Dis-

*"If we examine the nature of diseases, we will discover that they draw their origin from the passions and the sorrows of the soul. The Golden Age, exempt from them, was exempt also from disease; the Silver Age which followed still preserved its purity; the Bronze Age gave birth to the passions and the sorrows of the soul; they were in the process of formation and they still evidenced the weakness and delicacy of childhood. But they appeared in all their force and malignity in the Iron Age, and they spread throughout the world, in consequence of their corruption, the various diseases which have afflicted mankind for so many centuries. Ambition produces acute and delirious fevers; envy gives rise to jaundice and insomnia; from sloth came lethargy, paralysis and debility; anger caused choking, skin eruptions and pulmonary inflammation; fear produced palpitations and syncope. while vanity caused insanity; avarice, tinea and mange; melancholy produces scurvy; cruelty, gall stones; calumny and slander have caused the spread of measles, smallpox, and purpura; and to jealousy we owe gangrene, the plague, and hydrophobia. Sudden disgrace gave rise to apoplexy; lawsuits were causes of migraine and congestion of the brain; debts caused ethic fevers; annoyance of married life produced quartan fevers, and the lassitude of lovers who dare not separate were the cause of vapors. . . . Love in itself has produced more miseries than all the rest put together and no one should undertake to express them; but as it also produces the greatest good in life, instead of slandering it, we should remain silent, we should fear and respect it for ever."

I cited the whole chapter in its original French terms in my *Pensée Morale en médecine, Premiers principes d'une éthique médicale,"* Paris, Presses Universitaires de France, 1954, p. 35.

eases represent a first stage in the destruction of a world destined to crumble into ruin under the disastrous effect of man's infinite greediness, leaving him finally alone on earth.

Whatever we may think of these theories of moral thought, those which are linked with the names of Pinel, Esquirol, and Monakow are conceived by physicians, and for this very reason they represent in my opinion a glorious achievement of modern medicine in that they strive beyond analysis and experimentation toward a true science of man. In a sense it is Galen, a follower of Aristotle, who emerges as a precursor of these views.

Generally speaking, what is less in the foreground of the ethics of the Greeks is the element of conflict and of struggle. Far from passing through the crisis of conscience so characteristic of modern man, who braves decision and action—man, according to Aristotle, is just if he feels joy in accomplishing just actions; he is generous if he delights in generous actions and, the philosopher concludes: ". . . . actions which conform to virtue are agreeable in themselves."[22] Galen in his treatise "That the habits of the soul follow the temperaments of the body" sustains the thesis that the good and the bad are such as they are because of corporal temperament. To his adversaries who fear that the right to praise or to blame, to hate or to love, might be denied them, Galen replies that we are endowed with the innate faculty to prefer, to seek, to love the good, to turn aside from evil, to hate and to avoid it "without considering whether or not it was engendered."[23]

If it be true that Galen does not explicitly declare, as does Aristotle,[24] that we feel joy in accomplishing just actions, the love of the good none the less implies in his view the pleasure which we always feel in obeying our innate faculties. On the other hand, the attitude of modern man in relation to the good is utterly different. If a man happens to love the good, and if this love manifests itself by acts and not only by gratuitous admiration, then it is only after having endured conflict* and after having resisted the initial love of evil and of temptation. The dramatic explanation between desire and duty cannot be found in Galen. If drama there be, it does not take place in the con-

*It is true that Aristotle in his *Nicomachean Ethics* admits deliberation and choice (111, 5) and that, according to him, goodness and vice are based precisely on choice. However, he does not discuss the attitude of mind which is characterized by choice in *suspense;* this in my opinion, distinguishes modern man from the Greek. But Aristotle, like most Greeks, is mainly a metaphysician, and the *psychologic* effects which metaphysical data involve play no part in his preoccupations. This would mean that conflict, a psychological phenomenon of utmost importance, although derived from a metaphysical phenomenon, introduces a new and foreign element into the thought of antiquity.

sciousness of the Roman physician. But the terms which, for the physician, translate in the most evident manner the noncombative nature of Galen's concept of virtue, are those of diathesis and of disposition. This same nature was previously implied in the Platonic and Aristotelian definition of ethics as *wisdom* and *measure*, but also in the Platonic idea, used later by Aristotle, according to which justice and morals are the proper functions of the soul as the sight is that of the eye. Man to be virtuous and happy need only exercise his proper functions. But rising from the depths of this idea we see the danger of a *physiological* interpretation of ethics; we shall find this again in Galen. Aristotle in a most explicit manner defines virtues as acquired dispositions. "Moral virtue is the daughter of good habits." Thus it is neither by a natural nor an unnatural effect that virtues are engendered issues; we are predisposed by nature to acquire them conditionally on perfecting them by habit.[25] ". . . We become just, temperate and courageous by dint of practicing justice, temperance and courage."[26]

These Aristotelian and Galenic interpretations, however, seem to ignore the always-creative nature of any moral decision, to which they confer a somewhat dilatory element. In morals each law has, in a way, its given name,[27] since each moral act retains its legislative power only within the limits of the individual, irretrievable, and irreplaceable conditions under which it is performed. But that which seems to characterize Galenic and certain recent versions is the identification of nature with morals. It is difficult to understand how, then, a conflict can be engendered within the same power and, above all, how, beginning with a certain evolutive stage, purely instinctive and unconscious behaviors are able to engender conscience which, however, remains the vantage point for all comparative studies of ethical thought and conduct. Here are the limits of diagnosis, which remains a mental procedure instrumental in naming, identifying, and classifying the natural phenomena of disease, a procedure instrumental also in arriving at a mutual understanding at the bedside and in outlining the design of a preliminary treatment. But diagnosis is instrumental neither in sacrificing medical learning and experience in favor of an intrinsically moralistic approach toward causes and effects of diseases nor in preparing the patient for praise or punishment. Galen undoubtedly was an intelligent and resourceful psychopathologist, limited as this area seemed to be in his immense therapeutic activities. But it was an area that was promoted by the same observational and experimental reasoning which stood at the birth of scientific medicine and which still characterizes all its branches

REFERENCES

1. Galen, *De locis affectis,* II, 10.
2. *Ibid.*
3. Neuburger, M. *History of Medicine,* Playfair, E., tr. London, Frowde, Hodder, Stoughton, 1910.
4. Galen, *op. cit.,* I, 1.
5. Galen, *ibid.,* I, 2.
6. Riese, W. F. G. Gall et le problème des localisations cérébrales. *Hyg. Ment. 31:* 105-36, 1936.
7. Riese, W. Les discussions du problème des localisations cérébrales dans les sociétés savantes du XIXe siècle et leurs rapports avec des vues contemporaines. *Hyg. Ment. 31:*137-58, 1936.
8. Temkin, O. Gall and the phrenological movement. *Bull. Hist. Med. 21:*275-321, 1947.
9. Daremberg, C. *Oeuvres anatomiques, physiologiques et médicales de Galien,* Paris, Ballière, 1854, p. 49.
10. Aristotle, *De anima,* II, 41.
11. Galen, *Natural Faculties,* Loeb Classical Library. London, Heinemann; Cambridge, Mass., Harvard Univ. Press, 1947, vol. 3, p. 1.

11*a*. Riese, W. *The Conception of Disease, Its History, its Versions and its Nature.* New York, Philosophical Library, 1953, pp. 106-107.

12. Sarton, G. *Galen of Pergamon.* Lawrence, Kansas Univ. Press, 1954.
13. Riese, W. *A History of Neurology.* New York, M. D. Publications, 1959.
14. Riese, W. *La pensée morale en médecine. Premiers principes d'une éthique médicale.* Paris, Presses Univer. 1954.
15. Riese, W. and Bourget, L. Les gracieusetés à l'égard des maladies. Commentaire de Galien sur épidémies, vol. 6, sect. 4, div. 7.
16. Riese, W. La pensée morale de Maimonide. *Rev. Hist. Méd. Hébraïque 54:* 149-53, 1961.
17. Riese, W. *Galen on the Passions and Errors of the Soul,* Columbus, Ohio State Univ. Press, 1963.
18. Riese, W. La pensée morale de Galien. *Rev. Philosoph. France Étranger 153:* 331-46, 1963.
19. Riese, W. La théorie des passions à la lumière de la pensée médicale du XVIIe siècle. *Confin. Psychiat. (suppl.) 8:*1-74, 1965.
20. Riese, W. Le traitement moral de l'alienation mentale, histoire et principes. *Ann. Ther. Psychiat.* (publiées sous l'eglide de la Société Moreau de Tours par Henri Baruk et Jacques Launay) *3:*78-91, 1967.
21. Veith, I. Galen psychology. *Perspect. Biol. Med. 4:*316-23, 1961.
22. Aristotle. *Ethique de Nicomaque.* Voilquin, J. Paris, Garnier, p. 29.
23. Daremberg, C. *Oeuvres anatomiques, physiologiques et médicales de Galien.* Paris, Ballière, 1854, vol. 1, 85.
24. Aristotle, *op. cit.,* pp. 29, 145.
25. *Ibid.*
26. *Idem.,* II, 1.
27. Riese, W. and Réquet, A. *L'idée de l'homme dans la neurologie contemporaine.* Paris, Alcan, 1938.

GREEK MEDICAL AND PHILOSOPHICAL INTERPRETATIONS OF FEAR*

THOMAS S. HALL, PH.D.

Professor of Biology
Department of Biology
Washington University
St. Louis, Mo.

FEAR was a major motif of ancient Greek epic poetry and drama; it was a topic often treated by biographers and historians of the period and explicitly analyzed by philosophers and physicians. I shall focus on physiological and pathological aspects of fear as they appear in the thought of Aristotle, Epicurus, and Galen, examining these thinkers' answers to the questions: *What is fear? What causes it? What are its consequences?* We shall find that in answering these questions each author was influenced by certain broad explanatory assumptions that governed his thinking, not only about fear but about universal nature—about the cosmos in general, including what the Greeks liked to call the living microcosm, man.

ARISTOTLE

The general nature of fear. Aristotle was caught up in the tradition that the complexities of the cosmos are reducible to pairs of opposites such as hot versus cold, dense versus rare, potential versus real, and the like.[1] His predecessor, Plato, influenced by the same tradition, had made fear the opposite of hope, asserting that fear is the expectation of evil and hope the expectation of good.[2] Aristotle made fear the opposite of confidence and added that fear is the expectation of such evils as poverty, friendlessness, dishonor, pain, and especially death.[3]

To Aristotle or to a member of his circle we owe the thought-provoking suggestion that excellent men have a tendency toward sadness and, under certain circumstances, toward fear.[4] Excellence, Aristotle said, entails the ability to transcend such feelings through acts exhibiting virtue, including the virtue of courage.[5] Aristotle looked upon courage as a mean condition between the two opposites of undue

*Presented at the 46th Annual Meeting of the American Association for the History of Medicine held in Cincinnati, Ohio, on May 3, 1973.

fearfulness and undue fearlessness.[6] Fearlessness as such he did not regard as virtuous. Not to fear the gods and their works (earthquakes, for example) he regarded as insane and not to fear disgrace as ignoble.[7] A brave man does not, like a stone, feel no fear; he feels fear but overcomes it.[8] In acting thus virtuously he may attain a degree of happiness, since happiness is the habitual exercise of perfect virtue.[9] Plato's influence is apparent in these ideas but their precise formulation is distinctly Aristotelian.

The physical basis of fear. Aristotle divided the soul into three parts, which he spoke of—with variations of terminology in different works—as rational, nonrational, and nutritive.[10] He argued that courage, along with the other virtues, must reside in the nonrational part of the soul, because that part is the locus of feeling, and courage is a mean between feeling too much and too little fear.[11] Fear, then, is a feeling and, as such, an activity; in Aristotle's language it is a movement or kinesis of the nonrational part of the soul. Aristotle further tells us what he believes the soul itself to be: namely, the form of the body. Soul, in other words, is that dynamic organization of matter in certain things that permits them to engage in activities by which we recognize them as alive.[12] If we ask Aristotle what material configuration permits the activity that we recognize as fear, he answers: a cold configuration.

Aristotle was not the first, but he was the most influential early exponent of the idea that the heart is hot and that its heat travels throughout the body with the blood.[13] From this supposition it seemed to him to follow that animals with relatively little blood must be correspondingly cold and hence fearful. Among animals rendered fearful by the scantiness of their blood he mentioned the chameleon, which he supposed to have very little blood, and the cuttlefish, which he supposed to have none.[14] By the same reasoning he argued that animals—and men—with large and soft hearts must be fearful, because in hearts with copious contents the heat becomes diluted, like the heat of the hearth-fire in a very large room. Among large-hearted animals that he believed to be correspondingly fearful, Aristotle mentioned deer, rabbits, mice, and a curious quartet comprising the marten, the ass, the hyena, and the leopard. If the latter four seem not to be fearful that is because their underlying cowardice takes the outward form of vicious behavior, he said.[15] Finally, Aristotle considered the blood to be composed of two parts, one watery and the other earthy, the earthy part being that which makes up the substance of the clot. He argued that men and animals with relatively watery blood are correspondingly sensitive and, if the blood is too watery, fearful. Thus fearfulness is not only a cold configuration but also a wet one. The qualities of fearfulness and of sensitivity—intelligence, even—are, then, to some extent constitutionally related.[16]

Consequences of fear. In addition to developing these ideas about the nature and causes of fear, Aristotle's circle investigated its physiological consequences: pallor, trembling, pounding of the heart, thirst, diuresis, diarrhoea, and contraction of the genitalia, sometimes with the emission of semen. In fear and anger, they said, the blood in general—and with it heat—is contracted inward from the surface of the body toward the center. But in fear the blood and heat are also driven downward so that whereas in anger the heart is hot, in fear it is cold.[17] Moreover, in animals with scanty blood, changes in color may occur when such animals are frightened—as may be observed in the chameleon and the cuttlefish.[18] In the cuttlefish and other cephalopods there is also an involuntary discharge of ink, which Aristotle likened to the discharge of urine and excrement in higher animals when they are seized by fear.[19]

Cosmological aspect of Aristotle's physiological theory. Most of these notions about fear are traceable, at least in part, to Aristotle's preoccupation with the doctrine of opposites which, as he formulated it, reduced the contents of the entire sublunar cosmos to variations in the configuration and proportion of two pairs of contrary qualities: hot versus cold and wet versus dry. His attribution of fear to a cold and wet deviation from the mean was thus, in effect, an extension of cosmological assumptions to a physiological problem, the problem of the physical basis of fear. In other studies we have shown that the evocation of cosmological assumptions—"paradigms," in Professor Kuhn's fruitful use of that term—was characteristic of Aristotle's physiological theory in general.[20]

The point is illustrated by another cosmological doctrine, more peculiarly though not exclusively Aristotle's own: namely, his theory of causation. He classified causes in different ways in different works, separating them in some of his writings into *necessary* (inescapable) and *final* (purposive). He applied this distinction to an array of physiological phenomena, among them the discharge of pigment by the cuttlefish. This discharge has a necessary cause, he said, in the sense that it occurs involuntarily; it also has a final cause in the sense that it serves the purpose of protection. It thus did not escape Aristotle that fear is often advantageous. It should be added that if Aristotle applied cosmological ideas to the solution of biological problems, he also often reasoned in the reverse direction, using biological ideas in building his picture of the cosmos. He did so, for example, when he filled the universe with purpose. Early Greek biology and cosmology developed reciprocally, changes in either being able to induce corresponding changes in the other.[21]

Epicurus

The general nature of fear. Epicurus brought together within a single ideological framework his theories of ethics, esthetics, psychology, physiology, and physics. Among these the connecting link was, in his opinion, the atom. Dismissing the Aristotelian notion of contrary qualities as basic to everything, Epicurus invoked a pre-Aristotelian supposition that the cosmos and its contents were reducible to indivisible, impenetrable particles, numerous in kind and infinite in number. What have atoms—varying in their sizes, shapes, and movements in the void—to do with the subject of fear?[22]

The central concern of Epicurus, like that of Greek philosophers in general, was with the well-being of mankind,[23] to which the chief obstacle for most people, he thought, was fear.[24] The usual objects of fear, he said, were pain and whatever inflicts it, and hence ultimately the gods, because the Greeks generally held the gods responsible for the pleasure and pain that men experience, not only in the present life but also in the life to come.[25]

Epicurus urged a new approach to the avoidance of pain and hence the prevention of fear. He proposed that men should turn away from superstitious aspects of religion and seek well-being through the study of physics.[26] In doing so they would come to see that pain is not a visitation of the gods or a product of their vindictiveness or indifference; it is rather, a disarrangement of the atoms of which each individual is composed.[27]

Pain thus conceived is often preventable, not through prayer or propitiation of the gods but through avoidance of things that could lead to atomic disarrangements of the body (ranging from overeating to the stress of public office).[28] Further, at death the whole pattern of the atoms is irreversibly dissolved, whence there can be no life after death and no possibility of pain or of any other sensation.[29] Armed with the knowledge that this is the case, men may seek with confidence that freedom from fear and anxiety, that state of serenity (*ataraxia*) which Epicurus set forth as the primary goal of life.[30] To the extent that this esthetic goal is attained, moreover, men's ethical problems will diminish, since misconduct itself is largely the product of fear.[31]

The physical basis of fear. Epicurus composed the human frame of two interlocking networks of atoms, one representing man's body, the other representing his soul.[32] The soul contains four sorts of atoms, of which one sort are comparable to the atoms of breath or wind, a second sort to atoms of air, and a third sort to atoms of heat. The fourth sort of atoms are so mobile and minute that nothing comparable to them is found in the nonliving world.[33] Animals (and men?) in which heat atoms predominate are constitutionally fierce; those in which chilling breath predominates are fearful; those in which air predominates are calm.[34] The atoms of both soul and body are mobile but they are individually without sentience or awareness.[35] All cognitive acts are rearrangements of the patterns of movement of individually insentient atoms.[36]

Building on the premises just outlined, Epicurus accounted in atomic terms for cognition, recognition, association, and anticipation.[37] Both feelings and ideas could be painful, he supposed, and fear was in effect a painful anticipation of a painful feeling or idea.[38] Both the anticipative idea—the fear—and the anticipated evil came down, in his scheme, to disarrangements of ordinary patterns of movement of atoms.[39] Since Epicurus saw man and the universe as comprising, in the main, the same sorts of atoms,[40] we may view his interpretation of fear as an extension of his physical theory of the cosmos. I have already said the same about Aristotle; but the two drew different conclusions with respect to the welfare of man. Epicurus recommended that fear be anticipated and avoided, whereas Aristotle recommended that it be confronted and overcome.

Galen

Galen's medical theories owed much, as we shall see, to the physical and cosmological ideas of Aristotle. To these, however, he added some physiological suppositions that were peculiarly his own.

Fear as a deviation from the mean. Galen frequently compared the human body to a work of art.[41] The body and a statue are similar in certain respects, he said, and in other respects they differ.[41] The sculptor Polycleitus in his *Canon* specified the proportions of the ideally beautiful human body;[42] similarly, the physician seeks to specify the constitution ideally suited to health. In neither case will the ideal be realized in any actual person. In general, however, an individual approaches the optimum insofar as his constitution avoids disproportions and extremes.[43] In a well-constituted body the dynamic qualities —hot, cold, wet, and dry—are blended temperately.[44] The parts of the body are neither too large nor too small and neither too dense nor too rare; their conformation fits them properly together.[45] Structure is correlated with structure, function with function, and structure with function.[46] Each person departs idiosyncratically from this desirable mean, Galen said, but such deviations are pathological only if they interfere with the normal functions of the parts.[47]

Galen applied these principles to the soul as well as the body. He regarded fear, for example, as a faculty or habit of the soul and the healthy soul as intermediate between the undue fearfulness displayed by certain animals and the undue fearlessness displayed by others. Fear thus represented for Galen, as it had for Aristotle, a deviation from the mean.[48]

Fear and sadness. Galen praised Hippocrates for associating fear with sadness and for making sustained fearfulness and sadness the common symptoms of various forms of melancholy. Sad and fearful men, melancholy men, share certain characteristics: They hate their fellows and curse their own lives. Some of them long for death; some long for death but also fear it.[49]

Imagined evil. Galen accepted the Platonic position, adopted also by Aristotle and Chrysippus, that fear entails expectation of evil. In some unfortunate cases the evil is entirely imaginary. One of Galen's patients supposed himself to be made of a fragile ceramic; he managed his relations with others in such a way as always to be handled gently by them. Another patient was obsessed by the fear that Atlas would drop the world and everyone would be smashed. Another saw a terrible danger in being different from those around him. This even extended to the poultry yard where, according to Galen, he would crow like the chickens and flap his wings.[50] But what did Galen, see as the causes, the physiological correlates, of these unhappy conditions?

The causes of fear. Galen devoted a short treatise to the general thesis that the habits and traits of the soul are consequences of the temperament or blend of the body. Citing Hippocrates and Plato, he emphasized the effects on the soul of climate and of the things that we eat and drink, dwelling especially on the influence of wine, as well as of medicines and poisons.[51] Galen argued that the temperaments or blends of such things must alter the temperament of the body, which in turn must be able to alter the soul. How the body alters the soul he acknowledged to be a difficult problem—the solution depending on one's view of the nature of the soul and of the soul's relation to the body. Galen made a sensitive historical survey of the soul-body problem in earlier Greek thought and concluded that in all the major theories—pre-Socratic, Hippocratic, Platonic, Aristotelian, and Stoic—it had been implicit, and often explicit, that the blend of the body determines the faculties and habits of the soul. As for Galen himself, he accepted and, in his own view, went beyond the Aristotelian concept of the soul as the form of the body. This was true, he believed, of the soul's mortal part, which was ultimately nothing more than the blend of the dynamic qualities to which he believed the body reducible.[52] This assertion leads us to ask with what particular blend we ought to associate fear. Galen touches on this subject in his treatise *On Temperaments*.

For him, as for Aristotle, the ultimate reducibles were hot, cold, wet, and dry. Persons departing from the mean in a cold and dry direction, he said, display a characteristic syndrome. They are pale, soft, and hairless, and have inconspicuous veins. In mind they are fearful and sad. Thus, whereas with Aristotle fearfulness was a cold and wet disposition of the body, with Galen it was cold and dry.[53]

Coldness and dryness are traditionally earmarks of atrabiliousness or melancholia;[54] yet thus far we have heard nothing from Galen about black bile in relation to fear. This is a subject which he does not avoid but approaches with a certain caution. He seems to say that where emotions, fear included, amount to serious (pathological) disturbances, a special condition of the humors may be regarded as a cause. Such disturbances entail corruption of the animal faculties of the soul and are due to a dyscrasia or vitiation of the humors of the brain. The symptoms that implicate black bile in particular are sadness and fear. Persons so afflicted are sad without being able to say what has made them so. They often fear things that are in fact too trivial to be fearsome. It is not surprising that people are sad and fearful in whom black bile or an atrabilious exhalation has seized the brain, the seat of the soul. Among external influences none is so saddening and fearsome as darkness. Small wonder that darkness should produce the same symptoms in the brain.[55]

The consequences of fear. Galen considered the consequences of fear in a number of contexts and acknowledged that the sudden onset of fear could be fatal.[56] Modifying an Aristotelian idea, he believed that fear, anger, and other emotions had a motive effect on the blood. Anger drives the blood from the heart along with breath and heat, thus making the body warm at the surface. Fear has the opposite effect; it contracts the blood and leaves the body surface cold. The emotions likewise influence the pulse. Pulses in general may be 1) normal, 2) fast and strong, 3) slow and weak, or 4) mixed. Anger hastens and strengthens the pulse; fear slows and weakens it. When, as often occurs, fear and anger are present simultaneously, an irregular or mixed pulse results.[57]

To cite another example, Galen associated emotions, including fear, with fever. In many different works he developed a complex theory of fevers, which he classified as ephemeral, recurrent, or continuous, the latter frequently culminating in death. Ephemeral fevers may have either physical or psychological causes, according to Galen; they are often due to such psychic conditions as insomnia, anger, sadness, worry, and fear. It is important for the physician to determine which emotion has caused the fever in each case of this sort, since only thus can the fever be prevented from recurring. Galen gives a great deal of semeiotic information to help the physician decide.[58]

Galen also explained the way he believed fear could be responsible for trembling. Normally, a muscle is contracted by the influence of the motive faculty of the soul, this faculty reaching it by way of its nerves. Trembling occurs when this faculty is inadequate to its task. It occurs, for example, when a man tries to carry too heavy a burden or to lift too heavy a weight. We see these effects even in persons whose motive faculty is intrinsically strong. If the motive faculty is, for some reason, weak, a man may tremble even if his load is relatively light. The motive faculty is weakened, for example, by age, and it is for this reason that old people frequently tremble. Fear, too, can weaken the motive faculty and thus can cause various organs, especially the loose lower lip and the hands, to shake. In effect, Galen brings the interpretation of fear into line with one of his major explanatory assumptions: namely, that each part of the body possesses a particular "faculty" for performing its particular function.[59] In so doing, moreover, he squares his physiological theory with the Aristotelian theory of dynamic qualities. For, although he makes extensive use of his faculty theory, he denies that faculties have any existence of themselves. When we speak of, say, the peptic faculty of the stomach we mean merely that the stomach has a blend of dynamic qualities (hot, cold, wet, and dry) which permits it to digest the food.[60] We thus reduce the living microcosm, man, to the same basic terms we use in interpreting the cosmos.

Conclusion

These notes on Aristotle, Epicurus, and Galen are not intended as an exegesis of everything they thought or wrote about fear. Many factors affected these and other ancient thinkers in their treatment of the subject. Here I have emphasized chiefly the cosmological suppositions in the light of which these authors treated both physiological and pathological problems, including the problem of fear.

Two final points are worth making about the suppositions that were common to Greek cosmology and medicine. First, they were, in general, animistic: they ascribed all life phenomena to the presence in each individual of some sort of soul. Second, they were reductive: they reduced the complexities of the cosmos to a few first principles or to atoms. But there were many varieties of animism and reductivism in Greek thought, and these furnished each thinker with a special matrix, a kind of interpretive grid, within which to develop solutions to particular medical problems. The grid consisted of answers to certain general questions: Is the soul an incorporeal entity separate from but interactive with the matter composing the body? Or is the soul in some way immanent in matter itself? Is it merely a name that we give to the configuration, the special form, that matter assumes in things we think of as alive? Or, finally, is it a constellation of atoms which, though individually insentient, are collectively sentient and aware? Again, to what material ultimates is everything to be reduced? Are the ultimates *dimensional* in nature, that is, are they merely the shapes and sizes of atoms? Or are they, rather *dynamic*: are they the hot, the cold, the wet, and the dry? Interpretations of fear and other psychic and somatic manifestations depended on each author's answers to these encompassing questions, questions that transcend immediate problems and come to grips with human nature and the nature of the universe at large.

Acknowledgment

I am grateful to Professor J. D. Furley for his helpful criticism of this paper.

NOTES AND REFERENCES

Abbreviations. The titles of works of Aristotle are abbreviated according to the conventions used by Liddell, H. G. and Scott, R.: *A Greek-English Lexikon.* Other abbreviations: *DL,* Diogenes Laertius, *De vitis . . . philosophorum,* (*Book X Epicurus*); *LH,* Epicurus to Herodotus (in *DL*); *LP,* Epicurus to Pythocles (in *DL*); all are cited by section. *DRN,* Lucretius, *De Rerum Natura,* cited by book and line. *K,* Kühn, K. L.: *Claudii Galeni Opera Omnia.* Leipzig, Knobloch, 1821-1833, cited by volume and page.

1. The doctrine of opposites was among the deepest-rooted and most frequently invoked ideas in ancient science. For the development of this idea by Aristotle, see Anton, J. P.: *Aristotle's Theory of Contrariety.* New York, Humanities Press, 1957.
2. Plato: *Laches,* 198.
3. Aristotle: *Ethica Nichomachea,* 1115a-711 and 27.
4. Aristotle: *Problemata,* 953a10-13. For a discussion of Aristotle's treatment of the sad and fearful tendencies of outstanding persons, see Klibansky, R., Panofsky, E., and Saxl, F.: *Saturn and Melancholy.* London, Nelson, 1964, pp. 17-41. (The authorship of the *Problems,* now considered to be post-Aristotelian, has not been fully settled.)
5. Aristotle: *Ethica Eudemia.* 1230a21-36. In this treatise Aristotle makes virtue one of three cardinal goods of the soul, the others being wisdom and pleasure (see also *Magna Moralia,* 1183b19-1184b6). In these passages Aristotle acknowledges that there are also other legitimate ways of classifying "goods." (The *Magna Moralia* is now thought to be post-Aristotelian but to reflect Aristotle's thought reliably.)
6. *EN* 1115a3-1116a14 and *EE* 1228a20-b2. Courage is, in this formulation, brought into conformance with the other virtues (justice, temperance, etc.) which are, in general, mean states between extremes of feeling (*MM* 1186a10-1187a4).
7. *MM* 1185b24. Indeed, the man who fears disgrace is "sometimes called brave by shifting the word to a new connotation . . . ." (*EN* 1115a15). It is Aristotle's thesis that feelings are virtuous if they are rational, wise, and noble (*MM* 1185b1-13 and *EE* 1228b36-1229a11).
8. See, e.g., *MM* 1191a26, where we are also told that to be brave entails "feeling the fear but facing the danger." Again, "He who fears the right things for the right reason in the right way at the right time—but faces his fears with confidence," is brave (*NE* 1115b18).

9. *MM* 1184b22-1185a1 and 26.
10. Thus, at *MM* 1185a14-b13. In *de An* Aristotle sometimes spoke of the soul as having parts and sometimes as being endowed with, or defined by, faculties—rational, motive, sensitive, and nutritive (413b12-32 and 414a29-32).
11. *MM* 1185b5-14 (see also reference 6 above).
12. *de An* 413b11-14, 415b9-28.
13. *Juv* 969b6-30; *Resp* 474a25-b9; etc. The idea that the heart is hot was generally supported by later physiologists up to and including William Harvey.
14. *PA* 679a25-26 and 692a21-26; also *Rhet* 1389b30.
15. *PA* 667a11-23.
16. *PA* 650b14-35.
17. For the Aristotelians, it is a descent of the heat and blood that causes frightened people to experience a loosening of the bowels (which is caused, likewise, by drugs that have a heating effect). Further, in frightened persons, but not in angry ones, there is a rapid palpitation that gives a tingling sensation. We "boil" with anger but not with fear. Thirst, too, in frightened people is caused by a draining downward of the blood from the region in which thirst is felt. Trembling of the hand, voice, and lips can be attributed to the same cause. If it seems contrary to reason that descending heat should cause the genitalia to contract (usually they do so when cold) they explain this by supposing that while the heat descends it also moves inward, and the genitalia are external. These and other interesting speculations appear in *Pr* xxvii 947b10-949a20.
18. *HA* 621b28; *PA* 679a13-14 and 25-32. Aristotle notes further that changes in color serve a mimetic function useful for concealment in acts of predation. He says of the chameleon that bloodlessness is "at the root of the animal's habit of soul—he is subject to fear (to which his many changes in appearance are due), and fear is a process of cooling produced through the scantiness of blood and insufficiency of heat."
19. *PA* 678b36-679a28.
20. Hall, T. S.: *Ideas of Life and Matter.* Chicago, University of Chicago Press, 1969, vol. 1, pp. 104-19. On the role of paradigms, see Kuhn, T. S.: *The Structure of Scientific Revolutions,* 2d ed. Chicago, University of Chicago Press, 1970.
21. Thus, at *HA* 622a, where we hear that the sepia "employs its dark liquid *for the sake of* concealment as well as *from* fear" (Thompson D. 'A. W., translator). See also *PA* 679a28 ff, where we are told that "though this [discharge of pigment] is an effect *due to necessity* like the discharge of urine in others," yet "*Nature makes good use* of this residue at the same time for the animal's preservation" (Peck, A. L., translator). All italics added. On cosmology and biology, see Hall, T. S., reference 20 above, vol. 1, pp. 62-63.
22. *LH* 39-45, 61-62; *LP* 86; etc. The physics and cosmology of Epicurus was a development of ideas put forth by Leucippus and Democritus in the late fifth century B.C. For Epicurus in relation to Aristotle, see Solmsen, F.: Epicurus and cosmological heresies. *Amer. J. Philol. 72*:1-23, 1951.
23. *DL* 14; *LP* 85; *LM* 122.
24. *LH* 77; *LM* 127-28; *DL* 142-43, 149; *DRN* i 62-126 and v 146-94.
25. The point is made repeatedly; see, e.g., *DRN* v 1161-1240. Greek epic legends are pervaded by the supposition that individual pain and pleasure are brought about through the intervention of the gods. A. J. Festugière suggests that with the decline of Attic military and political dominance the discouraged Athenians, or some of them, moved away from the traditional belief that the gods were intimately involved in human affairs. A new view of the gods as indifferent and remote culminated in the doctrine of Epicurus. See Festugière, A. M. J.: *Epicurus and his Gods.* New York, Russell and Russell, 1955, chap. 1.
26. See reference 24 above; also *LP* 86, 97, 104, 111; *LM* 123-24 and 131-32.
27. *DRN* ii 963-72 and iii 246-57.
28. *LM* 128-32, where we learn further,

however, that not all pain should be shunned.
29. *DL* 21; *LH* 81; *LM* 124-25; *DRN* ii 1002-06.
30. *LH* 79-82; *LM* 122 and 127-28; *DL* 140-44.
31. *DL* 117-19; *DRN* iii 31-93.
32. *LH* 63.
33. At *LH* 63, writing to Herodotus, Epicurus acknowledges only three sorts of soul atoms: windlike, heatlike, and the very rare and mobile variety; to these his disciple, Lucretius, adds the fourth, airlike, kind (see *DRN* iii 177-287). At *LH* 27, Epicurus tells Herodotus that people who argue that the soul is incorporeal (Plato had so argued) are foolish.
34. So Lucretius, in *DRN* iii 288-322. Whether Epicurus believed human souls to differ in a comparable way is uncertain. For discussion, see Rist, J. M.: *Epicurus, an Introduction.* Cambridge, England, Cambridge University Press, 1972, p. 77 and Furley, D. J.: *Two Studies in the Greek Atomists.* Princeton, N. J., Princeton University Press, 1967, p. 200.
35. *DRN* ii 865-900.
36. *DRN* iii 350-58.
37. *DL* 31-33, 38, and 137; *LH* 46-53 and 66-67. *DRN* iv 722-960. For new insights into the Epicurean theory of cognition, see Rist, reference 34 above, chap. 5.
38. *DL* 137.
39. *LH* 81.
40. A possible exception to this statement is Epicurus' stipulation of a special sort of soul atom that is more mobile and minute than any found in things lacking souls. For discussion, see Rist, reference 34 above, p. 77.
41. *De naturalibus facultatibus, K* ii 27-30; *De usu partium, K* iv 346-62.
42. *De temperamentis, K* i 566.
43. *De optima corporis nostri constitutione, K* iv 737 and 745.
44. *De temp., K* i 572.
45. *De opt. corp., nos. const. K* iv 747-49.
46. *De usu part., K* iii 868-69. Also Hall, T. S., reference 20 above, vol. 1, p. 139.
47. *De temp., K* i 609.
48. *De temp., K* i 573 and 576.
49. *De symptomatum causis, K* vii 203.
50. *De locis affectis, K* viii 188-90.
51. *Quod animi mores corporis temperamenta sequantur, K* iv 801-22.
52. *Quod an. mor., K* iv 767-86.
53. *De temp., K* i 522 and 643.
54. The Hippocratic treatise *On the Nature of Man* (ca. 400 B.C.) made blood hot and wet, phlegm cold and wet, yellow bile hot and dry, and black bile cold and dry. See chap. 7 and 8.
55. *De causis morborum, K* vii 20-24.
56. *De loc. aff., K* viii 301 and *De methodo mendendi, K* x 841.
57. *De sympt. caus., K* vii 191-94 and *De causis pulsuum, K* ix 56-59.
58. *De crisibus, K* ix 696-97.
59. *De tremore, palpitatione, convulsione et rigore, K* vii 586-88.
60. Hall, T. S.: On biological analogs of Newtonian paradigms, *J. Phil. Sci. 35:* 9-10, 1968.

CICERO'S ESSAY *ON OLD AGE*

Saul Jarcho, M.D.

The recent proliferation of research on old age has already yielded a large crop of observations, hypotheses, opinions, and sociopolitical plans. It is to be expected that sound knowledge and improved social mechanisms will ultimately emerge. Until that happy time we may continue hoping to live long, although we know that longevity entails the statistical likelihood of penury, loneliness, and depression.

The plethora of new literature has produced nothing that even remotely threatens the fame of our greatest gerontological classic, Cicero's essay *On Old Age*. Even in the present age of sceptical analysis or systematic disparagement it is natural for an overwhelmed reader, whatever his age, to reread Cicero and to seek what enlightenment he can find. In a middle-aged physician who peers through trifocal lenses toward a future beclouded by committees and subcommittees, the temptation to reread the famous essay becomes irresistible.

In 44 B.C., at the age of 62, Cicero completed his dialogue *On Old Age*. His long career in rhetoric, poetry, oratory, and politics had come to a halt. He was burdened by debt and overloaded with domestic grief. For all these difficulties he sought solace in writing. In the space of about two years he wrote 11 works, most of which are still famous. Included among them is the treatise that forms the subject of the present discussion.

The essay on old age is cast in the form of an Aristotelian dialogue, in which two of the interlocutors, Publius Scipio Africanus Minor and Gaius Laelius, are limited to a few preliminary remarks, the main burden of the discussion being carried uninterruptedly by the third participant, Marcus Porcius Cato. The dialogue purports to have taken place in 150 B.C., when Cato was 84 years of age, about 50 years older than his two companions.

In a brief introduction Cicero, speaking in his own name, says—not quite credibly—that the composition of this book has been so delightful as to have erased the annoyances of old age, turning it into a happy time. The great discussion then begins.

At the outset Cato makes a series of memorable comments. He says that to those who lack the inner resources for happiness every age is burdensome. All men want to reach old age but reproach it when they reach it. The blame rests with character, not with age. In the presence of severe poverty old age cannot be taken lightly, even by a wise man; to a fool, even a rich one, it is necessarily burdensome. Unwise men attribute their own deficiencies and faults to old age.

There are four reasons, says Cato, why old age seems to be unhappy: it removes one from the active conduct of affairs; it weakens the body; it deprives one of nearly all physical pleasures; and it is not far from death. These four objections he considers in turn. Let the geriatric optimist take note that the treatment is wholly *defensive.*

The first objection, namely, that old age takes a man away from active pursuits, need not be regarded as very serious, according to Cato, since the most important deeds are done not by physical strength but by intellectual and moral qualities—precisely those qualities of character and judgment in which the old exceed the young.

This contention is both ingenious and specious. Old men, when they are removed from the active conduct of affairs, are usually extruded *both* from physical and intellectual participation. The young profess to admire the aged but their admiration is exceeded by their yearning for the status that age may bring. This must have been as true among ambitious young Romans as it is among ambitious young Americans.

Cato remarks that the greatest nations have been overthrown by the young and defended and restored by the aged. Youthful rashness stands in contrast with the prudence of age.

The second charge, that old age weakens the body, is rejected on several grounds. Cato does not need the strength he had during youth; those who are too weak to act can at least teach; and the old may take pleasure in the company of youths whom they have instructed.

At this point Cato offers noteworthy advice: we should resist old age; we should vigilantly compensate for its deficiencies; we should combat it as if we were fighting against a disease; and we should adopt a moderate regimen of life. Old age is honored only if it defends itself, preserves its rights, maintains its independence, and rules its own realm.

In refuting the third charge against old age: namely, that it deprives one of almost all physical pleasures—*quod privet omnibus fere voluptatibus*—Cato asserts that the deprivation is a boon if it takes away the most vicious defect of youth. He now quotes a remarkable speech made by one Archytas of Tarentum. This obscure guru allegedly said:

> No more deadly curse has been given by nature to man than carnal pleasure, through eagerness for which the passions are driven recklessly and uncontrollably to its gratification. From it come treason and the overthrow of states; and from it spring secret and corrupt conferences with public foes. In short, there is no criminal purpose and no evil deed which the lust for pleasure will not drive men to undertake. Indeed, rape, adultery, and every like offence are set in motion by the enticements of pleasure and by nothing else. . . .*

The suggestion that sexual impulses cause treason, sedition, and revolution, as well as ordinary coital misdemeanor, is probably uncommon in ancient literature, and impresses one as both medieval and proto-Freudian.

Cato adds that carnality impedes deliberation, that old age delights in mild pleasures, including those of conversation, and that the zeal for learning may increase late in life. The overarching benefit of old age is influence *(auctoritas)*.

Critics complain that the aged are moody, troubled, irascible, and difficult. Some old men are misers. These, Cato says—not quite accurately—are defects of character and are not attributable to age. Cato has conveniently overlooked the fact that the irascible old man *(senex iratus)* was so common as to have been a stock figure in Greek and Roman comedy; surely this is significant.

As to senile avarice, Cato sinks to an even lower level of incomprehension when he says: "As for avariciousness in the old, what purpose it can serve I do not understand, for can anything be more absurd in the traveller than to increase his luggage as he nears his journey's end." As if senile avarice were based on reason!

The final argument attacks the objection that old age is the close precursor of death. Death, says Cato, should be held of no account. Further, death occurs at every age, hence it should not be regarded as characteristic of old age. This fantastically specious example of lawyer's reasoning is not quite the nadir. The old man, Cato dares to assert, is

*Cicero: *De Senectute.* Falconer, W. A., translator. Loeb Classical Library. Cambridge, Harvard Univ. Press, 1923, reprinted 1946, page 49. Reprinted by permission of the publisher.

better off than the youth, since the old man has already reached what the young man desires; one wants to live long, the other has lived long. Ingenious.

But the same part of the essay that contains these pyrites also contains some valuable advice. Cato urges that whatever the amount of time that is given us, we should be content with it. Old men should not cling greedily to the little that remains but they should not give it up without a reason. Indifference to death, if taught in youth, will produce tranquillity in later life. And finally, Cato says, consolation is derivable from a belief in the immortality of the soul.

Such being the course of Cicero's defense, placed in the mouth of Cato, what is the reaction of a 20th century reader?

The essay contains many wise observations and several stirring thoughts. In the first place, Cicero points out that in the presence of poverty old age cannot be taken lightly; no amount of philosophy can overcome want. A second requisite is wisdom, or at least ordinary common sense; in the absence of this element not even wealth can make old age happy.

Throughout the dialogue Cicero insists that the blame rests with *character*, rather than with old age. To those who lack the internal resources for happiness, every period of life is burdensome. It is their own vices and their own faults that fools charge to old age. This is consistent with contemporary clinical experience. Further, one should take a positive attitude and resist senility by instituting a good daily regimen and by attempting continued mild activity.

Along with these admonitions, formulated clearly and expressed grandly, there are occasional failures and also several bits of sophistry, which I have pointed out in previous paragraphs. It is not astonishing that Cicero remained a lawyer to the end of his life.

The tone of the essay is one of seriousness, dignity, and nobility. The magnificent prose style, simpler than that of the perfervid orations, is well adapted to reinforce the impression of courage and gravity.

Perhaps, instead of picayune attempts to analyze each of Cicero's contentions, we should view the essay *On Old Age* as the attempt of a capable and noble man to cope with one of life's greatest problems and to provide solace for himself and others. Viewed in this way, the dialogue seems more than likely to retain its position as a beloved and admired treasure of the human race.

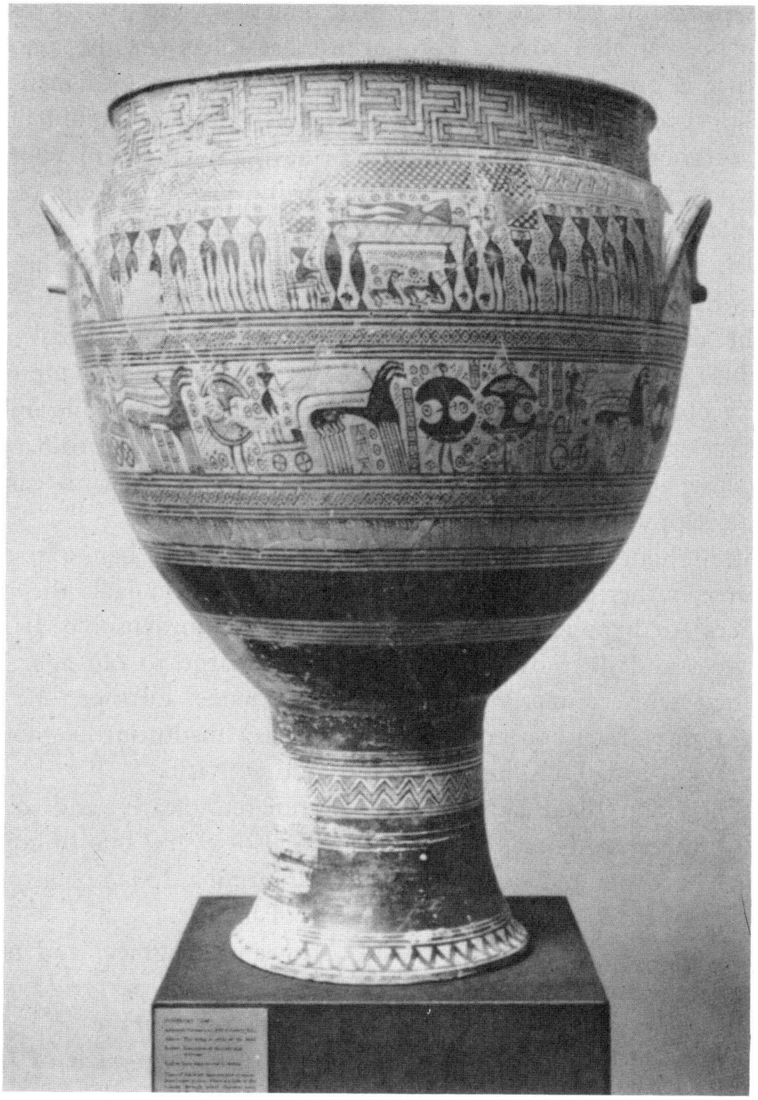

Fig. 1. Attic sepulchral vase, second half of VIII century B.C. In a panel at the center the deceased is depicted lying on a bier and surrounded by gesturing mourners. The lower panel shows a funerary procession of chariots and armed men. The vase is 72.3 cm. tall. Courtesy of The Metropolitan Museum of Art, Rogers Fund, 1914.

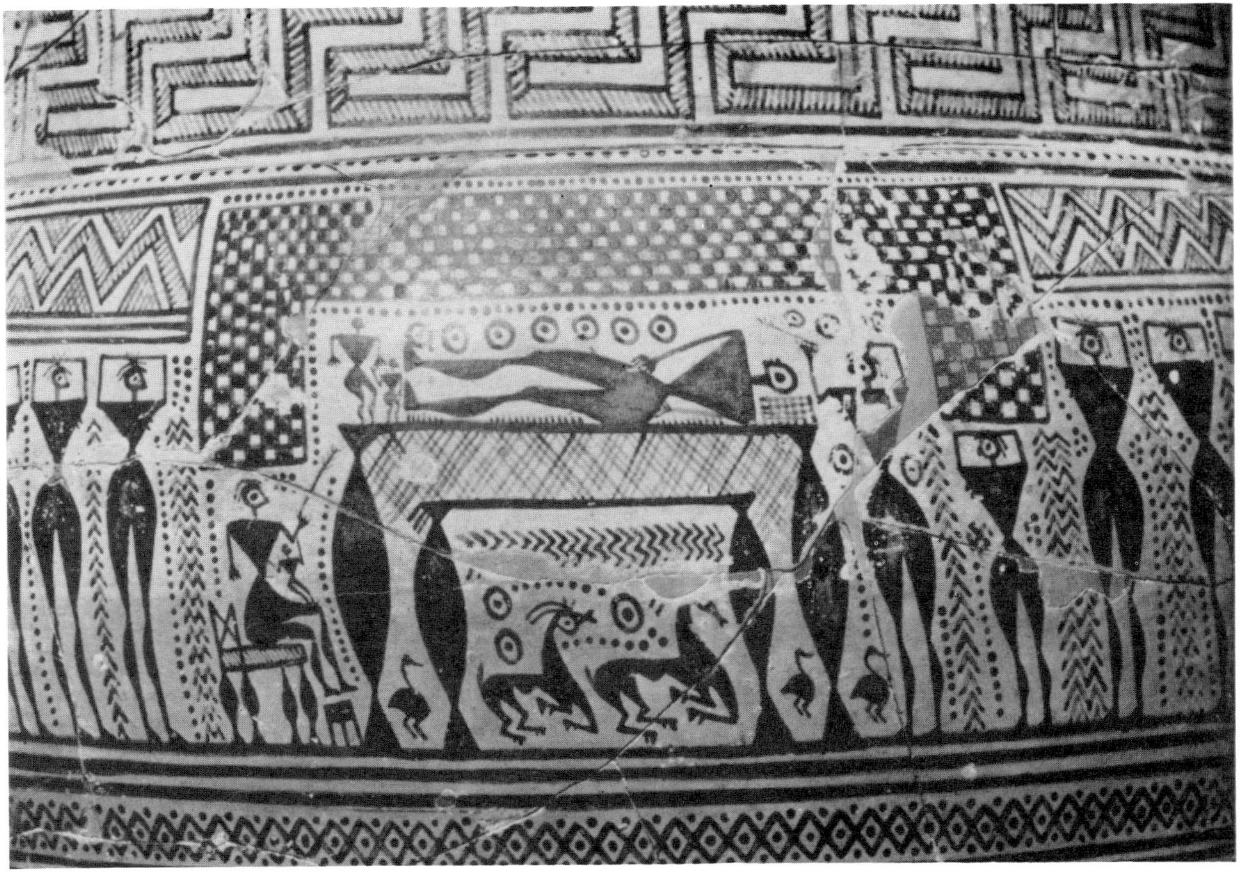

Fig. 2. Detail of Attic sepulchral vase, showing the deceased on his bier, surrounded by mourners. Courtesy of The Metropolitan Museum of Art, Rogers Fund, 1914.

THE MEDIEVAL CROSSBOW AS SURGICAL INSTRUMENT: AN ILLUSTRATED CASE HISTORY*

ROBERT IGNATIUS BURNS, S.J.

University of San Francisco
San Francisco, Calif.

School of Historical Studies
The Institute for Advanced Study
Princeton, N. J.

FROM prehistoric into modern times, physicians have had to cope with arrow wounds. The wars which ceaselessly punctuated man's progress ensured a stream of victims, to which hunting accidents added their share. Not long ago arrow wounds bedeviled American army surgeons during Indian wars,[1] and fighting in Vietnam has turned up a few cases. Treatment has varied according to the surprising variety of projectiles involved, the medieval crossbow offering a particular problem. Ranked as a kind of lesser artillery and manned often by elite corps, the ancient crossbow became a dominant weapon on 13th century battlefields, as technical advances improved its range and loading. The crossbow could be carried loaded, required little training or strength, and propelled its quarrel or bolt with frightening accuracy and force for eighty yards on direct aim and double or triple that on extreme range. Its metal bullet,

*This article was prepared during tenure of a grant from the National Endowment of the Humanities, Washington, D.C.

feathered with wood or leather and bearing one of several types of head, could penetrate deeply. Richard the Lion Heart popularized it in England as his favorite weapon, and died by it.[2]

The ecumenical council of Lateran II in 1139 and several popes, including the great Innocent III, expressed the general horror at the crossbow's bloody efficiency by forbidding it in Christian warfare under pain of excommunication; they allowed it only for the defense of Christendom against external enemies. The prohibition, ineffective like so many attempts at arms control, underlines the special problems the crossbow introduced to military medicine. Later in the century, at the French siege of Gerona, a crossbow sharpshooter called his shot and then fired from the town walls into the narrow window of a suburban church being used as a hospital, his bolt piercing both a wounded knight and his esquire.[3]

The medical problem posed by crossbows, both in higher incidence of wounds and deep penetration, was most acute on the Christian-Moslem frontier of Spain. In Spanish Islam, according to a treatise on military archery by Taybughā in 1368, "crossbows are a great favorite and are the weapons of preference."[4] This had certainly been true a century earlier, when battles often revolved around a fortification. At that time, as the Almohad empire fragmented in Western Islam, Spanish crusaders had surged down the lower half of their peninsula. On the east coast, ranks of Muslim crossbowmen defended town walls, while bodies of Christian crossbowmen from such renowned centers of crossbow archery as Tortosa matched them shot for shot. King James the Conqueror, who led Aragon's armies, nearly succumbed under the walls of Valencia as a bolt caught him across the forehead; blinded with a freshet of blood, he managed to hold his saddle and conceal the seriousness of his wound from the army, but his head soon swelled, and his skull, extant, carries along its front an impressive crease.[5]

King James's contemporary, Alfonso the Learned of Castile, has left his own testimony to the terrible crossbow, in a picture story about the siege of Elche, south of Valencia. Alfonso supervised the construction of a masterpiece as great as those of his contemporaries Aquinas, Dante, and the architects of Gothic cathedrals–though it is by its nature seldom seen. The *Cántigas* or "Songs in Praise of St. Mary" interweave a corpus of 1,262 miniatures with a matching corpus of troubadour poetry, all set to music.[6] Centering upon miracle legends of Our Lady, the themes

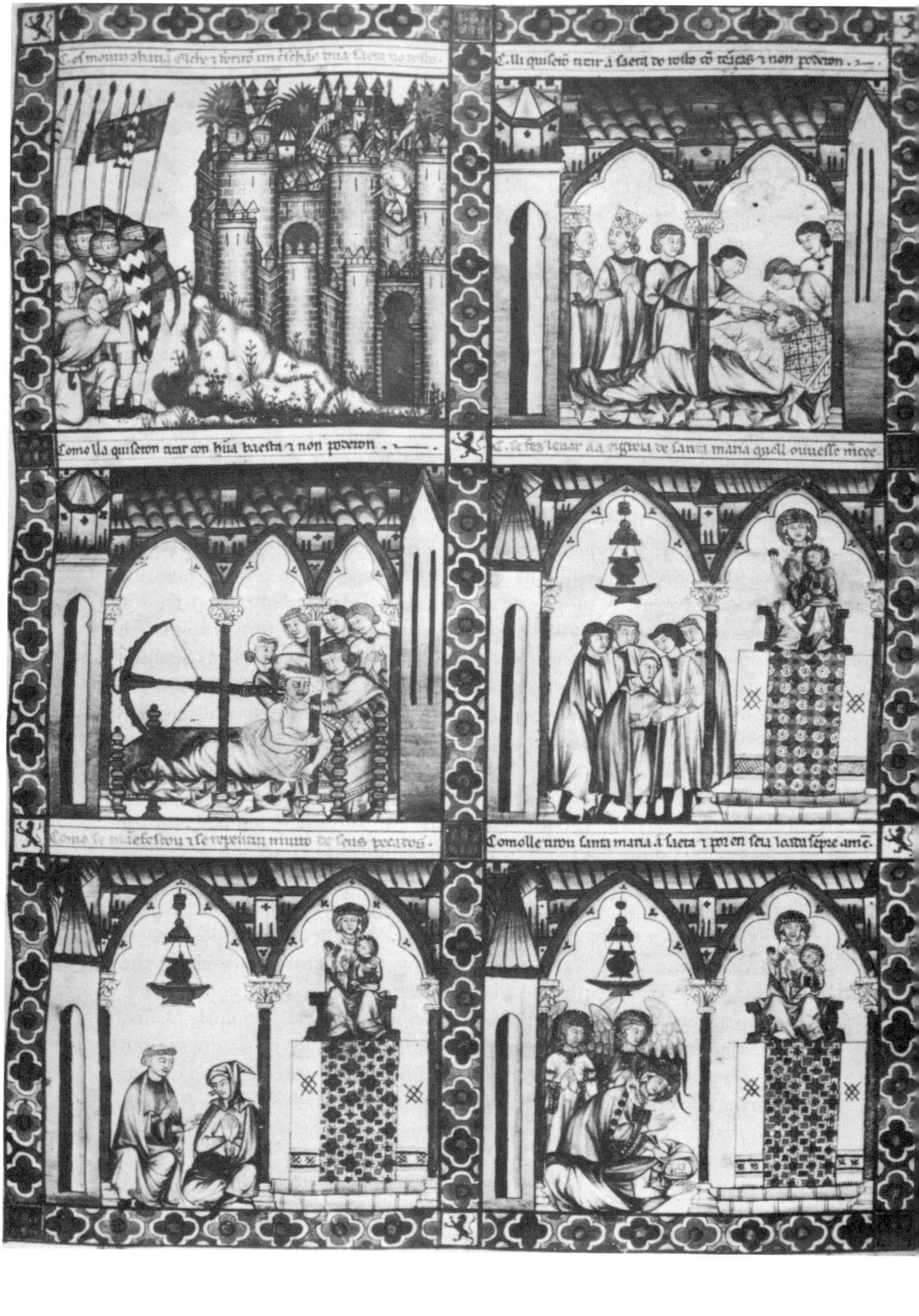

inevitably touch upon some medical problems. The almost anachronistically realistic style of the paintings heighten their value for historical study. The Elche episode shown in our illustration probably belongs to the definitive conquest of Murcia kingdom, tributary to Castile, by the combined forces of Kings James and Alfonso in 1266. The panels read like a comic strip, from left to right, down the page. The first picture shows a Muslim crossbowman hitting a citizen or possibly a commoner knight—any townsman who could maintain horse and equipment at his own expense. The bolt has taken him frontally in the neck, just below the right ear; short and heavy, it would have looked either triangular or square if seen in cross-section, with its tip an equilateral triangle when viewed from the side. Note the crossbow in the picture, the osmosis of military fashion in both armies, and the distinctive palms of Elche.[7]

In the second panel a body of surgeons attends the gentleman in his affluent home surroundings. Apprehension marks his face, as the senior surgeon applies forceps to draw the bolt. Perhaps lodged in bone, the bolt resists all efforts, but bleeding results. By panel three the medical men are resorting to a final expedient. The patient's head is bound, probably to staunch the bleeding; his disarrayed clothing suggests the ordeal he has been through; his countenance, swollen by now, betrays deep suffering; and he is clinging to a pillar of his house. A crossbow has been attached to another pillar, its cord connected with the bolt, seemingly by a forceps arrangement. Two physicians hold the patient's head in position, one supplying absorbent bandages under the wound. Obviously they plan to fire the embedded projectile in reverse, dislodging it by main force. Panel four shows the poor fellow, now much the worse for wear but firmly attached to his bolt, his case abandoned as hopeless, making his doctors help him to a nearby Marian shrine. The final panels portray his prayerful confession and his cure, while asleep, at the hands of the Virgin and her two attendant angels.

Until heavenly forces intruded, the patient had proved unlucky. Yet in terms of medical expertise, he lived in a fortunate country. Jewish, Christian, and Moslem physicians abounded; Aragon was soon to introduce legislation for examining and licensing doctors from all three communities. Montpellier, the birthplace of King James and home of his university, boasted the best medical faculty in Europe. One of the greatest physicians of Europe, the Valencian Arnold of Villanova, graced this area during the second half of the 13th century. During the siege of

Valencia, King James tells us in his memoirs, so many drugs from Montpellier and Lérida were on sale that the sick might think themselves in a large city. King Alfonso of Castile, patron of Islamic learning, also gave attention to medical education in his closet-code of ideal law, the *Siete partidas*. Thus the Elche victim could not have lacked competent diagnosis and care.[8]

The extractive methods employed in our illustration can be better understood when placed in the context of contemporary surgical practice, as revealed in a medical treatise such as Henri de Mondeville's *Surgery*. Compiled some 50 years later, it reflects the experience of the previous years. De Mondeville was physician to Philip the Fair of France. He cites ancient and modern authorities, including Villanova, and ranks himself with "the modern surgeons."

Like all university products of his day, he takes pride in his bookish background, dealing in syllogisms and erudition as handily as in experience. The first part of his second treatise in *Surgery* deals with foreign bodies embedded in the patient, with particular attention to arrows and crossbow bolts. He cautions against the traditional wisdom, which counsels leaving the object either because one fears hemorrhage or hopes for a facilitating suppuration or a rejection by the body; the "modern" physician has a range of instruments and techniques to ensure staunching of blood flux and to extricate any object.[9]

He knows that eventual lubrication cannot compensate for the damage bound to result from leaving the object, and that vital forces will decline before nature can reject it. He knows too that a few fortunates have been able to carry foreign objects for life, but he wryly reminds us that the majority with this problem are invisibly underground. The physician must not only counter such folk medicine, but must be resigned to gain little credit from these cases; if he does not operate, the friends of the dead victim cry negligence; if he does operate, his experimentation has caused death; if he succeeds, the layman credits nature and God, since the physician has merely removed an obstacle to health. Avicenna and others speak of magnets and "attractive medicines," but De Mondeville believes these merely masked a suppurative process in lightly embedded objects; and he suspects malpractice in some such cases, complicating a simple operation to win an easy reputation.

General rules in the case of arrows, he tells us, are three. First, one must choose or invent mechanisms most appropriate to the job at hand.

Not only are there many kinds of arrows, but military ingenuity is constantly challenging the surgeon with new species. What works in one case can wreak disaster in another, as when he himself diagnosed a wound to have been caused by a nonbarbed arrow. The position of the arrow, its degree of visibility, its composition in wood or metal, its size, the possibility of poison on it, the advisability of enlarging the wound, the location of the wound, and the complications of dirt and pebbles carried into it, all enter into the diagnosis. Above all, the physician must not simply wrench the thing out by force without such examination, nor allow his less experienced assistants to attempt this while he is on his way. The second rule is to extract as delicately and swiftly as possible, and the third is to staunch the flow of blood. As to particulars, he describes a half-dozen "engines of extraction"; and he gives practical instructions, such as to grasp the arrow as close to the body as feasible. If the patient is unlikely to survive, the physician should allow him time to prepare for death before precipitating the crisis; while priest and family rally around, the physician can be laying out his instruments, shaving the skin, and making similar preparations.

De Mondeville adverts to the bizarre method used in our Elche case. In explaining available mechanisms, he puts it last and briefly: "The crossbow is well known [and] is useful on occasion." Later, when dealing with the category of arrows visible externally, he lists the crossbow as an instrument of last resort, when all other expedients have proved ineffective. "I have never seen that means fail," he avers, "except once."[10] The Elche pictures, therefore, must illustrate a common medical practice, in its orthodox deployment, on a case far more stubborn than the normal. They illustrate as well a paradox which repeats itself in the intertwined history of warfare and medicine. The weapon which seems the ultimate horror of war can be turned to healing—in this instance to the healing of the damage it itself inflicted.

NOTES AND REFERENCES

1. Arrow wounds carried a higher death rate than those caused by any other weapon around 1860. See the medico-military reports cited in Burns, R. L.: *The Jesuits and the Indian Wars of the Northwest.* New Haven, Yale University Press, 1966, p. 226.
2. On the crossbow, see Patrick, J. M.: *Artillery and Warfare During the Thirteenth and Fourteenth Centuries.* Logan, Utah, Utah State University Press, 1961.
3. Desclot, B.: *Crònica,* Alentorn, M. C., editor, 4 vols. Barcelona, Editorial Barcino, 1949-1950, chap. 91.
4. Taybughā, al-Baklamishī 'l-Yūnānī: *Saracen Archery,* Latham, J. D. and Paterson, W. F., editors. London, Hol-

land, 1970, p. 9. On varieties of crossbow and Spanish preference for laqshah rather than the Frankish *jarkh,* see pp. 8, 9.

5. James I: *Crònica,* de Casacuberta, J., editor, 9 vols. in 2. Barcelona, Editorial Barcino, 1926-1962, chap. 266. Full background on Spain and this crusade is in Burns, R. I.: *The Crusader Kingdom of Valencia, Reconstruction on a Thirteenth-Century Frontier,* 2 vols. Cambridge, Mass., Harvard University Press, 1967; also in Burns, R. I.: *Islam under the Crusaders, Colonial Survival in Thirteenth-Century Valencia.* Princeton, N. J., Princeton University Press. In press.
6. In the manuscript collections of the Escorial Library, reprinted from Burns, R. I.: Christian-Islamic confrontation in the West: The thirteenth-century dream of conversion. *Amer. Hist. Rev. 76*:1,386-1,434, 1971, where a portfolio of companion episodes is also given, together with full information and bibliography on the *Cántigas.*
7. *Saracen Archery,*[4] pp. 29-30, 176 on bolts. On the commoner knight, see Lourie, E.: A society organized for war: Medieval Spain. *Past Pres. 25:* 54-76, 1966. On the Murcian war, see Fontes, J. T.: *La reconquista de Murcia en 1226 por Jaime I de Aragón.* Murcia, Diputación, 1967.
8. For background see Burns, R. I.: Los hospitales del reino de Valencia en el siglo XIII. *Ann. Estud. Mediev. 2*:135-54, 1965; also Burns, R. I.: *Crusader Valencia,*[5] vol. 1, chaps. 13, 15. For King James, see his *Crònica,*[5] chap. 265.
9. *Chirurgie de Maître Henri de Mondeville, chirurgien de Philippe le Bel, roi de France,* composée de 1306 à 1320, Nicaise, E., translator. Paris, Alcan, 1893, treatise II, *doctrina* I, chap. 1. See also Gurlt, E.: *Geschichte der Chirurgie und ihrer Ausübung,* 3 vols. Hildesheim, Olms [1898], 1964, II, 34-77, esp. p. 47; and Garrison, F. H.: *Notes on the History of Military Medicine.* Hildesheim, Olms, 1970, p. 81.
10. *Chirurgie de Maitre Henri de Mondeville, chirurgien de Philippe le Bel, roi de France,*[9] pp. 235, 237; "nunquam in extractione vidi modum istum deficere nisi semel."

MEDIEVAL MEDICAL MALPRACTICE: THE DICTA AND THE DOCKETS*

MADELEINE PELNER COSMAN, Ph.D.

Director, Institute for Medieval and Renaissance Studies
The City College
City University of New York
New York, N.Y.

SOMETIMES jocularly, sometimes seriously, modern critics maintain that all medieval medical practice was malpractice. While amusing, such judgment ignores not only the sophistication of much medieval medical and surgical practice but also the attempts and the achievements of medieval medical legislators to establish professional standards and to enforce these in practice. Therefore it is especially fascinating to examine documents of medicolegal case histories adjudged in their own time as malpractice litigations; and then to compare this evidence from the legal dockets with the contemporary legal dicta whose purposes were to legislate against such malpractice.

Such investigation of actual case histories and of official legislative documents has at least three salutory effects. First it permits the modern critic to apprehend what the medieval medical mind considered malpractice. Among the numerous types of malpractice pleas are suits brought because of lack of success of promised cure, excessive payment demanded for services, aggravation of an original complaint because of medical folly, death due to medical negligence and, even, "iatrogenic sequelae," in which the effects of cure and curer caused new injury to the patient.

Beyond allowing an understanding of malpractice, the cases and the dicta demonstrate better than almost any other type of source material the actual state of medieval medical and surgical practice. For unlike any other documents, malpractice case histories permit disease and modalities of cure to be examined from three separate vantage points: those of the patient, the practitioner, and the professional peers who sit in judgment. Thus the positive–good practice–is appreciated through its negative–malpractice. What is more, these malpractice cases pro-

*Presented at a meeting of the Section on Historical Medicine of the New York Academy of Medicine on October 27, 1971.

vide—better than any theoretical treatise, no matter how comprehensive or how brilliant—apprehension of the medical world as it was, not as it might have been or ought to have been. Thus for such subjects as medical fees, medical women practitioners or, of particular significance, astrology and zodiacal computations in medical and surgical practice, the case histories of the legal dockets and the accompanying legal dicta demonstrate the manner in which all of these functioned in actual practice, not merely in learned theory.

The third reason for this study is probably the most important. It intimates the startling relation between medieval medical authority and civil authority. By means of the medical and surgical guilds, the medieval practitioners achieved reformation of their profession from within and implementation of their regulations from without by powerful municipal and sometimes national cooperation. The malpractice case histories suggest the complex and effective procedures for complaints by a patient or his surrogate, by a fellow practitioner, or by a professional organization; procedures involving malpractice insurance; and procedures for adjudication of complaints. Almost all of these processes have shockingly complete internal checks and balances designed to secure equity for the patient, the practitioner, the profession and, not least, the citizens of the city.

To illustrate these three concerns with malpractice, actual practice, and medicolegal relations I have selected seven legal cases from the surviving documents of medieval London, ranging over the 150-year period from the mid-14th century through the late 15th. Arranged chronologically, they allow the tracing of certain developments and evolutions of ideas. With these seven major cases I have paired medico-legal legislative documents which indicate the theoretical tenets the cases demonstrate in practice. In addition to the seven major cases and their associated dicta, there are another seven minor cases which add significant details concerning malpractice outside as well as inside the City of London. To facilitate comprehension of these remarkable manuscript sources—written originally in Latin, Norman French, and Medieval English, and culled from London Guildhall archives, law-court registers, and various Public Record Office memoranda—I have designed two charts (Tables I and II) of these case histories detailing their sources, dates, trials, verdicts, punishments, significances, and related official documents. For the acknowledged habits of diagnosis,

TABLE I. SEVEN MAJOR MALPRACTICE CASES: THE DOCKETS AND THE DICTA

Case	*Date*	*Source*	*Plaintiff vs. defendant*	*Accusation*	*Verdict*	*Significance*	*Dicta*
1	1354	Guildhall *Letter Book G*	Thomas de Shene vs. John le Spicer	"Maiming" and neglect of jaw wound	Guilty	If had been expert and if had called counsel, then curable; since not, thus culpable	1369
2	1377	*Plea and Memoranda Rolls*	Walter del Hull vs. Richard Cheyndut	"Endangering" leg	Guilty	3 expert witnesses Punishment via fine and prison	1376
3	1382	Guildhall *Letter Book H*	Roger atte Hache and Mayor and Commonalty vs. Roger Clerk	Deceit and falsehood in treating woman	Guilty	Fee with downpayment Charm against fevers Public punishment	1376
4	1408	*Plea and Memoranda Rolls*	John Clotes vs. John Luter	Failure to cure and excessive fees	Guilty	"Goods" fee "Lepre" Direct adjudication by mayor	1390
5	1424	*Plea and. Memoranda Rolls*	William Forest vs. Simon Rolf, John Dalton and John Harwe	"Iatrogenic sequelae," maimed hand	Not guilty	Committee of Eight witnesses, chaired by Doctor Gilbert Kymer Astrological considerations	1410 1415 1423
6	1443	Mayor's Court files	1) George Baylle 2) John Roper vs. Matthew Rellesford	Worsening of: 1) "le stone" 2) "anoncomo" foot	Mainprised and case transferred	Fees with downpayments Suits for damages	1435
7	1464	*PRO Exchequer Records*	George Humphreyson vs. John Isyng	Ineffective treatment and excessive fee	Unknown	Countersuit	1461

TABLE II. SEVEN MINOR CASES

Case	*Date*	*Locale*	*Defendant*
A	1350	Devon	Pernell
B	1375	Chester	Thomas de Clotton
C	1385	Chester	John Leche
D	1387	London	Thomas Butolf
E	1417	London	John Severall Love
F	1433	York	Mathew Rutherford
G	1493	Unknown	Peter Blank

prognosis, and cure the seven major and seven minor cases offer splendid testimony.

CASE I

In 1354, assembled before the Mayor of London, the aldermen, and sheriffs, four surgeons swore their testimony against practitioner John le Spicer, who had treated Thomas de Shene for "an enormous and horrible hurt" of the left side of his jaw.[1] The surgeons were required to certify whether the wound had been curable at the time treatment had begun. Their answer: if John le Spicer had been expert, and if he had called in counsel and assistance to aid him, then the jaw would have been curable. Since he did neither, his lack of skill rendered the injury incurable.

This document is noteworthy in several ways. First, the highest civil authorities, the mayor and his council, judge the accusation of malpractice; second, their decision is based upon the testimony of four expert practitioners who had examined the patient and inquired into method of treatment, which they had adjudged deficient. The sworn testimony presupposes the third and fourth significant aspects of this case: that there were established criteria for treatment of certain wounds, and that there was available machinery for consultation by experts to advise and assist the individual practitioner in difficult cases. Finally, since the patient's wound had been curable in the past but would be incurable in the future, the treating practitioner was criminally culpable. Implicit is the practitioner's responsibility to cure what he has undertaken to cure and his legal accountability if unsuccessful.

The first case suggests an established set of standards, method of surveillance, and definition of responsibility expected not only of the practitioner but of his profession. Since the whole case is expressed in unremarkable Latin prose free of any references to the unusual nature of this court proceeding it would seem to represent an expected type and process of adjudication. No doubt it was. For in the very same Guildhall manuscript, although dated 1369, 15 years after the trial of Case I, is the legal document that describes the oath and investiture of the three master surgeons of the City of London, admitted in full ceremonial regalia, in full husting, by the mayor and aldermen.[2] Not only do the surgeons swear that they will faithfully follow their calling and take reasonable payment for their services, but that they would present to the mayor and aldermen the defaults of others who undertake cures; that they would be ready to attend the maimed and wounded at all times; that they would give truthful information to the officers of the city concerning such maimed, wounded, and others if they be in peril of death.

This means, of course, that it is the *duty* of the master surgeons to recognize malpractitioners and report them; to examine "questionable" cases, and report the results to civil authority. It implies, though it does not state, that patients who have desperate wounds or are in danger of death must be shown to the masters. Later documents, in fact, state that responsibility precisely.[3] Case I intimates the same. And the nature of the recording of this master surgeons' oath suggests that such might have been included; for not the least interesting word in this document is the persistent repetition of "etcetera," indicating that the procedure of investiture and components of the commitment were written down incompletely because they were familiar and formulaic.

Case II

But we need not speculate when still other documents most cooperatively reveal what some omit. Case II (A. D. 1377) is brought by Walter, son of John del Hull, pinner (a trapper of stray animals), against Richard Cheyndut,[4] practitioner, who had committed himself to cure Walter's "malady" of his left leg.[5] Three surgeons who at the mayor's order had examined the leg testified that because of the practitioner's lack of care and lack of knowledge the patient was in danger of losing his limb. The mayor asserted that only great experience, great care, and great expense might save the leg from permanent injury. Surgeon Richard Cheyndut thus was fined 50 shillings in damages by the jury and was jailed.

In this case not only is the expert testimony required and received by the mayor, and not only does the inquiry committee find the defendant surgeon guilty, but here is documentation of medieval punishment for malpractice. Damages must be paid to the aggrieved party, and the guilty party is imprisoned.

One year before Case II was heard, the mayor and aldermen granted an ordinance requested by the barber-surgeons.[6] This Norman French document is nearly one half a complaint against non-London surgeons and their poor practices and one half a petition for control against their abuses. It maintains that daily there come to London from "uppelande," that is, the north country or "the sticks," men who profess surgery and the curing of illness but who were never instructed in the craft. This is to the damage and deceit of the people as well as to the scandal of the good practitioners of the city. Thus the honorable Lordships are enjoined to prevent any stranger coming to London from "uppelande" from practicing until he is examined by London practitioners. To accomplish this two wardens are to be appointed, chosen by the craft, presented to the mayor, and sworn in by him, to regulate its practice. These masters are to inspect instruments, report "rebellious" practitioners to civil authority, and cause any in default of the ordinance to pay to the Chamber a fine of 40 pence. No franchises for practitioners are to be granted until attested before the mayor by examination as good and able. No foreigner shall be allowed to practice within the city or its suburbs. And this ordinance shall be enrolled in the Chamber of the Guildhall of London—where indeed it still is—"for all time to last."

In a Latin addendum following this document, the ordinance is granted as recorded, and Laurence de Westone and John de Grantone are chosen masters.[7] As in the Master Surgeon's Oath of 1369, this ordinance affirms the mutually advantageous relation between medical-surgical craft authority and municipal authority. For the sake of the citizens and the city, the London government is requested to assert, to dignify, and to enforce the code of professional behavior promulgated by the practitioners for the sake of patients and themselves. While the gist of this document is as much against "uppelanders" and foreigners

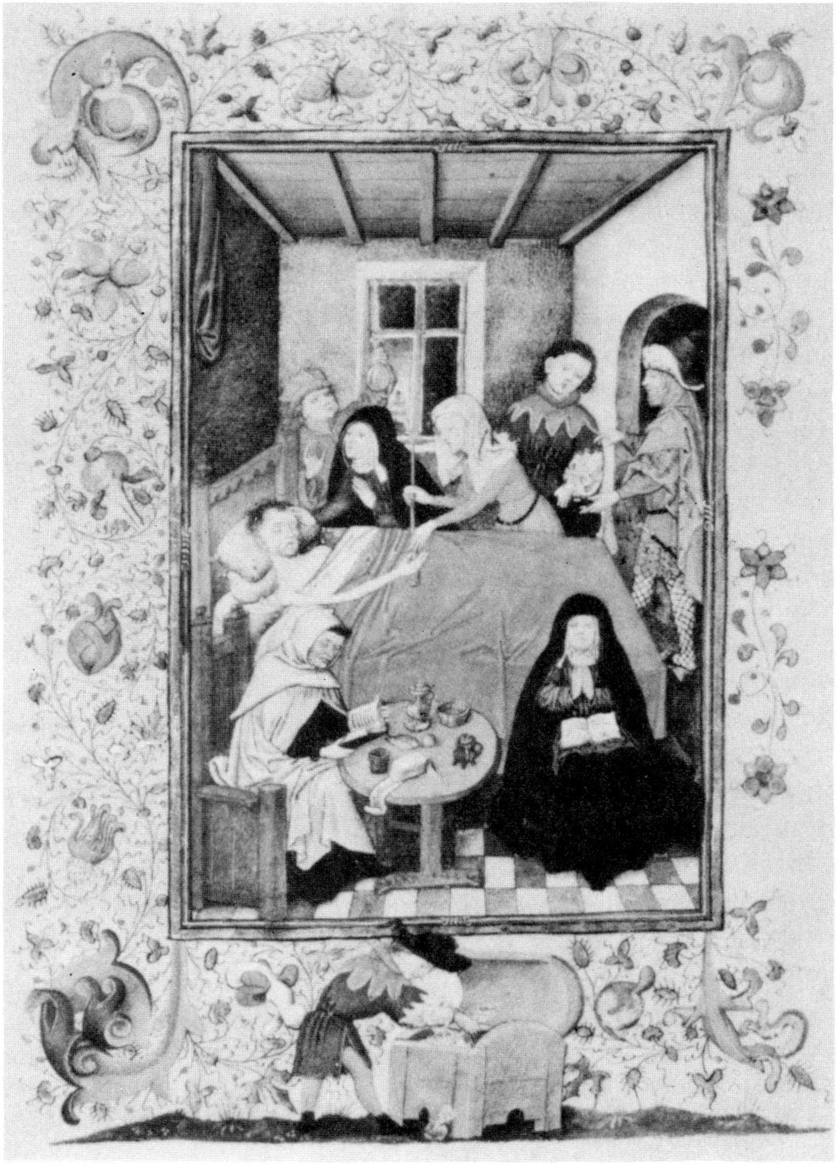

Fig. 1. Physician, rear left, at death bed of patient, in the 15th century illuminated manuscript, *Hours of Catherine of Cleves*. Reproduced by courtesy of the Morgan Library, New York.

intruding upon London practice as it is against malpractice in general, it is significant for its insistence upon examination and accreditation, with civil licensure, before admission to practice. And it specifically enumerates a fine for malpractice. Interestingly enough, this forfeiture is to be paid to the civil Chamber (in later years, as other documents testify,[8] the Guild of Surgeons will take its portion of all receipts from its members' perfidies). Internally appointed surveillance externally enforced by civil court is here augmented by monetary punishment.

Case III

The third case concerns not only false medical practice but a false practitioner. Roger Clerk of Wandelesworth is required to answer a complaint made before the mayor and by the mayor as well as by Roger atte Hache asserting deceit and falsehood.[9] Since no physician or surgeon "should intermeddle with medicines or cures" in London unless experienced and licensed therein, Roger Clerk, who was neither, and was also unlettered, came under false pretense to the house of Roger atte Hache to cure his wife Johanna, who was lying ill "with certain bodily infirmities" and fever.

After being paid 12 pence as downpayment on the larger sum to be paid upon healing, Roger Clerk placed an old piece of scratched parchment rolled up in a piece of gold cloth around the neck of Johanna, asserting that it would help her fevers and ailments. It did not. When confronted in court with the parchment still rolled up in its cloth, the false physician insisted that a charm against fevers was written thereon: "*Anima Christi, sanctifica me; corpus Christi, salve me; in isanguis Christi, nebria me; cum bonus Christus tu, lave me.*" When the parchment was examined by the court not one of these words was found. Since upon further questioning Roger Clerk was found to be illiterate, an infidel, and totally ignorant of the arts of medicine and surgery, and since it was necessary to protect the people from being deceived and aggrieved by such imposters, it was decided that Roger Clerk be led through the middle of the City, with trumpets and pipes playing (he being pulled by a horse), the said parchment and a whetstone for his lies being hung around his neck, and a urine flask being hung before him, and another urinal on his back.

The gullibility of those who would be deceived is splendidly depicted here, as in the amusing unity between Christian liturgy and

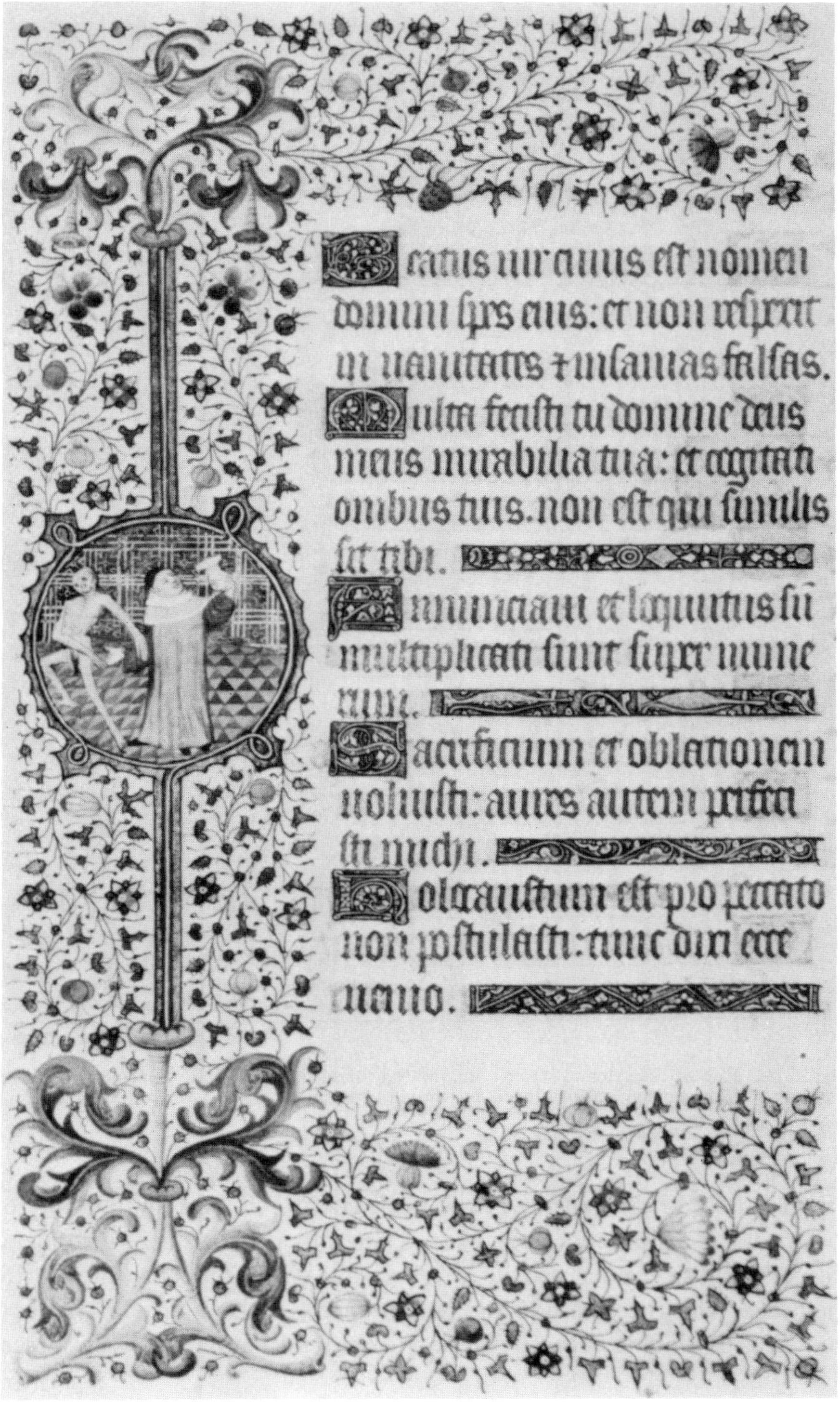

Fig. 2. Marginalia figure of physician and skeleton (Death?) in illuminated manuscript M 359. Reproduced by courtesy of the Morgan Library, New York.

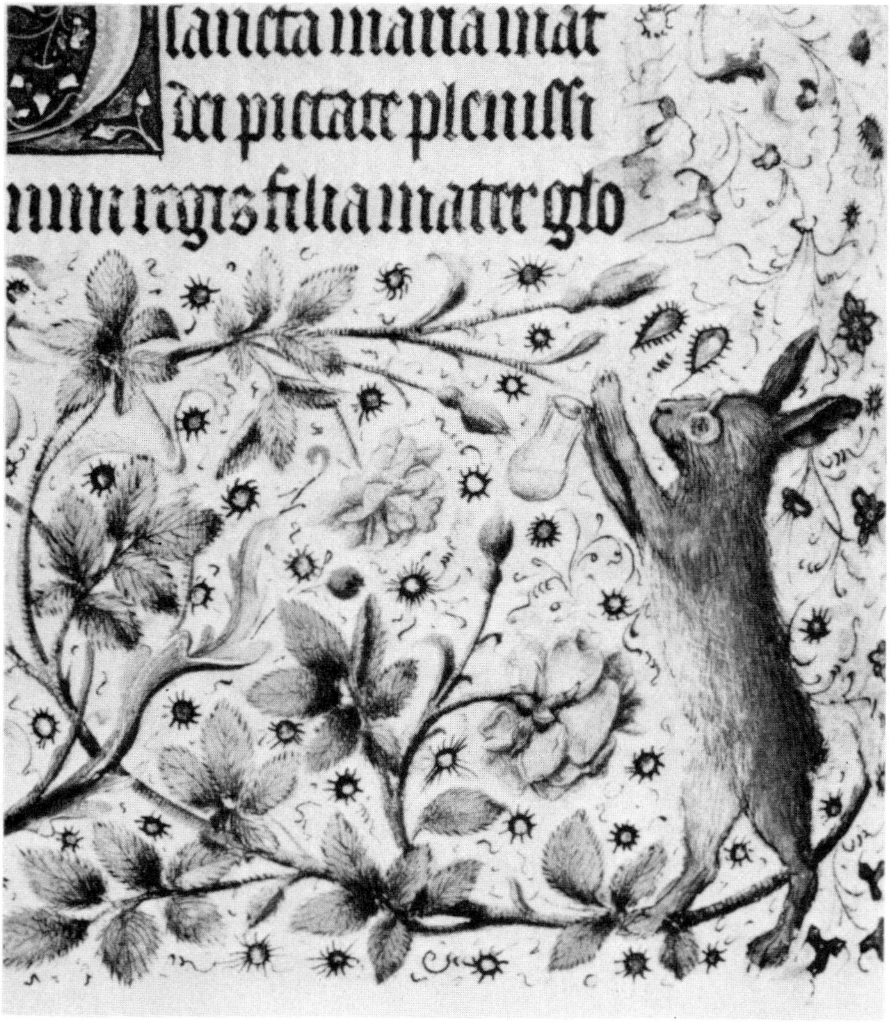

Fig. 3. A Rabbit Physician, from illuminated manuscript *Book of Hours,* Franco-Flemish, 15th century. Reproduced by courtesy of the Morgan Library, New York.

pagan amulet in the episode of the neck charm.[10-14] More important for the study of malpractice, however, is the impetus for suit. Not only is the false physician accused by the husband of the patient but also by the mayor and the commonalty (community) of London. The accusation thus is double: Roger Clerk violated not only one man's trust but London's civic code forbidding practice of the unlearned and the unlicensed. Very likely, that code was the ordinance of 1376 or its equivalent. Fascinating also is the reference to payment of fee, agreed to in advance: down-payment upon beginning treatment, the remainder upon healing. And the graphically depicted ignominious public punishment alludes to one of the major diagnostic tools of medieval medicine as well as the veritable insignia of the medieval physician, the urine flask for urinalysis[15-17] (Figures 1-3).

Case IV

Failure to cure and the exaction of excessive fees are the accusations leveled against John Luter, leche (physician), by John Clotes, who had come to him for cure of a disease of the face.[18] The document for this case asserts that the patient delivered to the physician: 15 serpentyns (semiprecious green jewels) of the value of 9 marks, a gold tablet of the value of 60 shillings, and a sword of the value of 6 shillings, 8 pence. These the defendant was to keep if he cured the patient of a disease called "lepre"; not only had the physician not cured the disease but he kept the fee, thereby causing the patient a loss of 20 pounds. The physician's response was that the patient had maintained he had the disease called "salsefleume," not "lepre"; on that basis he had undertaken the cure even though he knew the patient to be "leprous" and so told him. At the time of the transfer of goods-for-fee the physician promised cure only if the patient were not leprous. To this the mayor, Drew Barentyne, answered that the physician had taken the patient's valuables "fraudulently, deceptively, and injuriously." Afterward the defendant maintained that though he had not cured the plaintiff of "leprosy" he had taught him to make balsam and other medicaments and thus ought to keep his fee.

Numerous aspects of this case repay examination: the definition of disease, its diagnosis, the fee and the associated promises for cure, and the adjudication itself. Implicit in this case is the medieval recognition that certain diseases by definition were incurable. Thus "lepre" should not have been treated because it *could* not have been treated. "Salsefleume," however, by definition was curable and fairly could justify the promise of cure and payment for it. Definition of the patient's "disease of the face" proves to be the substance of the plea. Medieval medical and medieval artistic works present "lepre" and "salsefleume" as familiar attributes of description; Chaucer's repulsive, pustulous, lascivious "Summoner"[19] is a vivid reminder.

As interesting as definition is the method of diagnosis in this case. The practitioner excused his perfidy by accepting the patient's definition of his own disease! The fee composed of precious goods given in advance and kept upon success of treatment represents still another type and method of medical payment delineated by malpractice records. The last unusual quality in Case IV is its hearing: apparently by the mayor directly, with only his recorder present, with no mention either of expert medical witness or jury.

This last is especially surprising because of the legal milieu in which the case was tried. During this 150-year period the legal dicta concerning malpractice give ever-increasing responsibility and power to the practitioners' guilds and to their masters. This is accompanied by ever-closer interrelations between medical and civil authority. The Master Surgeon's Oath of 1390, for example, includes the commitment to serve the calling faithfully, take reasonable recompense, and examine patients for city authority when necessary; it embraces also the various other pledges familiar from earlier oaths.[20, 21] The use of "etcetera" again suggests the routine, indeed, formulaic nature of most of this consecration. However, certain additions to the expected points include increased surveillance by the masters over practice and increased reportage of medical circumstance to the officers of the city. The new master surgeons promise "to faithfully scrutinize" other men of their calling and present their defaults to the mayor and aldermen; likewise they will scrutinize all *women* of their calling and similarly report. This marks one of the first appearances of female practitioners in the official English dicta, although the history of women healers is venerable.[22-26] The masters also swear to give faithful information to the city administration as to those wounded or hurt, as well as to those in peril of death. Such reportage of prospectively desperate cases, which means that the practitioner had to alert the masters and they, in turn, the city officials, is especially significant. Probably it is an idea far older than its statement in 1390 (as Case I and its 1369 dictum suggest). It may well represent the origin of medieval malpractice insurance.

To illustrate this it is useful to interrupt the recital of the seven major cases in order to refer to one minor item, which actually is not a malpractice case but a 1417 writ of "recognizance" of great importance in the history of malpractice.[27] Case Letter E indicates that John Severall Love owes the chamberlain of London 20 pounds sterling as "recognizance." If he does not warn the wardens of surgery of the risk of maiming or of death of a patient under his care within four days of accepting the patient, the recognizance is to hold good; he will lose his 20 pounds. If he does alert them in time, he loses nothing. Provided that it is lawfully proved that John Severall Love has performed against the condition aforesaid, one half of the pledge will be forfeit to the city, one half to the faculty or craft of surgeons.

Thus, before attempting cure of a "high-risk" patient, the surgeon not only must report his case to the wardens of surgery but must surrender a monetary pledge to civil authority to insure his compliance with the medical-civil code. If recalcitrant, the practitioner pays, equally, the two institutions whose dicta he had violated. The timing of the pledge allows for a system for protecting the patient and a mechanism for guarding the practitioner. This recognizance is not a fine for malpractice after it is committed but advance payment required of the practitioner in case his unaided care is deemed malpractice. This assures the critically ill patient of expert consultation in the master-surgeon's examination, and it insures the practitioner against accusation that cure could have been effected if counsel had been called. Further, the practitioner is protected by the provision that he must be "lawfully proved" to have acted against the code if his money is to be forfeit. While not protecting the practitioner against all lawsuits brought by patients, it does protect him against some, such as the plea which caused Case I; and while not exonerating him in advance from all civil action which might be brought against him, such as that in Case III, this "recognizance" protects him against most. In effect the early 15th century London doctor had his prepaid malpractice insurance premium covering individual high-risk patients, administered jointly by craft and city, enforced by civic authority, and shared, if he defaulted, equally by profession and municipality.

This demonstration of proto-insurance procedure in practice in 1417 is partly corroborated in theory by two documents of 1415[28] and 1416.[29] A long Latin disquisition prefaces the familiar oath of allegiance sworn by the master surgeons in 1415 with a complaint against the inexperienced practitioners of surgery who undertake care of the sick and maimed, who thus obtain goods fraudulently, who are a menace to the sick, and who are a scandal to qualified practitioners. The manner of selection of masters as well as responsibilities of masters to scrutininze, correct, and manage the craft is followed by the selection of two sound, sagacious surgeons as masters: Richard Wellys[30] and Simon Rolf.[31] Directly following their oath of investiture, on May 3, however, the document stops. It is recommenced by another scribal hand under date of July 4, 1416, one year, one month, and one day after the master surgeons' oath, with this unhappy but not unexpected assertion: "Upon truthful information of certain trustworthy and discreet" practitioners of surgery it was understood that despite the ordinances against malpractice, inexperienced, indiscreet practitioners still were treating those in peril of maiming or death without alerting and consulting with the master surgeons. Accordingly the mayor and aldermen agreed that since "in these times" many more dread the loss of money than are amenable to the dictates of honesty or of conscience, a penalty paid to the Chamber of London "in form underwritten," would be forfeit by the medical miscreant so often as and when he violated the ordinance. Six shillings, 8 pence would be shared, 5 shillings to the Chamber, 20 pence to the craft.

Such monetary sanction appears in documents earlier and later for other offenses. Whether this was a "fine" paid upon judgment of guilt or whether this was a "recognizance" paid in advance "in the form underwritten" the records do not tell. That reportage by practitioners to guildmasters was enforced by pecuniary penalties is definite. John Severall Love's debt to the city chamberlain may represent the next step in enforcement after the 1416 dictum: payment in advance of guilt in order to prevent guilt. Medical malpractice insurance thus may have had its beginnings in medieval prophylaxis against malpractice.

Case V

Our return to the seven major malpractice cases introduces Case V, one of the most fascinating documents in English malpractice history.[32] No doubt it was considered significant in its own time as well, for it was arbitrated before the mayor and aldermen by a learned committee of eight expert witnesses, including the master physicians and the master surgeons, under the chairmanship of Dr. Gilbert Kymer,[33] churchman, rector of medicine, and chancellor of Oxford University. The plea is "iatrogenic sequelae," a new injury caused by surgical intervention in an original condition. The defendants are surgeons: John Harwe, John Dalton, and Simon Rolf; this last just nine years earlier had been the surveying master surgeon of London. The plaintiff is William Forest who, suffering an injury to the muscles of the thumb of the right hand and bleeding frequently and profusely, was treated by the three major surgeons. They, to prevent exanguination and death, and with the patient's consent, cauterized the wound. The patient then sued his surgeons for maiming his hand. Not the least remarkable aspect of this case is its depiction of the role of astrology in medieval practice.[34-39] Here is the award of the committee, their words translated from Latin:

> William Forest, plaintiff, when the moon was dark and in a bloody sign, namely under the very malevolent constellation Aquarius, was seriously hurt in the said muscles on the last day of last January and he lost blood enormously even to the ninth day of February last past, the moon remaining in the Sign Gemini. That the said Simon Rolf himself staunched the blood successfully at the beginning and that afterwards the said John Harwe helped by John Dalton . . . artificially arrested it when the bleeding had recurred six times with great vehemence from the aforesaid wound even to (syncope) and as if William Forest would die. And that on the seventh occasion William was thought to be in danger of death owing to the excessive loss and quickly deciding that he would suffer mutilation of his hand rather than death, the said John Harwe with the express consent of the said William, who was thus bleeding, when other remedies had failed, stopped the bleeding with the cautery, as beseemeth, and saved his life and freed him from the bonds of death. Wherefore we praise, we award and we decide that the aforesaid John Harwe, John Dalton and Simon Rolf individually by themselves and by any of them, especially John Harwe, acted well and surgically in what they did in the aforesaid treatment and that none of them made any mistake in any way in this matter. Wherefore we absolve them and each of them and especially John Harwe, from being impleaded by the same William Forest in the aforesaid matter by imposing perpetual silence on the same William in this affair. Moreover we find that they themselves are so free from the fault attributed to them and

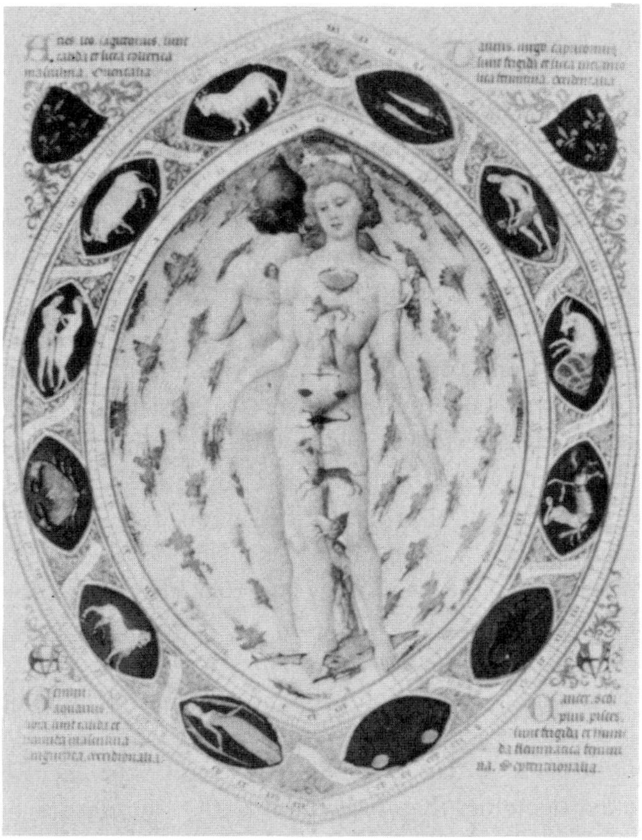

Fig. 4. Astrological Man, with zodiacal insignia which "control" physiological features, and with constellation signs and numerals which were thought to predict and aid diagnosis, prognosis, and treatment. From the *Très Riches Heures* of John, Duke of Berry, 15th century, Chantilly.

to any of them and especially to John Harwe, defamed maliciously and undeservedly, that as far as in us lies we restore to them unsullied their good name so far as their merit demands and deserves in this affair.

We further declare that any defect of the aforesaid hand, or mutilation or the ugly scar, so far as our industry avails to decide it, is due to the aforesaid constellation or to some peculiar defect or injury of the said William owing to the original wound.[40]

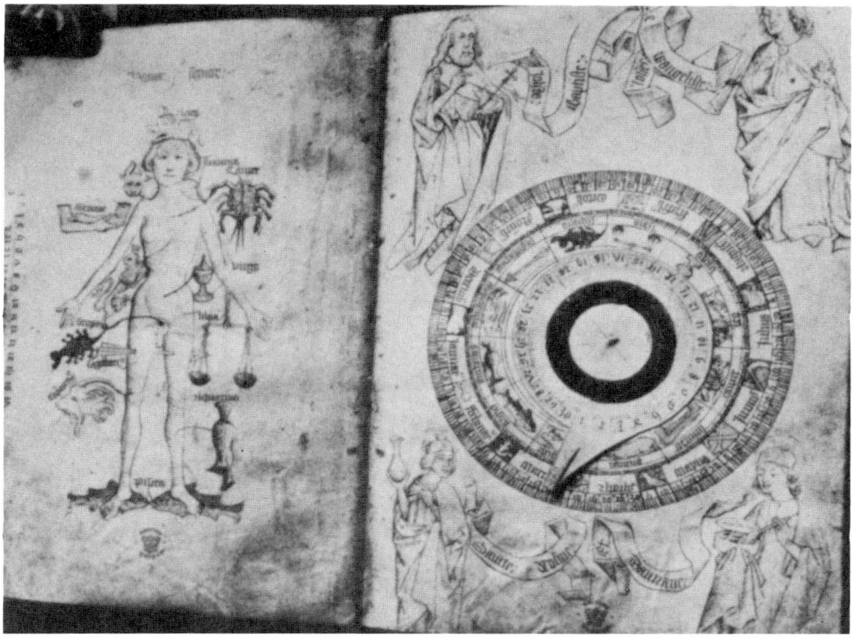

Fig. 5. Manuscript leaves from *The Guild Book of Barbers and Surgeons of York.* Astrological Man, on left. On right, Volvella, concentric spinning disks with zodiac symbols, for computing appropriate times for surgery and administration of medicines, 15th century. Courtesy of the British Museum.

Marvelous is the tripartite justification for any disfigurement or mutilation: the inauspicious constellations, the inherent defect of the patient, and the nature of the original wound. While medieval empirical judgment required emphasis on the patient's demeanor and on the type of his injury, the astrological computations explained the inexplicable: the inefficacy of otherwise expert care. Just how the medieval practitioner achieved his unity between often sophisticated scientific knowledge and celestial zodiacal computations is illustrated in figures 4 through 6.

In addition to astrological fascination, Case V suggests that the contemporary legal documents might reveal information on the importance and complexity of its examining committee, led by the estimable Dr. Gilbert Kymer. Indeed, it appears that William Forest's maimed

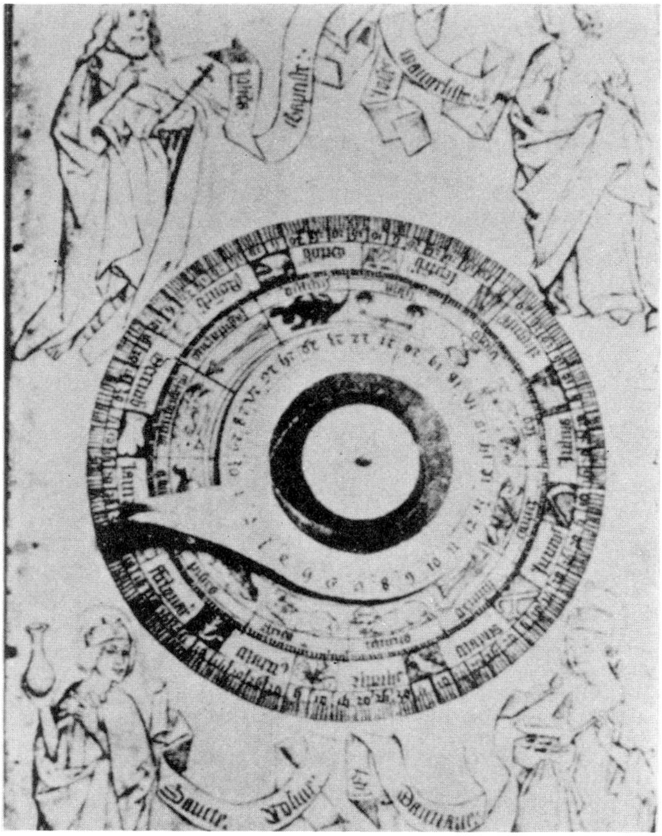

Fig. 6. Volvella, close-up of figure in Figure 5. Note Saints John the Baptist and John the Evangelist in upper margin and Saints Damian and Cosmos, the patron saints of medicine and surgery, in lower margin. Damian carries an ointment (or feces) box while Cosmos bears a urine flask.

hand marked one of the first legal tests of the Conjoint Faculty of Physicians and Surgeons. For in 1423 a petition proudly worded in English, the first of these malpractice documents written in the vernacular rather than in Latin or French, was presented to the mayor and aldermen and quickly granted by them.[41] To prevent malpractice in medicine and surgery a joint college of the two crafts was to be ordained, with medical practice under the aegis of two surveyors of medicine, and surgical practice under two masters—the two houses united under a single rector of medicines. The document itself is a treasure of theoretical and practical information, including methods of examination of professional candidates for licensure; reportage to authority of dangerous cases; provisions for conviction by peers and civil punishment of medical malefactors; procedures for medical care of the indigent; inspection and control of apothecaries; surveillance over medical and surgical practice by peers as well as surveyors; and a system of fines and forfeits shared equally by the municipal chamber and the professional faculty.

Yet more important than these provisions is the list of petitioners who introduced them and later, upon appointment, implemented them. These are: Doctor Gilbert Kymer, rector of the conjoint college, the two surveyors of medicine, and the two masters of surgery. All gave learned testimony in Case V. Or, better, all testified but one, Master Surgeon John Harwe,[42] for he was one of the accused. It appears that William Forest with the maimed hand had the audacity to sue two of the most important surgeons in England: Simon Rolf, master in 1415, and John Harwe, master in 1423, as well as surgeon leader of the new joint faculty. Possibly John Harwe was called to the case upon consultation required by the law of reportage of cases in danger. Nevertheless, the magnitude of his official surgical appointment explains the frequent references in the documents of the case to exonerate from blame "especially John Harwe." Then as now, professional distinction granted little immunity and less peace.

Case VI

The London Mayor's Court Files for 1443 document Case VI, which really is two cases here joined because of their common qualities.[43] Both patients complain that their original conditions deteriorated under medical ministration; both claim not simply return of fees but damages for suffering wrought; both agreed in advance to pay the surgeon a specific fee, and one made down payment of half the fee before treatment; both accused the practitioner of ignorant mistreatment; and, indeed, both accused the same defendant, Matthew Rellesford.[44] Whether this surgeon was proved guilty of worsening George Baylle's "stone" or John Roper's "anoncomo" of his left foot, the records do not tell. Noteworthy, however, is this glimpse of a practitioner who by professional ineptitude, litigious personality, or selection of contentious patients twice drew lawsuits in the space of one year.

For Case VI the paired dictum is of greater interest than the record of the docket. In a small vellum volume dated 1435 a long treatise of laws for the regulation of the craft of surgery appears in detail so startlingly complete that not only is professional practice controlled but private behavior as well.[45] Minuscule considerations of corporate meetings, guild dinners, personal quarrels, charitable acts, deportment during masters' meetings—all of these are detailed and fines are assigned to all prospective offenses. The document is an exemplification of responsible self-government. For the honor of the craft, for its probity, and for its perpetuity, the ordinance regulates all aspects of academic, practical, and ceremonial function, while clearly appreciating the humanity and the foibles of its individual members. Here is an example of the human and professional checks and balances inherent in each provision.

As in many of the past dicta, this proposition, advanced in A.D. 1435, requires each practitioner with a case likely to result in death or mutilation to report it to the masters and receive consultation. In the ordinance of 1416 a fine was added for enforcement and, in the document of Doctor John Severall Love (1417), a prepaid "recognizance" was required to assure compliance. The document of 1435 goes even further to ensure equity. All must show such dangerous cases to the masters or suffer a penalty of 13 shillings, 4 pence. However, if the *master* did not appear when called, he was to be fined 6 shillings, 8 pence. Or if the master, upon consultation, attempted to take the patient out of the private practitioner's hands to treat him himself, he was bound to pay restitution of the expected fee to the aggrieved surgeon as well as to pay a fine to the craft for the filching of patients.

This document is written by those who know men as well as instruments. In their provisions concerning the uses and abuses of power, in their delineation of punishments for all levels of professional and personal corruption, they demonstrate a concern as humane as it is practical. To account for the vagaries of human achievement they establish for the craft a probation period before tenure and a statute of limitations for achieving professional accreditation. To account for the unpredictability of human failure, they allot a portion of the craft's dues and fines for the support of their fellow surgeons who had fallen into poverty. To account for the unexpected, they predict, prescribe, and proscribe not only major professional actions but those trivia of personality that contribute to the image of the practitioner held by the patient, by the fellows of his calling, and by the municipality. Few compilations of rules legislate so pervasively and so justly.

Case VII

The seventh and last of the major cases is amusing for the method by which an accused practitioner institutes countersuit against his patient. While the document leaves unsaid as much as said, it appears that Gilbert Humphreyson, who had suffered an injury to his hand, brought complaint against his surgeon for ineffective treatment and excessive fees.[46] John Isyng, the practitioner, retaliated by accusing the patient before the local authorities of stealing a horse from Anthony Woodville, the second Earl Rivers. The patient, maintaining that this was vindictive nastiness, begs the earl to intercede in the case and dismiss the charge. We do not know whether the noble lord came to the rescue nor whether the surgeon was deemed guilty of malpractice, nor do we know what happened to the allegedly stolen horse. But the significance of this case to the history of malpractice is its depiction of protection of the practitioner by means of legal counterproceedings.

Paired with Case VII is a legislative document of 1461 which essentially and specifically reconfirms privileges and responsibilities granted in earlier decrees.[47] Rather than pursue its repetitions of familiar pledges, it will be pleasant to examine briefly the seven minor cases, in order to determine what qualities they add to knowledge of malpractice in medieval England (Table II).

Most of these seven cases, which I have labeled Cases A through G, occurred outside London. Not too surprisingly, these records often are less detailed than those which had the ready perquisites—the official scribes and their parchments—to memorialize the minute acts of a proud city. For London long has had a tradition of civic pride, and its pride in turn is its venerable civic tradition. Yet these minor cases are often instructive when they demonstrate similarity to dockets of London, thereby implying that what was considered malpractice in the metropolis was similarly malpractice in the towns. These minor cases are even more useful when they differ from the major cases, especially with respect to punishment for malpractice and with respect to royal intervention in the implementation of the regulations. The minor cases are most interesting when they introduce notions undefined by the seven major reports.

An example of this last proposition is Case A, in which Pernell, a woman physician from Devon, is accused of causing the death of a miller of Sidmouth because of her ignorance and poor practices.[48] Apparently judged guilty, she was punished by outlawry, physical outcasting. However she received royal pardon and was thus freed from stigma. Here is a significant reminder that not only did women practice medicine in medieval England, but like their male counterparts, they also malpracticed—or were so accused. The punishment of expulsion from town is far harsher than most thus far discussed in the major cases occurring in London, and the cancellation of punishment by royal intercession is unexpected. This same circumstance, of the king intervening to reverse the punishment of malpractice, appears again in Case C, where the locale is Chester.[49] There John Leche,[50] who was actually a court physician who had originally practiced in Chester, was sued by a woman for damages because of her husband's death after a surgical operation. The physician was fined his "goods and tenements." From this great forfeiture the king pardoned him.

These two cases raise interesting possibilities. Since I know of no instance in the years between 1350 and 1500 in which the monarch interfered in the malpractice jurisdiction of the city of London, and since these Devon and Chester cases represent comparatively severe punishment for guilt, it is reasonable to surmise that: 1) towns other than London had little complex machinery for the adjudication of malpractice; 2) whatever procedure did exist was not as carefully instigated or as carefully controlled by professional guilds, as London's was; and 3) in the absence of strong guild and powerful municipal authority, the national authority, the king, was the only arbitrator to whom appeal was possible.

Case B, again from Chester, is a straightforward accusation of a practitioner for causing death by his ministrations.[51] One element marks it as unusual. Because of the death of Roger, son of Robert, Thomas de Clotton is accused by the Earl of Chester. That it is the nobleman bringing suit, rather than a relative or other commoner associated with the patient, may have meaning beyond the possibility that the deceased or his father were servants to the earl. Here again surmise, not fact, suggests that the processes for complaint against malpractice, just as the procedures for adjudicating them, were less comprehensive outside London than inside, and that the commoner might well have needed, or believed that he needed, the aid in litigation of the friendly local nobleman.

Case D has a London venue and is a garden-variety accusation for failure to cure.[52] Similar to it is Case G, for which no locale is known. Of interest here is the description of the patient whose malady was uncured—one of the infrequent references to children in these documents.[53] Simon Lynde, a stationer, accuses practitioner Peter Blank for failing to cure the diseased eye of a child.

Case E is that remarkable writ of recognizance referred to earlier as one of the prototypes for modern medical malpractice insurance.[54] The last of the minor cases, lettered F, amusingly reverses fault for failure of cure.[55] The testimony of Matthew Rutherford, accused of careless treatment of a cleric's left leg, and attached for damages amounting to 40 pounds, maintains that cure was ineffective not because of professional inadequacy but because of defiance by the patient. The cleric, Brother Richard of Guisborough, uncooperatively threw away his medicines and persisted in eating inappropriate and unwholesome foods!

Clearly these seven minor cases and the seven major malpractice cases, as well as the official edicts associated with them, demonstrate as much about medieval medical practice as they do about malpractice. First, they distinguish definitively between proper practice and inadequate practice, and between accidental error and willful or mindless evil. Such malpractice accusations as maiming, neglect, endangering limbs, deceit and falsehood, failure to cure, excessive fees, iatrogenic sequelae, worsening of original complaints, death due to medical ineptitude—all these define standards and expectations of the perfect, of which these complaints are the opposite. Further, this apprehension of what constituted malpractice was shared by three constituencies: the patients, the individual practitioners, and the professional guild organizations. Uniting the interests of these three groups against medical malpractice were the civic authorities, who simultaneously gave allegiance to them and required obedience from them.

The second contribution of the malpractice dockets and the malpractice dicta is the depiction of certain aspects of medieval medicine and surgery as they were, not as they might have been. Habits of actual practice, not theory, and habits of accepted proper practice, are superbly delineated. These practices include diagnoses, each followed by definition, in order to distinguish between diseases or wounds which were curable as opposed to those considered incurable, for which care could not be begun; treatment planned, executed, and justified according to astrological computations; and fees for professional services granted in money or in valuables, agreed to and paid in advance, in installments, or on cure. Such accepted and acceptable practices were mutually understood by the same three constituencies: patient, practitioner, and profession. Yet again, the municipality united the concerns of these three in legislation and in its vigilant enforcement.

This pervasive presence of city authority is the third lesson of the malpractice documents. The professional medical and surgical organizations themselves proposed and then petitioned for reformation of their craft. Their self-regulation, however, was enforced by the power and ceremony of strong civic government. Intricate relations evolved between professional and civic responsibility, as in the reportage of "high risk" cases by the practitioner to the masters and hence to the highest officials of the city. The same was true of the systems of fine, forfeiture, recognizance, the "precursor of malpractice insurance," administered jointly by craft and city, and financially beholden to both. From this medicocivil unity the benefactors were the three constituencies: the patient as citizen, the practitioner as craftsman, and the guild as component institution of the city. Cases and edicts both contain one phrase which appears with insistent regularity: "the common profit," the common good, the mutual advantage. Malpractice must be reported for the common good, punished for the common good, and eradicated for the common good. Advantage accrued to the three constitutencies mutually. Of this common profit the city was arbiter and guardian.

Remarkably, the only medieval documents which depict a medical idea or medical event from all three vantage points of patient, doctor, and professional peers are the malpractice records. Of the thousands of medieval medical manuscripts and related fragments extant, some are theoretical treatises, some are accounts of medical procedures, some are complaints of theoretical follies, some are legal edicts from the courts of kings. All are dedicated to one or two of the three constituencies.

None unites theory with practice to address all three—except these dockets and dicta of medieval medical malpractice. Apparently perverse is this notion of learning the truth by investigating its opposite, error. These fascinating materials suggest the utility of perversity. Perhaps they prove that eccentric old rule, one fundamental law of historical dynamics: accentuate the negative in order to redefine the positive!

ACKNOWLEDGMENT

Figures 5 and 6 are reproduced with the gracious cooperation of Dr. Harry Bober, Avalon Professor in the Humanities, New York University, New York, N.Y.

REFERENCES

1. London Guildhall: Letter Book G, folio XVIII. English translation appears in Riley, H. T.: *Memorials of London and London Life*. London, Longmans, Green, 1868, pp. 273-74.
2. London Guildhall: *Letter Book G*. folio CCXIX. Translation, Riley, H. T., op. cit., p. 337.
3. See Master Surgeons' Oaths for 1390 and 1424, MacKinney, L.[15] and Talbot, C. H.[26]
4. Talbot, C. H. and Hammond, E. A.: *The Medical Practitioners in Medieval England*. London, Wellcome Hist. Med. Library, 1965, pp. 141, 150, 218, although there is no formal entry for Richard in this biographical register.
5. London Guildhall: *Plea and Memoranda Rolls*, Roll A 22, February 13, 1377. See Thomas, A. H.: *Calendar of Plea and Memoranda Rolls, A.D. 1364-1381*. Cambridge, Cambridge University Press, 1929, p. 236.
6. London Guildhall: *Letter Book H*, folio XXVIII. Translation, Riley, H. T., op. cit., pp. 393-94.
7. These surgeons are not listed or mentioned in Talbot and Hammond's register.
8. For example, the 1423 and 1435 dicta. Talbot, C. H.[26] and Talbot and Hammond, op. cit., pp. 283-84.
9. London Guildhall: *Letter Book H*, fol. CXLV. Translation, Riley, H. T., op. cit., pp. 464-66.
10. Bühler, C. F.: A Middle English Medical Manuscript from Norwich, In: *Studies in . . . Honor of Professor Albert Croll Baugh*, Leach, M., editor. Philadelphia, 1961, pp. 285-98.
11. Meyer, C. F.: A Middle English leechbook and its XIV century poem on bloodletting. *Bull. Hist. Med. 7*:388-90, 1939.
12. Jones, I. B.: Popular medical knowledge in XIVth century English literature. *Bull. Hist. Med. 5*:405-51, 538-88, 1937.
13. Robbins, R. H.: Medical manuscripts in Middle English. *Speculum 45*:393-415, 1970.
14. Forbes, T. R.: Verbal charms in British folk medicine. *Proc. Amer. Phil. Soc. 115*:293-316, 1971.
15. Mackinney, L.: *Medical Illustrations in Medieval Manuscripts*. Berkeley and Los Angeles, Univ. Calif. Press. 1965.
16. Randall, L. M. C.: *Images in the Margins of Gothic Manuscripts*. Berkeley and Los Angeles, University Calif. Press, 1966.
17. The Morgan Library Manuscripts. No. 917 F 180; No. 359 F 143V; No. 358 F 20V.
18. London Guildhall: *Plea and Memoranda Rolls*, Roll A 40, November 15, 1408. See Thomas, A. H.: *Calendar of Plea*

and Memoranda Rolls, A.D. 1413-1437. Cambridge, Cambridge University Press, 1943.

19. Chaucer, G.: Prologue, *The Canterbury Tales,* 11, Robinson, F. N., editor. Boston, Houghton, Mifflin, 1957, pp. 623-68.
20. London Guildhall: *Letter Book H,* folio CCXLVIII. Translation, Riley, H. T., op. cit., pp. 519-20.
21. Sharpe, R. R.: *Calendar of Letter Books.* London. Francis, 1907, book H, p. 352.
22. Hughes, M.: *Women Healers in Medieval Life and Literature.* New York, Kings Crown Press, 1943.
23. Power, E. Some women practitioners of medicine in the Middle Ages. *Proc. Royal Soc. Med. 15:*1922, pp. 17-34.
24. Bonser, W.: *The Medical Background of Anglo-Saxon England.* London, Wellcome Hist. Med. Library, 1963.
25. Kittredge, G. L.: *Witchcraft in Old and New England.* Cambridge, Mass., Harvard University Press, 1929.
26. Talbot, C. H.: Women Doctors and Surgeons in the Middle Ages. Presented at the New York Academy of Medicine, February 23, 1972.
27. Corporation of London Library: *Journal I,* folio 19 V. Translation, Riley, H. T., op. cit., p. 651.
28. London Guildhall: *Letter Book I,* folio CXLIX. Translation, Riley, H. T., op. cit., pp. 606-8.
29. London Guildhall, op. cit.
30. Talbot and Hammond, op. cit., pp. 283-84.
31. Loc. cit., pp. 326-26.
32. London Guildhall: *Plea and Memoranda Rolls,* Roll A 52, September 10, 1424. See Thomas, A. H.: *Calendar of Plea and Memoranda Rolls, A. D. 1413-1437.* Cambridge, Cambridge University Press, 1943, pp. 174-75.
33. Talbot and Hammond, op. cit., pp. 60-63.
34. Wickersheimer, E.: Figures medico-astrologiques des ixe, xe, et xie siècles. *Janus (Arch. Int. l'Hist. Med.) 19:*157-55, 1914.
35. Pagel, W.: Prognosis and diagnosis: A comparison of ancient and modern medicine. *J. Warburg Inst. 2:*396, 1938-1939.
36. Bober, H.: The zodiacal miniature of the Tres Riches Heures of the Duke of Berry: Its sources and meaning. *J. Warburg Courtauld Inst.:* 1-34, 1948.
37. Gunther, R. T.: *Early Science in Oxford.* Oxford, Oxford University Press, 1925.
38. Gunther, R. T.: *Early Science in Cambridge.* Oxford, Oxford University Press, 1937.
39. Cosman, M. P.: Medieval medical malpractice and Chaucer's physician. *N.Y. J. Med.* 1972. In press.
40. Gask, G. E.: *Essays in the History of Medicine,* Power, D'A., translator. London, Butterworth, 1950.
41. London Guildhall: *Letter Book K,* folio LXII, Power, D'A., editor. Smith, J. F.: *Memorials of the Craft of Surgery.* London, Cassell, 1886, Appendix B.
42. Talbot and Hammond, op. cit., pp. 154-55.
43. City of London, Mayor's Court: File III, No. 165, and No. 161.
44. Talbot and Hammond, op. cit., p. 213.
45. The Barbers' Company ms., *tempus* 13, King Henry VI, Power, D'A., editor. Op. cit., pp. 60-69 and Appendix C.
46. Public Record Office: *Exchequer Records,* E/315/486, folio 10. Talbot and Hammond, op. cit., pp. 157-58.
47. The Barbers' Company ms., *sub* 1461. Power, D'A., op. cit., p. 60.
48. Public Record Office: *Calendar of the Patent Rolls, A.D. 1348-1350.* London, His Majesty's Stat. Off., 1931, p. 561, Talbot and Hammond, op. cit., p. 241.
49. *Calendar of the Patent Rolls, 1381-1385.* London, His Majesty's Stat. Off., n.d., p. 182.
50. Talbot and Hammond, op. cit., pp. 161-62.
51. *Chester Plea Rolls, tempus* 48, Edward III. Talbot and Hammond, op. cit., p. 424.
52. Talbot and Hammond, op. cit., p. 424.
53. Public Record Office: *Early Chancery Proceedings,* bundle 187, No. 89. Talbot and Hammond, op. cit., p. 246.
54. Corporation of London Library.[27]
55. Edwards, W.: *The Early History of the North Riding.* London, 1924., p. 161. Talbot and Hammond, op. cit., p. 214.

NICHOLAS COPERNICUS, M.D.

LEONARD J. BRUCE-CHWATT, M.D.

Professor of Tropical Hygiene
London School of Hygiene and Tropical Medicine

JOAN M. BRUCE-CHWATT

London, England

"I believe that of all things human nothing better could befall me than the friendship of this great and learned man..And if at some time my efforts in this respect will be found useful to the common wealth to whose good we ought to devote our endeavours, acknowledgement should be rendered to this Doctor." George Joachim Rhetieus in *De Revolutionibus Narratio Prima*, the first summary of Copernican theory, published in 1540, three years before the publication of the first edition of the original treatise of Nicholas Copernicus.

IN February 1973 the scientific world celebrated the 500th anniversary of the birth of Nicholas Copernicus and many articles have been devoted to his astronomical work, which culminated with the publication of the revolutionary book *De Revolutionibus Orbium Coelestium*. It is often overlooked that Copernicus was also a qualified and practicing physician, and it is this aspect of his life that will be emphasized in the present short essay.

Nicholas Copernicus* was born in Torun, Poland, on the Vistula River on February 19, 1473. Torun was one of the towns of Pomerania that had formed an alliance in order to escape from the military domination of the Teutonic Knights, who settled in northeastern Poland in the 13th century.

The incorporation of the Alliance into the Kingdom of Poland led to war with the Teutonic Order. At the end of this 13-years' conflict (1454-1466) the whole of eastern Pomerania and the ecclesiastical do-

*The surname has many spellings such as Copernic, Coppernic, Cupernick, Coppernik, Copphernic, Kopernik, Koppernik, Koppernigk, Kopperlingk, Kupernick. Nicholas himself usually signed his name Copernicus.

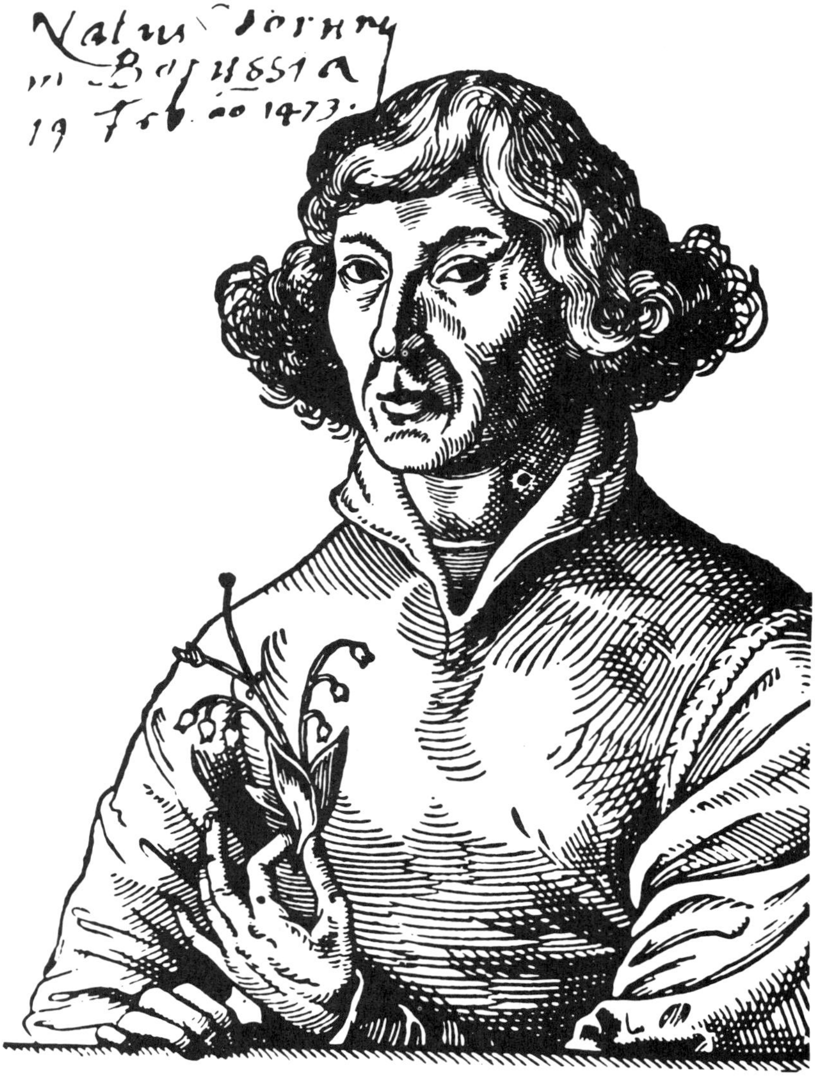

Fig. 1. Nicolas Copernicus. A contemporary woodcut showing the astronomer holding lillies of the valley (*Convallaria maialis*). The plant has medicinal properties and has been used as a cardiac stimulant. Reproduced by permission from Adamczewski, J.: *Nicolas Copernic et son époque*. Warsaw, Poland, Interpress, 1972. Photograph by J. Baranowski.

main of Warmia was given the name of Royal Prussia and rejoined the Polish Crown.

Nicholas Copernicus the Elder, a merchant of Cracow, moved to Torun and married Barbara Watzenrode (Weczelrode). The Watzenrodes had come from Silesia a century earlier and were well established among the Torun patriciate. Barbara's brother was Lucas Weczelrode, bishop of Warmia.

Having lost his father at the age of 10, Nicholas, with his elder brother Andreas, came under the protection and guidance of their uncle the bishop, a man of great influence and means. The two boys spent some years at the cathedral school in Wladislavia and in 1491 went to the famous University of Cracow. There Nicholas studied philosophy, then closely associated with mathematics, and was already passionately interested in astronomy. This subject was taught by Albert of Brudzewo, famous for his commentaries on Aristotle and a supporter of the geocentric system of Ptolemy. At the same time Copernicus learnt drawing and painting and was already dreaming of a journey to Italy. In 1496, having been elected canon at the Cathedral of Frombork (Frauenburg), Nicholas was enabled by the generosity of his uncle to go to Italy, where he entered the University of Bologna.*

There he studied canon law, philosophy, mathematics, and astronomy under the famous Domenico Maria Novarra. From Bologna he transferred to Padua; here, it would seem, he began his medical studies. According to notes left by Comnenus Papadopoli (*Historia Gymnasii Patavini*), Nicholas studied philosophy and medicine under Professors Nicholas Passerus and Nicholetus Vernia Teatinus. In the Archives of the medical faculty of the University of Padua it is noted that in 1499 Professor Teatinus awarded the crowns of philosophy and medicine to his Polish student. In 1499 Copernicus also spent some time teaching mathematics in Rome. These studies were interrupted for a while when

*While in Bologna, Copernicus joined the student's fraternity known as "Natio Germanorum," the most influential and fashionable of its kind. This was the origin of a bitter controversy between Polish and German scholars, both claiming Copernicus as their own national.

The debate is largely pointless: the ancestors of Copernicus were of mixed Slavonic and Germanic origin. Copernicus himself, a fervent Catholic, was a loyal subject of a Polish King. Although he left a few letters written in German, his cultural background and heritage were Latin and Greek.

Thorvaldsen's beautiful monument to Copernicus, standing in the center of Warsaw, was one of the few that escaped destruction during the bombing of the Polish capital in 1940-41. Its inscription, "To Nicholas Copernicus, his compatriots," was changed during the occupation of Poland to: "To Nicholas Copernicus, the German Nation." Today the original inscription has been restored.

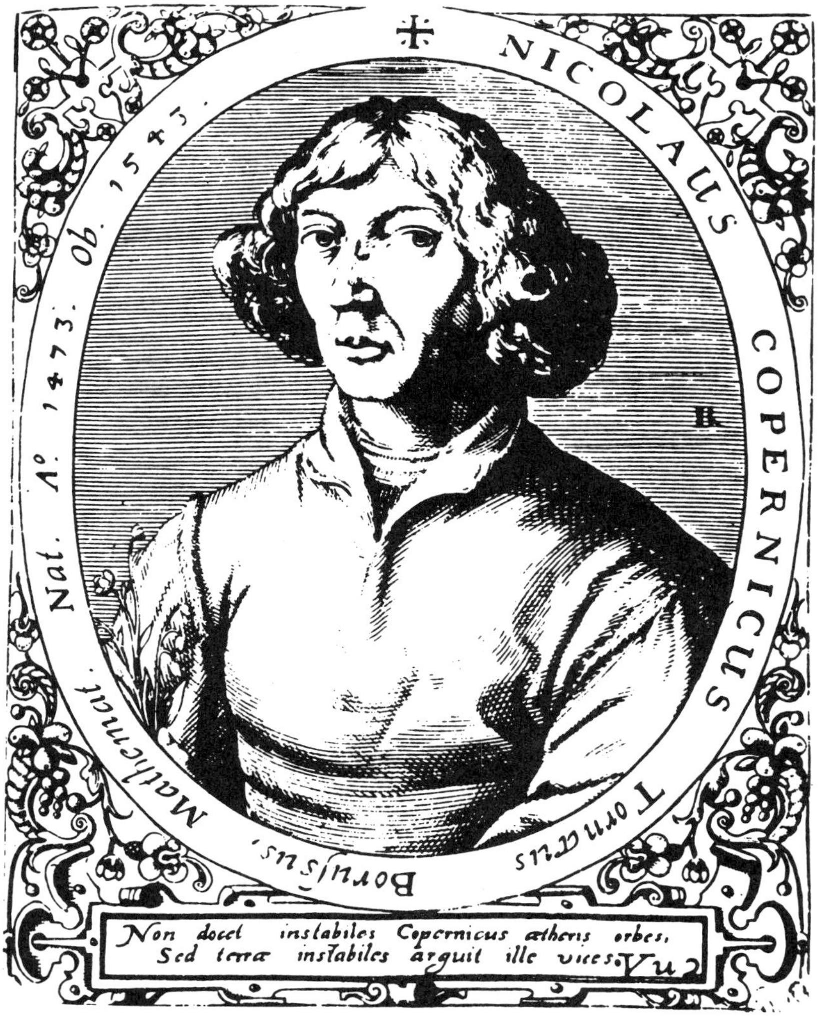

Fig. 2. Nicolas Copernicus. A contemporary engraving. Reproduced by permission from Adamczewski, J.: *Nicolas Copernic et son époque*. Warsaw, Poland, Interpress, 1972. Photograph by J. Baranowski.

he was recalled to Poland in order to obtain the consent of the Chapter of the Cathedral at Frombork to return to Italy for completion of his medical studies. Being a "*clericus minorum ordinum*" he had been able to undertake the study of medicine without special dispensation from either bishop or pope. His dependable uncle arranged for Nicholas to obtain, in addition to the Warmian canonry, the office of "*scholasticus*" at the Church of the Holy Cross in Wroclaw (Breslau). This ensured him a regular income and financial independence.

In 1501 Copernicus returned to Padua, passing through Florence, where he admired Leonardo da Vinci's celebrated anatomical drawings. Records of the University of Padua testify that Copernicus was regularly enrolled as a Polish subject (*Patet ex polonorum*) studying medicine, law, and philosophy.

The formal outcome of the years of study in Italy was the doctorate in canon law taken in 1503 at Ferrara. Copernicus' decision to take his degree at the small University of Ferrara was probably due to the fact that a newly promoted doctor at Bologna or Padua was expected to celebrate the event in style. In Ferrara the degree itself was less expensive and the burden of lavish hospitality could be avoided. This choice confirms the opinion that Nicholas had a retiring, pedantic, and thrifty nature—so different from that of Andreas, an improvident rake.

In 1505 Copernicus returned to Poland and spent some time in Cracow before finally settling in Warmia. His duties as Canon at Frombork left him free to pursue his astronomical work and to practice as a physician. Much of his time was spent at Lidzbark (Heilsberg) with his uncle, the stern and powerful bishop to whom he became secretary and private physician.

In 1512 Lucas Watzenrode fell ill on his return from Cracow and died so suddenly in Torun that poisoning was suspected. Copernicus, who was not present at his uncle's deathbed, soon left Lidzbark and moved to Frombork, the site of the Chapter. He was active in the administration of the diocese and in 1521, after the end of hostilities with the Teutonic Knights, was responsible for the monetary reforms that helped to restore commerce and industry.

It is in the field of astronomy, however, with his immortal work *De Revolutionibus Orbium Coelestium Libra VI*, that Copernicus' greatest achievement lies. Working in a small observatory set up in a tower of the castle, with instruments of his own invention and construction, he made the 27 astronomical observations upon which his theory was based. The work itself was completed in 1520 and circulated as a manuscript, but Copernicus hesitated to publish a book so controversial and revolutionary; he was at last persuaded by his friends

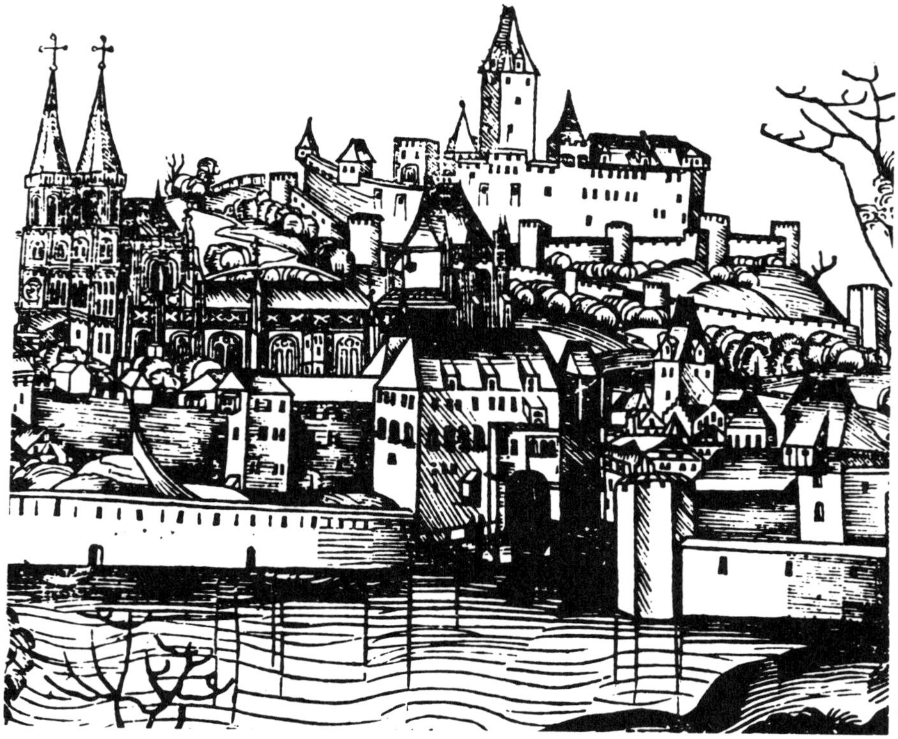

Fig. 3. Padua in the 16th century. From "Cronica mundi" by Hartmann Schedel. Reproduced by permission from Adamczewski. J.: *Nicolas Copernic et son époque.* Warsaw, Poland, Interpress, 1972. Photograph by J. Baranowski.

to agree to the publication of the work, the culmination of 30 years of observations. The book was dedicated to Pope Paul III who, in accepting the dedication, gave it his approval. The first copy, from the presses of John Petrinus of Nüremberg in 1543, was brought to Copernicus when death was already at his bedside. In 1542 Copernicus had suffered a cerebral hemorrhage followed by partial paralysis. In January 1543 Bishop Johannes Dantiscus mentioned in one of his letters that Copernicus was dying. But the end did not come until May 24, 1543, and Tiedemann Ghisius, the only intimate friend of Copernicus, tells us that the great scholar glanced at the book and touched it before closing his eyes forever. His tomb in Frombork bears the inscription

"*D.O.M.R.D. Nicolao Copernico, Torunensi, Artium et Medicinae Doctori, Canonico Warmiensi, Praestanti Astrologo Instaurati Martinus Cromerus Episcopus Warmiensis, Honoris et ad posteritatem memoriae causa posuit MDLXXI.*" This inscription recalls not only Copernicus the astronomer but also the physician. What, then, is known of the medical studies of Copernicus or his practice as a doctor?

Guided as he was by his interest in science, why did Copernicus choose Padua for his medical studies? Padua was at that time known as the Athens of the Renaissance. Lying within the Republic of Venice, that shining light of Europe, the University of Padua, which bore proudly the title of "*pupilla degli occhi della Repubblica Veneta*" (pupil of the eyes of the Venetian Republic), was also recognized as "Queen and Mother of the Renaissance. Home of the Muses, Meeting Place of the Nations, Sanctuary of Science." Since 1315, when Mondino, under an edict granted by the enlightened Emperor Frederick II, carried out the first dissection of a human cadaver, the renown of the schools of Padua and Bologna had spread far and wide. Toward the end of the 15th century the practical study of anatomy was officially authorized by a papal bull of Sixtus IV, himself a former student of Bologna and Padua. This authorization, confirmed by Clement VII, contributed greatly to the development of medical studies in Italy. Although dissections were carried out only once a year and only 20 students could be present at the dissection of a man (30 in the case of a woman), the reputation of these medical courses drew crowds of young men eager for scientific knowledge. It was at Padua, too, that Giovanni Batista da Monte first began the practice of clinical teaching at the patient's bedside.

Medical studies at that time were closely linked with the study of philosophy and lasted four to five years. During the first year most of the time was spent on the study of Avicenna's *Canon.* The second year was devoted to the *Aphorisms* of Hippocrates and to his *Liber prognosticorum.* The third year was taken up by Galen's *Microtegne*, Philaretos' *De pulsum negocio*, the *Liber urinarum* of Aegidus Carbonensis, and to works of Aristotle, Pliny, and others. After the first two years the degree of bachelor was awarded and, two years later, the licentiate. The doctorate was granted after special ceremonies and on payment of a large fee. Graduation was a church ceremony, proclaimed by the ringing of bells and conducted in the presence of the entire faculty.

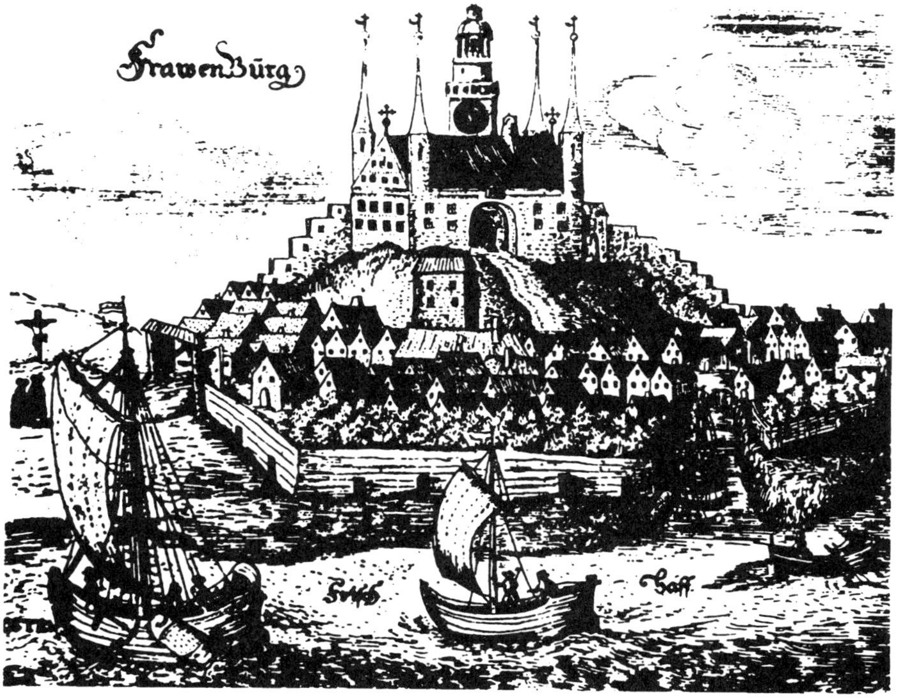

Fig. 4. Frombork (Frauenburg). From an engraving in C. Hartknoch: *Alt und neues Preussen, 1684.* Reproduced by permission from Adamczewski, J.: *Nicolas Copernic et son époque.* Warsaw, Poland, Interpress, 1972. Photograph by J. Baranowski.

When Copernicus returned to Padua in 1501, he had most certainly completed the first part of his medical studies and now he once more set to work with a will, attending lectures and winning the respect and friendship of his professors. One of these, Alessandro Achillini of Bologna, physician and philosopher, commentator on Aristotle and Averroës, developed a firm friendship with Copernicus based on their common interest in medicine and their passion for astronomy. Other great professors at the faculty of Padua were Marcus Antonius de la Torre (for whom Leonardo had drawn his anatomical studies), Bartolomeo Montagnana the Younger, Antonio Gazzi and Girolamo Gubbio who, in addition to medicine, taught astronomy privately. Among his fellow students Girolamo Fracastoro,* the famous poet-doctor of the Renaissance, was also a pupil of Achillini. Whether Copernicus actually finished his medical studies and obtained his doctorate does not appear to be recorded officially, although most of his biographers assume that it is unlikely that he would have failed to do so.

Copernicus led the quiet, uneventful life of a canon at Frombork, continuing his studies but also caring for the needy or the sick and dispensing medicines which he prepared himself. Soon the fame of Copernicus the doctor spread far and wide. In May 1519 a strange epidemic, apparently of plague, broke out in northern Warmia and Nicholas Copernicus directed the campaign, giving advice to the other doctors and to the populace. This was also a time when the little principality suffered from marauding bands of Teutonic knights. Many physicians came to him for his opinion on difficult cases and called him to attend their more illustrious patients. As physician to the Chapter he attended Bishop Fabian Reich until his death. Fabian's successor, Mauricius Farber, left 12 letters in which he begged Copernicus to attend him in Gdansk (Danzig) and expressed his admiration and gratitude for the medical care he received. One of these letters, dated 1528, reads as follows: "*Quum dissenteria in senioribus pericolosa esse solet, rogamus ut fraternitates Vostri nostros Dom. Joannem Tymmerman Cantorem et Doctorem Nicholaum Copernic ad nos in Heilsberg sine mora mittant.*"

In January 1532 Bishop Farber, having recovered from his illness, wrote to John Benedict, physician of King Sigismond I of Poland, expressing his admiration for the medical care he had received. Later the bishop, suffering from "colica ventosa," requested the Chapter to release his favorite physician once more. "*Rogamus vostra Fraternitate nostro DOM. Doct. Nicholas Copernic ut quanto potest fieri citius huc ad nos veniat conversaturus . . . super adversa corporis nostri valetudinae.*" But in 1537, in spite of all this care, the bishop of Warmia died in the arms of his physician and friend.

Three years later the bishop of Chelmno (Kulm), Tiedemann Ghisius, invited Copernicus to visit him in Lubawa (Libau). After a successful cure, Copernicus received a warm letter of thanks from his grateful patient. The fame of Doctor Copernicus soon reached Prince

*Girolamo Fracastoro was also a mathematician. He constructed an improbable alternative to the Ptolemaic universe based on concentric spheres and published it in *Homocentrica,* Venice, 1538.

Albert I of Prussia, then a vassal of the Polish king, and Copernicus spent four months in Koenigsberg, the capital of East Prussia, treating Albert's friend George Kuhnheim.*

There are other mementoes of the medical activity of Copernicus. Five medical books formerly belonging to him are in the library of the University of Uppsala; they contain many marginal notes in his own hand which confirm the opinion that Copernicus was an observant and keen clinician throughout his life.

In the book *Bartolomeo Montagnane Consilia Medica*, 1499, on a margin of a paragraph quoting Avicenna's remark that ignorance of the physician may lead to the death of his patient, there is a cryptic note in Copernicus' hand: "*In Dantisco a. 1526 augusti die*" and then *exemplificatio aurea*," followed by "*si dosis ab auctoribus non ponitur.*" It is likely that Copernicus saw in Gdansk (Danzig) a striking case of illness that needed unusual doses of drugs.

One of the notes on the margin of a page in *Mesue Johannes Opus Medicinale cum Expositione Mondini*, published in Venice in 1502, contains the following note in Copernicus' hand: "Composition of a wine sublimate for stomach ache according to Frater Bernard. Take two pints of wine sublimate, 4 drachms of figs, cinnamon, cloves and saffron 5 drachms each. Mix and pass in a clean vessel. Use commodiously with moderation. God willing this should help." Another page carries a prescription written in an unknown hand; it refers to the illness of the sister of a cleric who suffered from prostration and stomach trouble: "*Rotule stomacales in abiectione et defectu appetitum cibo admisceando domino N. Copernico autore anno domini 1532 die Saturni XXIII februarii gravissime decumbente Sorore magistri achatti freunth Canonici Warmiensis et plebani ecclesi Elhygensis.*

"Rp Corallorumr rubr.
Cinamoni am zj.
Specierum diarod abbat zijs
Zucceri albi lbs/libram semi/
Aq destill.p.s. et fiat confecto in rotulum."

*In the otherwise blameless personal life of Copernicus some biographers mention an embarrassing episode. It concerned Anna Schilling, a distant relative who was employed by Copernicus as his *focaria* or housekeeper. Johannes Dantiscus, the successor of Bishop Lucas Watzenrode, objected to Canon Nicholas (then 63 years old) having Anna Schilling in his house. After a timid attempt to oppose the bishop, Copernicus complied with his wish and sent Anna away.

According to Birkenmajer, one of the biographers of the great astronomer, there is evidence that Copernicus wrote a treatise on medical philosophy, and Abbot Broscius left a Latin note: "*Itaque Copernicus materiam morbi contumacem pondus vocabat: potentiam vero, praesidia medicamentorum quibus materia contumax moveratur. Neque mediocris ingenii est colligere dato ponderi movendo quae serviat potentia.*"

It is difficult for us to realize today the boldness and the far-reaching effects of Copernican thought on the science, philosophy, and theology of the 16th and 17th centuries.* But Copernicus the man will appear to us a somewhat unfamiliar but not less appealing figure if we remember that he was not merely an austere scholar, but a good administrator and a practicing physician whose achievements in astronomy have eclipsed the remembrance of his medical vocation.

ACKNOWLEDGEMENT

We thank the Interpress Publishing House, Warsaw, Poland, for permission to reproduce the four figures illustrating this paper from the book *Nicolas Copernic et son époque by* Jan Adamczewscki, 1972.

*Albert Einstein on Copernicus: "The Copernican system made a clean sweep of the view which thought of the entire firmament as revolving round the earth and humanity. That was probably the severest shock man's interpretation of the cosmos ever received. It reduced the world to a mere province so to speak instead of being the capital and centre." Quoted by Count Harry Kessler: *Diaries of a Cosmopolitan*. New York, 1927.

GENERAL REFERENCES

Adamczewski, J.: *Nicolas Copernic et son époque*. Warsaw, Interpress, 1972.

Armitage, A.: *Copernicus, Founder of Modern Astronomy*. London, Allen & Unwin, 1938.

Birkenmajer, L. A.: *Mikolaj Kopernik*. Cracow, Biblioteka Narodowa, 1900.

Brozek, L.: *Copernican Bibliography*. Poznan, 1949.

Bruce-Chwatt, L. J.: *Presse Méd.* (Paris) *67*:1523, 1959.

Curtze, M., editor: *Reliquiae Copernicanae*. Leipzig, Täubner, 1875.

Hipler, F.: *Die Biographen des N. Kopernicus*. Braunsberg, Peter, 1873.

Koestler, A.: *The Sleepwalkers*. London, Hutchinson, 1959.

Mizwa, S. P.: *Nicholas Copernicus*. New York, Macmillan, 1941.

Polkowski, I.: *Life of Mikolaj Kopernik*. Gniezno, Towarzystwo Przyjaciol Nauk, 1873.

Prowe, L.: *Nicolaus Coppernicus*, 2 vols. Berlin, Weidmann, 1883-1884.

Rudnicki, J.: *Nicholas Copernicus*. London, Quatercentenary Celebration Comm., 1943.

Schmauch, H.: *Nicolaus Kopernicus*. Kitzingen/Main, Holzner, 1953.

Sliwinski, M.: Dr. Copernicus. *World Health*, 12-15, 1973.

Szperkowicz, J.: *Nicolaus Copernicus, 1473-1973*. Warsaw, P.I.W., 1972.

HISTORICAL NOTES ON THE BETHLEM ROYAL HOSPITAL AND THE MAUDSLEY HOSPITAL

Patricia H. Allderidge

Archivist

The Bethlem Royal Hospital
Beckenham, Kent.

The Maudsley Hospital
London

England

The Bethlem Royal Hospital is one of the five Royal Hospitals of the City of London, the other being St. Bartholomew's, St. Thomas's, Christ's Hospital, and Bridewell. Although ostensibly royal foundations of the 16th century, all but the last two were actually refoundations, and Bethlem, when it was "granted" to the City, had not only been in existence for three centuries but had been under the patronage of the City for more than two.

The Bethlem Royal Hospital was founded in 1247, although at the time its founder neither intended nor foresaw the centuries of charitable work which lay before it. Simon Fitzmary, an alderman and twice sheriff of the City of London, granted all his lands in the parish of St. Botolph without Bishopsgate to the Church of St. Mary of Bethlehem, with the object of establishing a priory where the rule and order of that church would be professed, where divine service could be celebrated for the souls of Fitzmary and of his friends and relations, and where the bishop of Bethlehem and members of the order could be received whenever they should come there. The deed confirming this grant was dated October 23, 1247. The land conveyed in it, in Bishopsgate, is now covered by part of Liverpool Street station. The name "Bethlem," with its innumerable variants of which the most notorious is "Bedlam," is a corruption of "Bethlehem," and came into use early in the priory's history.

The house's development over the next century is obscure, but it did not prosper, and in 1346 the master and brethren were obliged to petition the City for help in the running of their affairs. As a result it was put under the supervision of members of the Court of Aldermen, and its association with this body of governors thus long precedes the arrangements made in the 16th century.

By now it had acquired the designation of "hospital" or "hospice," which indicates that it was already providing a harbor for wayfarers, and perhaps also a refuge for the infirm. By the end of the 14th century the second of these functions had become established; moreover there is documentary evidence that in 1403 six of the patients residing there were men deprived of their reason *(sex viri mente capti)*. From this time on, Bethlem's ministrations to the mentally ill have continued unbroken.

Until the dissolution of the religious houses Bethlem retained its monastic status, but with the dispersion of the religious orders which ran them, the hospitals were no longer able to care for the City's poor. In 1538 a movement was begun which ended in the purchase of the hospitals by the City. Bethlem does not seem to have featured in the negotiations at first, but was included in the charter of 1547, by which its government and that of St. Bartholomew's was vested in the mayor, aldermen, and citizens of London.

In 1556 an order of the Court of Aldermen directed that Bethlem be administered by the governors of Christ's Hospital, but in 1557 the hospital was annexed to Bridewell; one set of governors and one treasurer were appointed for both hospitals, an arrangement which lasted until the introduction of the National Health Service.

Bridewell, a new foundation of Edward VI, was intended as an institution for employment of the idle and for correction of the disorderly. It developed along two separate lines, as a prison and as a place for the training of apprentices, and the latter part of it finally emerged, after much 19th century reform, as a school. This still exists as King Edward's School at Witley in Surrey.

Bethlem's next major upheaval came in 1674 when it was decided that the hospital house, still occupying the original site in Bishopsgate, was "old, weak and ruinous," and also too small and cramped—it never held more than 50 to 60 patients—and should be rebuilt elsewhere.

A site was obtained on lease from the City that backed onto London Wall and looked north over Moorfields (now approximately occupied by Finsbury Circus); and on this the new building, capable of holding 120 patients, was erected between April 1675 and July 1676. Later additions enlarged the accommodation to more than 250. The architect was Robert Hooke, and his design, French in spirit and palatial in concept, was much and justly admired by the Court of Governors, by connoisseurs, and by the general public; but its elegant exterior belied the life inside, and the period of occupation at Moorfields must go down as the most regrettable in the hospital's history. This was the era when tourists thronged the galleries at weekends and bank holidays, and when the name of Bedlam acquired its well-known connotations.

Until the 18th century Bethlem was the only public institution of its kind in the country, and this attracted an attention and gave it a contemporary reputation which, if deserved, has subsequently done much to obscure another fact; that the only alternative form of treatment, in private "madhouses," was frequently far worse and moreover had to be paid for. As it was a charitable hospital, one of the conditions of admission was that neither the patient nor his friends (which included relatives) could afford to pay for private care, and the governors never turned away a deserving person for whom there was room. Whatever might be said of the officers and servants, whose conduct frequently led to abuses, the governors on the whole and according to their lights administered the hospital in accordance with its charitable purpose. Their lights may have been a little dim; but given the prevailing social attitudes and state of medical knowledge, there would certainly have been little hope for many of their patients, wherever they had been; and a high proportion were, in fact, discharged cured.

For a long time only those who were considered curable could be admitted, and a bond had to be entered into for their removal, whether cured or not, whenever the hospital should see fit to discharge them. A patient who had not recovered after 12 months was deemed incurable, and his friends, or the parish overseers, were requested to take him away.

In the 18th century, however, a fund was set up for incurable cases, largely supported by an estate in Lincolnshire bequeathed specifically for this purpose by Edward Barkham, who died in 1733. Two wings were added to the building (then at Moorfields), and patients who had been discharged uncured could be readmitted when a vacancy occurred if it was plain that they could not be cared for outside.

The speed with which the Moorfields hospital was erected turned out to be no cause for congratulation, having been achieved through a total disregard for the most elementary precautions and for most of the accepted techniques of building. Within 100 years it was beginning to fall apart. The site had been an unfortunate choice, being part of the old city ditch, which was in effect a rubbish pit of long accumulation. No foundations had been provided, which further encouraged subsidence; the bricks were bad, the timbers too short, the walls not properly tied, and the roof too heavy. By the beginning of the 19th century no floor remained level, no wall upright, and the front, according to the architect's report, waved out of line and inclined north and south according to the direction in which it had settled. It was "dreary, low, melancholy, and not well aired," and nothing could be done about it.

It was therefore decided to move again and, after much difficulty, a site was found in St. George's Fields, Southwark, formerly occupied by the notorious Dog and Duck Tavern. Because of the terms of the Moorfields lease, it was necessary for the City to exchange this land for the old site, for the remainder of the term of 999 years which had been created in 1674; and as a result of another exchange made this century, the lease is still in operation today.

The new building was begun in 1812 and completed in 1815. The surveyor for the hospital, James Lewis, was responsible for the design, which he adapted from the three prize-winning plans in a national competition; though the dome, later to be its best known feature, was not added until 1844-1846 by the then surveyor, Sydney Smirke. The central part of this building now houses the Imperial War Museum, the wings having been pulled down. The fabric of the Moorfields building was sold off at a series of auctions.

A feature of the new hospital was the provision of separate blocks to accommodate so-called Criminal Lunatic patients. Bethlem had from time to time received patients by order of the government for over a century, but the attempted assassination of George III by James Hadfield in 1800 and changes in the law consequent on this case had brought the need for a separate establishment into prominence. The rebuilding scheme gave an opportunity for such a provision. The government, in addition to its grant toward the rest of the building, paid for the whole construction of the Criminal Department and thereafter contributed annually a portion of the officers' salaries on this account, as well as the maintenance costs of the inmates. While the Secretary of State, later the Home Secretary, retained over-all responsibility for the department, it was run as an integral part of the hospital, and this system continued until Broadmoor was built. The women were transferred to Broadmoor in 1863, the men in 1864.

A number of improvements were made in the new hospital from the outset, but the period of real reform began in 1852 when the first resident medical superintendent, Sir Charles Hood, was appointed. Within a short time the wards were comfortably furnished, entertainments and excursions were organized for the patients, and kindness and understanding rather than coercion on the part of the attendants became a reality throughout the hospital, instead of the unfulfilled ideal which it had so often been in the past. Equally important, Hood initiated a properly organized system of lectures and clinical instruction, which led to the rapid rise of Bethlem's reputation as a teaching center.

At about the same time there was a change in the type of patient admitted. It was felt that the county asylums (established under an Act of 1808) were now able to provide for the pauper classes, who previously formed a large proportion of Bethlem's admission; and a greater need for special provisions was arising in a different quarter. Under Hood's guidance, therefore, the emphasis came to be laid increasingly on the admission of middle-class patients whose loss of livelihood prevented them from paying for private treatment, and for whom the alternative of a county asylum would mean the additional distress of "going on the parish." Evidence of genuine poverty was still required in each case, though the Charity Commissioners later agreed to a relaxation of the rules so that paying patients could also be taken. Treatment remained the same for all, but this did away with the anomalous situation in which possession of means, rather than lack of them, might preclude anyone from getting the best treatment available.

The need for more space was partly met in 1870 by the opening of a convalescent establishment at Witley in Surrey, and this continued in use until the whole hospital moved to Beckenham. An outpatients' department was also opened in 1919, and in 1924 the hospital was admitted as a medical school of the University of London, a status which it retained until 1946.

A restricted site, increasingly urban surroundings, and buildings designed in an age holding very different views about the needs of psychiatric patients, saw the hospital ready to move again in the 1920's. In 1924 the Monks Orchard estate at Beckenham, on the Kent Surrey border, was bought. The new buildings, designed by J. A. Cheston and C. E. Elcock, were begun in 1928 and opened by Queen Mary in 1930. The four wards—Tyson, Fitzmary, Gresham, and Witley—are housed in separate units, each having its own large garden. The old mansion house of Monks Orchard, completed in 1854 by Lewis Loyd of the banking firm of Jones Loyd & Co., was pulled down, but its terraced garden can still be seen in the garden of Witley House.

The hospital's greatest administrative change since the 16th century came with the introduction of the National Health Service in 1948. The link with Bridewell was severed after nearly 400 years' duration and another was immediately formed, with the Maudsley Hospital in Denmark Hill. The two are now administered jointly by a single Board of Governors as one postgraduate Teaching Hospital, known formally as The Bethlem Royal Hospital and The Maudsley Hospital, and informally as The Joint Hospital. Together with their medical school, the Institute of Psychiatry, they comprise the only postgraduate institution in this country devoted wholly to the teaching of psychiatry.

The Maudsley Hospital

The Maudsley Hospital owes its foundation to the intiative and persistence of one man, Henry Maudsley.

The third of four brothers, Henry Maudsley was born at his father's farmhouse, Rome, in the parish of Giggleswick, W. Yorks, on February 5, 1835. His father, Thomas Maudsley, described himself as yeoman, and his mother, Mary Bateson, was the daughter of a farmer at Scale Hall near Lancaster. His mother, had she lived, would have liked to see him become a clergyman, but she died when he was still a child.

His school education was received at Giggleswick School, which he thought did him little good, and afterward as a private pupil for two years with the Rev. Alfred Newth at Oundle, from which he benefitted more. His greatest educational debt, however, he acknowledged to his aunt Elizabeth Bateson who, amongst other things, introduced him to poetry at an early age.

After matriculating at London University in the first division, he declined "to go in for honours." He decided on a medical career, and was accordingly apprenticed to University College Hospital for five years. If Maudsley's own words are to be believed, this did not do him much good either, though he owned the fault to be largely his own. When the man to whom he was nominally apprenticed left for private practice, his experience moved him to say that "he never had but one pupil and would never have another," and his successors "made no pretence of meddling" with their apprentice. Maudsley felt that his own attitude at this period was adequately summed up by a remark attributed to the professor of physiology, that "Maudsley has great abilities but he has chosen to throw them into the gutter."

Despite all this he gained the gold medal and first place in all six of the classes in which he competed, and in his London University examinations gained a scholarship and gold medal in surgery and three more gold medals; these 10 medals he later, with what one feels to be typical practicality, exchanged for a gold watch.

Having chosen surgery for his career Maudsley applied for a House Surgeonship at the Liverpool Southern Hospital, but lost it because a letter was delayed in the post. "Disheartened and disgusted by this contretemps," he turned to psychiatry in order to gain the necessary experience to qualify for service in the East India Company. A temporary post at the Wakefield Asylum was followed by a short and uncongenial spell at the Essex County Asylum until—the lure of India now apparently diminished—he was appointed medical superintendent to the Manchester Royal Lunatic Asylum at the age of 24: "a somewhat rash appointment," he wrote 50 years later.

After three years Maudsley returned to London and thereafter, in his own words, his life was spent "in getting such practice in lunacy as I could, which increased gradually, and in writing the books which I published in succession." Or, since he was too modest to say so, in becoming one of the most eminent psychiatrists of his day.

In 1907, through his intermediary Dr. (later Sir) Frederick Mott, who was then pathologist to the London County Asylums, and director of the Pathological Laboratory, Maudsley offered £30,000 to the London County Council toward establishing a hospital under the following conditions: the hospital was to be for early and acute cases only; it was to have an outpatient department; it was to be equipped for 75 to 100 patients, 50 to 75 pauper patients, and the remainder paying patients; and it was to be in a central position, within three to four miles of Trafalgar Square.

Due provision was to be made for clinical and pathological research (the suggestion was made to move the staff and equipment of Mott's laboratory at Claybury to the new institution if this was considered suitable). This hospital, laboratory, and teaching side of the institute were to be recognized as a school of the University of London, for the study of mental diseases and neuropathology.

The London County Council was to have entire charge, control, maintenance, and upkeep of the institution, except for appointing medical officers and in matters relating to education and research; it was suggested in this connection that three nominees of the London University should be co-opted with the Asylums Sub-Committee of Management of the Institution. Only cases certified as insane or convalescent after cure of insanity, or cases brought by practitioners for advice and treatment were to be received at the institution.

It was about nine months before the Council was able formally to accept the offer, as there was some doubt as to whether their statutory powers would allow compliance with some of Maudsley's conditions: but Maudsley was resolute, the Asylums Committee was in agreement with him about the desirability of the whole project and, finally, it was agreed to go ahead with the building of a hospital at an estimated cost of £50,000 to £60,000. An Act of Parliament was later obtained to cover points which had been in doubt.

The next problem was that of a suitable site, which in 1910 was still "engaging the earnest attention" of the Asylums Committee, and the purchase of the site in Denmark Hill was not completed until 1911. Maudsley believed the delay to be caused by lack of enthusiasm among the "moderates" on the Council, and declared that "the cost of getting the thing done after the Council had accepted the proposal, was a greater burden than the money"; but he was then in his 70's and naturally anxious to see his plans come to fruition, and perhaps he exaggerated a little.

One can see Maudsley's point, however, in noting that the contractors did not move onto the site until August 1913. Even now the way was far from smooth and, after five months, work was brought to a virtual standstill by a building trades strike, which in its turn was ended only by the outbreak of war.

Maudsley lived to see his hospital built and used, though not for its intended purposes. With his complete concurrence the buildings were handed over, as completed and equipped, for use as a military hospital, first under the Fourth London General Hospital and afterwards as a separate unit. The hospital was used for the treatment of nervous disorders arising from war service. The original plan for moving the pathological laboratory from Claybury and installing it under Mott's direction at the hospital was carried out in 1916; part of the laboratory was loaned to the War Office for research. Work done at the hospital during the war was said to have had Maudsley's entire sympathy, and he appreciated the research contribution made by the laboratory.

Henry Maudsley died on January 24, 1918. The Maudsley Hospital was demobilized in 1919, and then loaned to the Ministry of Pensions for similar work. Vacated in October 1920, the hospital still seems to have been beset by an inbuilt delaying mechanism, and protracted negotiation with the government followed, concerning the settlement of accounts for dilapidations and reinstatement. It was finally opened by the Minister of Health on January 31, 1923, 15½ years after Maudsley's offer had first been put forward.

Dr. Edward Mapother was appointed the first medical superintendent, and Dr. F. L. Golla took over the directorship of the pathological laboratory. Recognition as a medical school of the University of London was granted in 1924, and chairs in psychiatry and the pathology of mental disease (later redesignated neuropathology) were instituted in 1936, to be occupied first by Mapother and Golla respectively. The number of chairs has subsequently risen to nine.

Major building extensions took place in 1932, 1936, and 1939; but on the outbreak of World War II the buildings were all evacuated, the hospital dispersed to Mill Hill and Sutton, and the laboratories to West Park Hospital. Lectures were continued at the otherwise empty hospital, and clinical teaching was carried on at Mill Hill and Sutton. On its return to normal after the war the program of postgraduate education was enlarged.

In 1948, just before The Maudsley Hospital's amalgamation with The Bethlem Royal, the British Postgraduate Medical Federation on behalf of the University of London took over the administrative and financial control of the medical school, which was renamed the Institute of Psychiatry. The Institute moved in 1967 to a new building in De Crespigny Park, adjacent to the Maudsley Hospital, but it remains the medical school of the Joint Hospital, and even the physical separation is more apparent on paper than in practice. At the highest level, the theoretically distinct governing bodies share many members in common; and joint appointments, joint committees, and interchange of services strengthen the mutual dependence which is indispensable to both parts of the institution.

PAULUS ZACCHIAS ON MENTAL DEFICIENCY AND ON DEAFNESS*

PAUL F. CRANEFIELD AND WALTER FEDERN

The Rockefeller University
and
The New York Academy of Medicine
New York, N. Y.

PAULUS ZACCHIAS (1584-1659) was a papal physician and the author of the first extensive modern treatise devoted to medicolegal problems. The treatise contains a chapter that deals with mental deficiency which is followed by a chapter dealing with deafness. These chapters are offered in translation because they form a very useful summary of the opinions about mental deficiency held by the classical authorities upon whom Zacchias relied. The translation follows the first edition: Paulus Zacchias, *Quaestiones Medico-legales* [Rome, 1621], Tomus Primus, Liber II, Titulus I, Quaestio VII (De Ignorantibus, Fatuis, Stolidis, Obliviosis & Memoria Orbatis) and Quaestio VIII (De Mutis and Surdis).

The footnotes to the text of the translation require special explanation. The two chapters which we have translated contain very condensed references to Zacchias's sources. These references have been

*This article is based upon research supported by a grant from the National Institute for Child Health and Human Development (HD-01198). The article is based on a first draft written by the authors prior to the death of Dr. Federn in 1967; much of the article was written while Dr. Cranefield was executive secretary of the Committee on Publications and Medical Information of The New York Academy of Medicine. Dr. Cranefield is now associate professor at The Rockefeller University, New York, N. Y.

expanded and appear as footnotes to the translation. Even in their present form they fall short of a high standard of bibliographical detail. Nevertheless they will lead the reader to the source of the material more readily than the original citations. The first footnote may be taken as an example. Zacchias had "Card. comm. 6. Aphor. 51." We have changed the text to read "Cardanus"[1] and have added a footnote which reads "Cardanus (Girolamo Cardano, 1501-1576), *Commentarius in Hippocratis Aphorismos*, Liber 6. Aphorismus 51, *Opera*, 1663, vol. 8, 523, 1st ed, 1564." This expanded citation more fully identifies the author, gives the exact location of the passage, gives the date of the first edition of the work referred to, and also notes where the passage may be found in the 1663 edition of the *Opera* of Cardanus. To give full details would make the annotations excessively long but the present annotations are much more useful than the original citations given by Zacchias. An occasional footnote identified by a number and a letter (e.g., 3*a*) is used to add a citation or comment which does not appear in the original text. In those footnotes which have been designated by numbers only, all material is essentially an expansion of Zacchias's citation, with the occasional addition of the source of a modern translation of a quotation. All of the text has been translated but we have not translated the summaries which precede each chapter since they add little if anything to the text.

The text is straightforward and does not require extensive commentary. There are some aspects of it which are nevertheless of special interest. References to mental retardation are not at all common in the medical literature prior to the time of Zacchias; nor can one say with certainty that the condition was regarded as a clinical entity prior to that time. It thus seems worthy of mention that Zacchias is in fact discussing the phenomenon which we would call mental deficiency or mental retardation. Apart from some passages about those who have suffered from a failure of memory, the text deals with persons of inferior ability to learn. Zacchias is explicit, for example, in saying that those about whom he writes ought not be called crazed. Many of the earlier authors who mention diminution of intelligence lump together congenital mental deficiency with a great variety of acquired conditions including senility, postpsychotic apathy, and deterioration following prolonged and severe epilepsy. The fairly clear-cut limitation of the condition by Zacchias is thus important in itself.

Zacchias offers a rather simple and unsophisticated classification of mental deficiency according to the severity of the defect. The least severe degree he suggests calling obtuseness; he later indicates that the obtuse may be taken as having no more judgment than a child of 14 years. These "slow learners" may be allowed to marry; interestingly he supports this opinion by a ruling of the Rota. He also holds that the obtuse cannot be held wholly free from responsibility if they commit crimes. A more severe grade of mental deficiency is illustrated by "those who are properly called fools by all." These, Zacchias says, seem to exist below the condition of human nature. They cannot be instructed in anything but trifles, but they can speak, even though their speech may be foolish and childish. The most extreme form of the condition is represented by persons Zacchias describes as mindless. Such persons are excused from the penalties of the law if they commit crimes and they are also debarred from civil actions, including, by implication, marriage. Those of the second grade ("properly called fools by all") may perhaps marry, but this must be left to the discretion of a judge.

It would be an exaggeration to say that the classification given by Zacchias corresponds in any precise way to the later classification into moron, imbecile, and idiot, but a rough comparison of those classes with the *obtuse*, the *foolish*, and the *mindless* is not entirely inappropriate. While Zacchias uses his classification largely in the interests of deciding legal questions, he also makes it clear that he was aware of the possibility of alleviating the condition of the obtuse by education.

Zacchias's chapter on the dumb and the deaf offers some curious and interesting ideas. That congenital deafness leads to defective intelligence has been known since the time of Aristotle; even today it affects intelligence unfavorably unless special educational procedures are applied early and skillfully. The congenitally deaf are to be treated as being in the class of the most severely retarded and "regarded in all things like as infants and madmen." They cannot be allowed to make a will even if they wish to make a pious bequest!

By far the most important statements in the two chapters are those concerning the reasons why the congenitally deaf ought not to be allowed to marry. Quite apart from various religious objections, Zacchias says that the congenitally deaf should not be allowed to marry because "there is evidence that they beget children like themselves, and now it profits the commonwealth that sound and in every respect perfect people are born, not so strikingly impaired ones." This statement is peculiarly important. It means that Zacchias was aware of the hereditary factor in congenital deafness and it means that he was willing to adopt a "eugenic" position. In the interest of the commonwealth, he says explicitly that those whose children may be imperfect should not have children. This is not, of course, a particularly early statement of a eugenic point of view. What is interesting and important is that Zacchias, holding this view, did not apply it to the mentally retarded of *any* degree. He did debar from marriage the severely retarded, but he did so on religious grounds (inability to understand the sacraments), not on eugenic grounds. It seems clear that Zacchias, who did recognize a hereditary factor in deafness and who did believe in the application of eugenic concepts, did not believe that heredity plays a major role in the transmission of mental deficiency.

Without granting Zacchias any extraordinary sophistication we may well note that there is no doubt or difference of opinion among modern geneticists about the existence of hereditary factors in deafness while there is a great deal of doubt and controversy about the role, if any, played by heredity in mental retardation.

Question VII
On the Ignorant, Foolish, Stupid, Forgetful, and Bereft of Memory

The impairments of reason with which we have dealt before are not properly numbered among the dementias. Among the dementias proper (or among those persons who do not possess the sound reason required by the human condition) the first place is taken by those persons commonly called fools. There are several kinds of fools, however, according to the greater or lesser slowness and indolence of the mind and intellect. Cardanus[1] set up only two kinds of folly, in one of which the victim does not recognize the things which should be recognized. Such persons may be those whom the jurists call witless (Ripa)[2]; according to Cardanus they are called rude because everything they do or say is done or said without grace or wit. For that reason the ancients called people of this sort by the term blite because it is a herb of dull and insipid taste and has no pungency (as Pierius Valerianus[3] reports). Hence this herb is rightly termed foolish by Martial[3a] in this poem: "That insipid beet, the noon meal of artisans, may acquire flavor."

The other kind of folly according to Cardanus is that kind in which the victims do not reason correctly from things which they have recognized, and he would limit the term folly to this sort. But the kinds of folly and of fools are far more differentiated. In some persons one merely discerns some laziness and indolence of intelligence which renders them unfit to obtain by the use of their intellect things which other people obtain easily (either on their own, or with nature dictating or by a little application). Those things include the first beginnings of education, some mechanical skills, manners, some civic regulations, the civil care of one's own body, the natural cunning common to all, and alacrity in domestic affairs. Such persons we call ignorant and unlearned, not because they are the opposite of persons whose knowledge comes from a skillfully acquired education, but because (as I have said) they are incapable of arriving at a natural and less than mediocre knowledge of things. Persons like these formerly were called Boeotians, which was the origin of the proverb, "a Boeotian intelligence," for a man of gross and dull intelligence; whence Horace:[4] "You would swear he was born a Boeotian in thick air."

Such persons might better be called obtuse, and this kind of folly might better be called obtuseness, as Cardanus[1] calls it. Among the jurists, the Rota[5] calls these undiscerning and witless. This ignorance or obtuseness is the rudiment and beginning of folly, but it is not truly folly and, as Galen[6] asserted, people should not be called fools on account of it. Plato[7] said that ignorance is dementia of the soul, and if we say that he spoke of this ignorance then I should say that Plato meant nothing but what we have said above.

Persons afflicted with obtuseness of this sort are reckoned among those whom we ordinarily term simpletons or people of a coarse grain or gross mind; in addition we call them slow, dolts, buffoons, clowns (and about these see Budaeus[8]), and by comparison blocks, etc. Plautus[9] reviews terms of this sort very nicely:

> Of all the silly, stupid, fatuous, fungus-grown, doddering, drivelling dolts anywhere, past or future, I alone am far and away ahead of the whole lot of 'em in silliness and absurd behavior!

In imitation of which Terrence[10] says:

> Any one of the terms used for a fool is a cap for my head, block-

head, wooden-pate, ass, leaden-wit—not one of them fits him, for his folly is in size too large for any of 'em.

But while we are dealing with terms, it should be called to mind that the word crazed is by no means appropriate to describe a fool, even though it is used by a number of jurists (Decius,[11, 11a] Thesaurus[12]) unless the term is understood in a broad manner or applied to fools of the third kind. Neither should fools be called insane, as Bartolus[13] declares. A number of jurists divide fools into those who have as much judgment as a child of 14 years and those who in judgment hardly equal a 10-year-old child (Thesaurus,[14] and of the physicians, Aetius[15]). It is the former group to which the first class of folly, termed by us ignorance and obtuseness, belongs. Ripa[2] meant the same when he said that among fools there are some who are only rude and obtuse while others are entirely mindless and without sense. But of the jurists, Menochius[16] distinguished more diligently between the kinds of fools. He does not proceed by our method, though, but by one which seemed to him to serve his cause better.

The first kind of folly does have its signs: for ignorant persons of this sort or (to use the word of the jurists) macaroons, are known by the fact that they are of slow intellect in all things, whence they are quite incapable of learning even childish elements of education. They are also devoid of natural courage, wherefore they stand in awe of their elders' frowns and threats even after attaining manhood. This vain awe of their elders causes them to dread to execute things which are not only permitted by their greater age but are for that reason exceedingly becoming to them to do. For instance, Melitides, having taken a wife did not touch her lest she accuse him before his mother, as related in the Adagia.[16a] Anything whatever is palmed off on them quite easily, and they are persuaded of vain and infeasible things by what sometimes deceiving friends have said. Persons kept down by this ignorance also, as I have said, give witless answers to questions. To say it in a word, where an effort of the intellect is needed, they perform everything slowly and without measure, and not at the proper occasion or time. On the other hand, they excel in an exquisite memory of things, as Fracastorius[17] reports. This as a rule happens naturally so that those who are slow of intellect are most retentive of memory, as is known to the philosophers, and noted among the jurists by Tiraquellus.[18] Though on the whole they are of moderate judgment, at times they have in certain things a not mediocre judgment as, among the jurists, Corsettus[19] notes.

It should be noted, however, that this defect as a rule is innate, while the other kinds of folly usually spring from both old age and disease. Though this kind of folly, called ignorance or obtuseness, can occur in old age and in disease, in such instances it always tends toward the worse, that is, toward perfect folly or toward death, as in cold diseases, whenever the sick already are close to death.

Besides, since folly is nothing but a coldness of the brain, having its origin in paucity and lack of heat and spirits (Galen[20] and Aetius[15]), it is clear that the brain's cooling or lack of heat can have many grades, whence a greater or a lesser faculty will arise. In the first grade of folly, therefore, it should be believed that there is in the brain a moderate cooling compared with the others (in whom however the coldness always increases, while the heat itself dwindles). To those, therefore, who attain this grade only, many of the sanctions of the laws and many decrees of the jurists ought not to apply. Indeed, though these do not obtain perfect use of reason, they are not alien from it [reason] to such a degree that they cannot apprehend by long use some things familiar to normal people. Thus in certain cases I do not see why they ought to be restrained from testifying, especially about those things which they have seen since, as I have said elsewhere, they may have an exquisite memory. About things which they have heard, some doubt could be allowed, since a greater soundness of reason is required in signifying the latter than in signifying the former, for the sense of sight is more direct and moves the imagination even more than the sense of hearing does, as has been said earlier.

I think they are rightly allowed to make a will, for of these I deem that Decius[21] correctly understands the teachers, moreover, the Rota[22] makes it plain by what follows that it speaks of this sort of fool. No less does it seem to me in accordance with the law that such persons are by no means prohibited from entering into religion and from making profession, because whatever use of reason there is in them can be adequate to these things, for a dementia that hinders profession has to be such as to take away every use of reason. (The same Rota.[23])

Nor do I believe that marriage should be forbidden to these persons, because even with such obtuseness of intelligence continuing unchanged they can obtain the power of the sacrament and the goal of marriage. This also is the view of the same Rota.[24] Nay, in my opinion, they can more easily be admitted to marry than to enter into religion, for in marriage nature itself cooperates somewhat and teaches ignorant persons also. Now from other things which require soundness and perfection of the intellect (for instance ordination, succession to fiefs, administration of a guardianship or of a public office) they should be debarred by right, it seems.

Furthermore, whether they should be excused for crimes can be difficult to decide. It is a fact that these persons can easily apprehend the nature of crimes at least from habit, even if they cannot do so from intellective cognition, since these children, especially those close to puberty, with whose intelligence we said the intelligence of these persons should be put on a par, easily recognize that crimes are bad by their own nature and therefore should be shunned. Yet it would seem that it should be said that just as children of this sort are excused for most things, so fools of this sort ought to be excused, since we stated that they have no greater judgment than the aforesaid children.

I hold the opinion that for a few crimes fools should not be excused the same way as children are; I am speaking of these fools only, not of the others. The reason is that though we like to compare these fools to children of fourteen years with respect to the use of reason, fools can advance in some things through habit since the power of habit is very great and it is capable of instructing not only these fools but even animals devoid of a rational soul. Well, then, if children close to puberty are able to deceive (lex Pupillum, i.e., Corpus Juris, Digesta, Liber I, Tit. XVII,[25] Num. CXI; Zabarellus)[26] much more should these persons be considered able to deceive. Now where deceit is present, and malice, guilt takes effect. Guilt, however, ought to be accompanied by punishment, by an argument opposite to that which states that where there is no guilt, there is no punishment (Angelus a Gambellionibus, quoted by Zilettus).[27] In the same way, where there is no deceit no crime deserving of punishment is thought to exist either (Menochius).[28]

There follow in the second grade those persons who are properly called fools by all, both by the jurists and by physicians (for extremely few or, rather, none I know of has expressly mentioned the first sort). These persons not only have indolent and slow intellect, but seem to exist below the condition of human nature with respect to the use of reason. They are hardly taught to speak and are known to be incapable of those things which human nature itself is wont to dictate on its own. Neither do they advance in reasoning with age, but they are distinguished from seven-year-old infants by nothing but their speech, in which they seem for a while to be prompter. But by their very speech they make plain that they are fools, whence they have therefore been called fools *(fatui)*, because by talking *(fando)* they show their imperfection (Bartolus).[29] This sort are of an altogether childish intelligence and delight in childish things, as for instance: "To play at odd or even, to ride on a long reed [hobby-horse]."[29a]

Otherwise they are thought to be incapable of anything and can not be instructed in anything save some trifles; for they have very little intellect and are also devoid of memory. That is because the brain's coldness, and its lack of spirits, is both greater and more constant in these persons: for folly is nothing else but either diminution or loss of memory at the same time as of reason, as Paulus[30] holds. Consequently it is of these that the dictum of the jurists should be understood, viz., that a person who has a disordered memory should be presumed to be a fool (Alexander;[31] Grammaticus;[32] Caevalus[33]). For in these persons the natural heat of the brain is so modest that it cannot serve any function of the brain. Hence we say correctly in common speech that a fool has no brain, as Galen[34] attests. Plautus[35] says facetiously: "Oh, no! You cleaned out all the brain from my cranium!"

In worse condition, though, are those persons in the next class, in whom neither any reason nor any memory at all is found. They reveal their folly both by words and by deeds, do not learn anything at all, nor advance in anything by civil habit, and in sum do not tell good from bad, appropriate from inappropriate, vice from virtue. (This does not take place in the same way as it does in the others about whom we spoke above). Therefore they are properly called stupid and mindless, and metaphorically stones, inasmuch as they seem to be devoid of all sense like stones. This term we use whenever we charge somebody with stupidity, as Plautus[36] did facetiously: ". . . for no flint's as foolish as you, that love her," and:[37] "My master is circumcompassed with an elephant's hide, not a human being's and he has no more sense than a stone. *P.* I know that, myself."

This affection was called by the Greeks *anonia*, just as the one mentioned earlier was called by them *morosis*, though in the authors both terms are accepted for the same affection. However, to the same extent as those mentioned earlier, these persons—though both classes are at times affected by greater or lesser folly, since some gradations of both ailments according to severity are allowed—are altogether rightfully debarred from all civil actions and are entirely excused for crimes.

About the former, though, it should be seen whether they can marry, since they preserve some shadow or rudiment of human intellect and are not entirely devoid of memory. Nor do they entirely lack human sense and passions like those whom we reviewed before. And because, as I have said repeatedly, the range of folly of this sort is great, I deem it correct to leave these decisions to the discretion of a judge, along with many other problems that can arise concerning this class of fool.

Now there can be doubt whether such persons ought to be permitted to draw a will. The reason for the doubt is that in him who disposes of his property an entirely sound mind is not required, but rather it is required that he should not be deranged. (Joseph Ludovicus;[38] and the Rota.[39]) This very matter though, like the things mentioned earlier, I remit to the discretion of the judge, for he will easily discern whether a fool is so devoid of sense and human passions that he by no means recognizes those who are closely connected with him, and who are his benefactors, or contrariwise; and so the judge will easily state a just opinion.

After the fools there are persons who are called forgetful, and wanting in memory. Between them, however, it is meet to make an important distinction. Let us say, then, that by "forgetful persons" we understand those who retain the memory of things with difficulty. By "persons wanting in memory," however, we mean those who do not retain any memory at all of things that have passed, either a long time or a short time ago, at least while they suffer from this condition. I prefer to distinguish them even though they seem not to differ except in degree, because to the latter group many things apply that by no means apply to the former. The latter should be regarded in every way as nothing less than fools of the second grade of folly. The reason is that as soon as the affection by which memory is impaired intensifies greatly, reason is also ruined (Galen;[40] Forestus[41]). It is from a dwindling of memory at the same time as of reason that folly arises, as I have already said.[30]

Now this affection as a rule arises from long and severe diseases, as Pliny[42] relates of Messala Corvinus. Pestilential diseases also provoke this illness; Lucretius relates that it occurred in a severe plague:[43] "And there were others who fell into oblivion of all things, so that they could not even tell who they were." Among the jurists, Menochius[44] has noticed this.

Besides, since in the former group memory has not been impaired in a manner that also impairs reason it should be said that many things may be allowed them that cannot be allowed the latter. The former ought not to be prevented from drawing a will; the latter contrariwise. The former should not be prohibited from entering into religion and making profession, the latter very much so. The former should be permitted to marry, to contract, to obligate themselves, to administer their property, and other things of this kind; the latter by no means. In some other things, though, the former perhaps should not be admitted (for about the latter there should be no question). These things I would lay before the jurists, who are to see whether such persons can be ordained licitly, since because of this defect they are not equal to many things to which a person who is to be ordained ought to be equal. The jurist may also determine whether these persons ought to be admitted to the exercise of public offices, since in public office both prudence and an exquisite memory of things are needed. Finally, the jurists may determine whether these are capable of testifying; for how would they be capable of doing so, who remember the things they have seen and heard either not at all or with the greatest difficulty? Wherefore, since it is mostly old people who are subject to this defect, may they notice how cautiously old people are admitted to testify, especially of things that have passed a long time since. Furthermore, since we have been talking of forgetfulness, let us discuss that question of the jurists in which they inquire how much time it takes for forgetfulness to be induced. Although a number of jurists (quoted by Menochius[45]) have tried to define the limit of forgetfulness on this point, it is plain that they have exerted themselves in vain. The reason is that there are a great many things that make people more and less forgetful, namely the temperament of the body and especially of the back of the head, sex, age, the constitution of the parts, the quality and the regulation of one's life, the exercise of memory itself, and other things of this sort. For with respect to sex it is clear, for example, that women are more forgetful than men, as the same Menochius[46] notes. This should be regarded as happening in consequence of the moister temperament of the former, which is fluid and less capable of retention; hence forgetfulness will be more easily induced in a woman than in a man. With regard to age, it is known that old people have very little memory of things; for this is first encroached upon by old age, as shown by experience and as Seneca notices,[47] and before him Aristotle.[48] But for these things he who wants more may read Mascardus.[49] As for temperament, persons who have a dry one have a more retentive memory, persons who have a moist one have a less retentive memory (Aristotle[48] and Averroes[50]); as a result of which it can hardly, if at all come to pass that people are strong in judgment and memory at the same time (Plato,[51] Forestus[52] and, of the jurists, Caevalus[53]). Regarding the conformation of the parts, those who have larger upper parts than lower parts are less strong in memory, as Aristotle[48] testifies. Finally, with respect to the quality of one's life, those who attend to affairs are easily forgetful, as the same Menochius witnesses.[54] Forgetfulness, then, can be induced more easily or with more difficulty, according to the diversity of these and similar things, to which the condition of the deed and of the event is to be added, since extraordinary deeds and great things are not presumed to be readily forgotten (the same Menochius);[55] and forgetfulness is more easily induced in the case of a strange deed (Verallus);[56] consequently the same Menochius prudently determines that this part of the question is remitted to the discretion of the judge, who must however take into consideration both these and many other things.

Question VIII
On the Dumb and the Deaf

We must consider the dumb and deaf separately, for it seems that we cannot correctly include them among the mindless or among the fools, and yet it cannot be truly affirmed that they are of sound judgment. For the present we speak of the dumb and deaf who are such from birth. About the others it is wrong to have doubts: for in my judgment no distinction should be made between them and those persons who both are of a sound mind and hear well and speak (provided you make one little bit of exception, as you will find at the end of this *Question*).

Besides, everybody knows that those who are deaf from birth are at the same time dumb. However, it has never come to my knowledge that one dumb from birth hears, so that conversely he who is dumb from birth at the same time is also deaf. My opinion is seconded by the lex Discretis[57] and the gloss there on the word raro.[58] Now the cause of both facts should be believed to have its origin in a dwindling of the nerves that are common to both senses. So Andreas Laurentius[59] judges after having denied the cause adduced by others, which is that the deaf are also dumb because they cannot learn a language or speak. Though if one concedes another cause of deafness from birth (about which Hieronymus Fabritius[60] writes), it would seem that this cause adduced by others [and denied by Laurentius] could act. That cause, about which Fabritius writes, is some thick extra tunic which has grown in the ear in front of the membrane that is called the tympanum; perhaps such deafness need not hinder speech. Consequently, I have not been greatly astonished at what Vallesius[61] relates about a friend of his, a monk, who taught those deaf from birth to speak. I do not believe that this could succeed with all the deaf, but with those about whom Fabritius writes, I believe it could.

Now while it should by no means be questioned that all the dumb and deaf from birth are deficient in prudence and vigor of mind, yet there are among them those of greater or lesser judgment, prudence, and vigor of mind, as of the jurists, Bartolus[62] maintains. But speaking of them as a whole, the same jurists, for instance Bartolus,[63] Cujacius,[64] Vantius,[65] Farinacius,[66] assert absolutely that one who is dumb and at the same time deaf from birth is put on a par with an infant and a madman, and is treated as absent. The distinction made by a few, however, that those who understand by nods do not lack prudence (Bartolus),[67] should not be understood to mean a prudence sufficient to render them fit for all things, but only for a few things of minor moment. Not without an evident reason, however, such a person is put on a par with a madman, which is double, one sensory, the other physical [physical here seems to be equivalent to our psychological]. The sensory one is the dwindling of the nerves, on account of which they are hindered both in hearing and in speaking. Now this dwindling presupposes a dwindling of the brain, which is the instrument of the intellect, whence without doubt intellection deteriorates, as it happens in madmen and in the mindless.

For that dwindling of the nerves is the true cause of both defects (rather than that the hindered hearing takes away speaking) is demonstrated by the very babes who hear most exquisitely yet do not speak, since they are hindered by the softness of the nerves that serve speech, which owing to their softness are not capable of being moved in order to articulate the voice. On the other hand, if you let a child that hears well hear nobody speak, as long as he can articulate and speak on his own, he will speak in his own manner when he has grown older. It is not necessary, then, that he who hears well also speaks. Nor, on the other hand, is it necessarily true that he who hears nobody speak does not speak because he cannot learn to speak.

The other cause, which is physical, I deem to be the fact that human intellect is perfected from day to day. On its own, the intellect is rude. It can be perfected only by habit and by learning, which is obtained from hearing. As a result, deprivation of hearing makes the intellect ruder; and if the deprivation of hearing is innate, it prevents instruction of the intellect.

It should be noted that this imperfection of the intellect in those who are dumb and deaf from birth is entirely irreparable. It cannot be hoped under any circumstances that they will obtain a sounder mind. According to their age, though, they can be said to have greater or lesser intellect, so that a number of things ought to apply to them when they are younger which perhaps will not apply when they grow in years. Yet they should be regarded in all things as infants and madmen, as I said above; for the perfection of intellect which they require on account of their age is not so great that they can ever be equal to anything.

Since, then, the imperfection of their intellect is irreparable to such a degree: just as infants and children, as long as they are of that age, and madmen, as long as they persist in their madness, are prohibited from all actions, the same opinion should be held about the dumb and the deaf (the lex Discretis, i.e., Corpus Juris, Codex, Liber VI, Tit. XXII, Num. X).[68] In particular they are not permitted to make a will, as is found in the same law and in the lex Qui in potestate, (i.e., Corpus Digesta Liber XXVIII, Tit. I,[69] Num. VI) surdus[70] (Decius;[71] Nepos a Motalbano);[72] which fact the teachers amplify to make it the procedure even in the case of pious bequests (Baldus).[73] They cannot contract a marriage (Abbas,[74] Jason[75]) and much less enter into religion;

(Brunellus[76] and others quoted by him; he himself, however, maintains the opposite).[77] It seems troublesome, though, to advocate his opinion, since such persons (even those who are of a more vivacious nature and endowed with some prudence) except for a rude and gross understanding of things which they have by nature, cannot obtain the power of marriage and the end and the purpose of that sacrament, to wit, the procreation of children for the glory of God. Now nature by itself does not dictate this, unless implicitly, but merely the enjoyment of coitus and of the expulsion of semen. Therefore animals, to which these persons are akin with respect to their understanding, copulate to no other purpose but in order to excrete semen, just as they also urinate and defecate, goaded by the quantity of urine and of feces, as Galen[78] teaches. Since, however, in my opinion a person who contracts a marriage, or whatever else, ought to recognize the true and real purpose of this action or contract, and since these persons do not recognize this purpose, but rather another, feigned one, which is insinuated to them by nature, I do not see how they ought to be permitted to contract a marriage; for one does not contract unless he wants to do so, and with the dwindling of the will the assent ceases. With the purpose not being recognized it cannot be said that one acts by choice and voluntarily; it is by chance, then, that he will contract, since his action lacks an end. Not to mention the fact that the deaf and dumb ought to abstain from marriage not only because they do not understand the end of marriage, but also for the good of the commonwealth, because there is evidence that they beget children like themselves, and it profits the commonwealth that people sound and in every respect perfect are born, not such strikingly impaired ones. Now apart from these things they are restrained from testifying, as is evidenced by Mascardus.[79]

Next, about those whose dumbness and deafness is acquired, one could hesitate whether they should be regarded as fit for all things. First about the merely dumb, who have lost their speech by accident, in my judgment one need have no doubts whatever about their abilities; this opinion is supported by the same lex Discretis,[68] Ubi autem. Their dumbness does not prevent them from doing whatever things other people can do. This has been asserted in the case of the limits of donation by the text in the law Qui id quod, (i.e., Corpus Juris, Digesta, Liber XXXIX, Tit. V,[80] Num. XXXIII), Mutis,[81] and by the gloss there which Maranta[82] adduces. One chance, though, you are to except, namely when the dumbness results from a defect of the brain; for such dumbness is always attended by some folly and diminution of intellect or at least ignorance; these persons, then, should be dealt with more cautiously,

Now about the deaf, doubts are occasioned by what the philosopher has said, from whom Valescus[83] borrows it. This is that hearing is the gate of the mind; thus, complete deafness without diminution of mind and intellect seems hardly to occur. In my judgment, in people of rude intelligence and a base condition, the intellect suffers greatly on account of their complete deafness; of others, inasmuch as they were very much in their right minds before their deafness, though on account of their deafness henceforth it [the intellect] is injured, I would say that it is not injured to such a degree that they need to be forbidden anything on account of this cause; the same lex Discretis[68] favors this view.

REFERENCES

1. Cardanus (Girolamo Cardano, 1501-1576). *Commentarius in Hippocratis Aphorismos,* Liber 6, Aphorismus 51, *Opera,* 1663, vol. 8, 1st ed., 1564.
2. Ripa (Giovanni Francesco de Santo Nazario de la Ripa, 14??-1534). In legem ex facto. *Digesta,* Liber 28, tit. 6. De vulgari & pupillari substitutione, lex 43, Num. 82.
3. Pierius Valerianus (born as Giovan Pietro della Fosse, 1477-1560). *Hieroglyphica,* Liber 58. Fol. 423vo of the ed. of 1567, 1st ed. 1556.

3*a*. Martialis. *Epigrammata,* Liber 13 (Xenia), 13. Ker, Walter R. A., transl. Loeb Classical Library.

4. Horatius, *Epistalarum,* Liber secundus, Epistula 1, line 244.
5. Decisiones Sacrae Rotae Romanae, Melitensis Testamenti, Friday, February 17, 1612, coram Manzanedo. *D. Prosperi Farinacii I.C. Romani Sacrae Romanae Rotae Decisionum ab ipso selectarum, nec unquam alias impressarum Tomi quatuor.* Aurelianae 1621, vol. 1, pp. 440-41. Reverendissimo P.D. Manzanedo. Meliten. Testamenti. Veneris 17 Februarij 1612. (Argumentum. Testamentum a demente conditum non valet, & qualis debeat esse ista dementia, de quo tempore, & quomodo probanda.) P. 441, Num. 5. [This decision is also found, as Decisio XXXIV, in the *Decisiones S. Rotae Romanae, ad praedictas materias spectantes,* a Cl.D. Lanfranco Zacchia collectae, which form an appendix to Horst's folio-editions of the *Quaestiones Medico-legales.* Lanfranco Zacchias (16??-1685) was a grandson of Paolo Zacchias. Unfortunately, his collection is not comprehensive.]
6. Galenus. *Commentarius 2. in Hippocratis Prorrheticum I,* textus 60(?) (In Kuehn's ed. it is 94, in Kuehn's ed. of Hippocrates, it is 92; see Kuehn, XVI, 696.)
7. Plato. *Sophistes,* cap. 15.
8. Budaeus (Guillaume Budé, 1467-1540). *Annotationes in XXIV pandectarum libros* (1508), in *Digesta,* Liber. 21, tit. 1: de Aedilitio Edicto, et redhibitione, et quanti minoris, lex. 4.
9. Plautus. *Bacchides* ("The Two Bacchises"), Act V, scene 1, Nixon, P., transl. Loeb Classical Library.
10. Terentius. *Heautontimorumenos* ("The Self-Tormentor"), Act 5, Scene 1. Sargeaunt, J., transl., Loeb Classical Li-

brary.

11. Decius (Filippo Decio, 1454-1536). *In legum Humanitatis,* Codex. Liber 6, Tit. 26. De Impuberum & aliis substitutionibus, lex 9, Num. 1, Gloss in Institutiones, Liber 2, tit. 12: Quibus est permissum facere testamentum, Praeterea, on the word Furiosi.

11*a*. Cf. Zacchias, II, 1, 9 De melancholicis, Num. 13/14.

12. Thesaurus (Gasparo Antonio Tesauro, 15??-16??). *Decisiones Pedimontanae,* 1610. Decisio 92, Num. 2.

13. Bartolus (Bartolo da Sassoferrato, 1314-1357). *Tractatus de testimoniis,* Num. 98. *Opera,* 1552, vol. 3, p. 178.

14. Thesaurus (as in note 12). Num. 4.

15. Aetius. Sermo 6, cap. 22. *Tetrabiblos,* 1535, vol. 1, p. 249.

16. Menochius (Giacomo Menochio, 1532-1607). *De Arbitrariis Judicum Quaestionibus et Causis, Centuriae sex,* 1569. Liber 2, cas. 529, Num. 2 ff.; pp. 920-21, ed. of 1691.

16*a*. Erasmus of Rotterdam. *Adagia,* 1515. Chil. IIII, Cent. IIII, 69, pp. 976-77, ed. of 1612.

17. Fracastorius (Girolamo Fracastoro, 1483-1553). *Turrius sive de intellectione dialogus,* Liber 1. Opera omnia 1573 & 1584, fol. 127ro; *Opera,* 1555, fol. 173ro.

18. Tiraquellus (Andre Tiraqueau, 1488-1558). *De Legibus Connublialibus,* 1513; after 1524 the title continues: *et jure maritali,* Gloss. 5, Num. 24.

19. Corsettus (Antonio Corsettus, 14??-1503). *Singularia,* Num. 2, on the word Testamentum, 1477.

20. Galenus, Liber 4, de praesagitione ex pulsibus, cap. 8; IX, 407 Kuehn.

20*a*. Galenus, Liber 2. De symptomatum causis, cap. 7; VII, 200-01, Kuehn.

21. Decius (cf. note 11). *In legem Furiosum.* Codex, Liber 6, tit. 22. De his qui testamenta facere possunt, vel. non, lex 9, Num. 8 & 11.

22. *Sacrae Rotae Romanae decisiones novissimae,* decisio 384, Num. 5, pars 1, tom. 1. Decisio XI in Lanfranco Zacchia's collection, which is not necessarily identical with the Decisio 384 here mentioned, in any case says the same thing: Romana Haereditatis, Veneris 15. Novembris 1592. Coram R. P. D. Penia. Num. 5.

22*a*. The above is found also in *Melitensis Testamenti* (see note 5).

23. *Rota,* as in note 22, dec. 134, Num. 1, pars 2.

24. *Rota,* as above, decis. 107, Num. 29, pars 2.

25. *Lex Pupillum, Digesta,* Liber 50, tit. 17. De (diversis) regulis juris antiqui, lex 111.

26. Zabarellus (probably Francesco Zabarella, 1360-1417). *De homicidiis casualibus & voluntariis,* cap. si furiosis, Num. 3.

27. Angelus a Gambellionibus (Angelo Gambiglioni, 15th cent.). Quoted by Zilettus, (Giovanni Battista Ziletti, 16th cent.). *Consilia,* cons. 95, Num. 1.

28. Menochius (cf. note 16). *Consiliorum sive Responsorum,* liber primus, consilium 28, Num. 13, vol. 1, p. 146, ed. of 1628; 1st ed., 1572.

29. Bartolus (cf. note 13). *Tractatus de Testimoniis,* Num. 98.

29*a*. Horatius. *Sermonum,* Liber secundus, sermo 3, line 248.

30. Paulus Aegineta. *Medicina,* Liber 3, cap. 11, p. 146, ed. of 1551.

31. Alexander (Alessandro Tartagna, 1424-1477). *In legem Cum servus,* para. constat, Digesta, Liber 30. Liber 1: De legatis et fidei commissis, lex 39, para. 7. See also *In legem si cum dotem,* para. si maritus. *Digesta,* Liber 24, tit. 3: soluto matrimonio, lex 3, para. 7.

32. Grammaticus (Tommaso Grammatico, 1473-1556). *Decisiones,* 1547, Decisio 2, Num. 1.

33. Caevalus (Geronimo de Cevallos, 16th? cent.). *Quaestiones Communes contra Communes* (Speculum aureum opinionum communium contra communes?), in the preface, Num. 98 (1602).

34. Galenus. Liber 3, de locis affectis, cap. 4.

34*a*. Galenus, Liber 3, de Placitis Hippocratis & Platonis, cap. 4 (V, 310-11, Kuehn).

35. Plautus. *Mostellaria* ("The Haunted House"). Act V, scene 1, line 1110. Nixon, P., transl. Loeb Classical Library.

36. Plautus, *Poenulus* ("The Little Carthaginian"), Act I, scene 2, lines 291-2. Nixon, P., transl. Loeb Classical Library.
37. Plautus. *Miles Gloriosus* ("The Braggart Warrior"), Act II, scene 2, lines 235-36.
38. Joseph Ludovicus (Giuseppe Ludovisi, 15??-16??). *Decisio Perusina prima,* Num. 14, pars I. In: *Decisioncm seu Diffinitionum causarum perusinarum et provinciae Umbriae pars prima,* 1572.
39. *Decisiones Sacrae Rotae Romanae coram J. Cavalerio,* 1629. Romana Donatio de Gualteruciis, 1622, Monday, December 12, coram Cavalerio [Decisio 50 in Lanfranco Zacchias's collection, Num. 5].
40. Galenus, *De locis affectis,* Liber 3, cap. 4 (VIII, 460, Kuehn).
41. Forestus (Pieter van Foreest, 1521-1597). *Observationum et curiationum medicinalium libri tres,* 1590, Liber 10, observ. 1, p. 13.
42. Plinius. *Naturalis historia,* Liber 7, cap. 24. Loeb edition, vol. 2, p. 564. Actually, Zacchias is not quoting Pliny, but rather Caius Iulius Solinus, *Polyhistor,* cap. 1, para. 104, ed. of 1777, p. 34. The reason for his mistake was that he took the quotation at second hand from Menochius; see note 44.
43. Lucretius. *De rerum natura,* Liber 6, lines 1213-14. Rouse, W. H. D., transl., Loeb Classical Library.
44. Menochius (as in note 16), Liber 2, cas. 26, Num. 5, p. 170 of ed. of 1691.
45. Menochius, as above. This refers to note 44, but not merely to Num. 5 but to the entire Casus 26, the title of which is: Tempus quod sit, quo causatur oblivio, & quid in ea re a judice observandum sit.
46. Menochius. Ibid., Num. 3.
47. Seneca ("Rhetor"). In the preface to his book of Declamations, i.e., *Controversiae,* Liber 1, p. 51 in vol. of the Elzevir ed., 1639, of the work of his son, the philosopher Seneca.
48. Aristoteles. *Liber de Memoria & Reminiscentis,* cap. 2.
49. Mascardus (Guiseppe Mascardi, 15??-1588). *De Probationibus.* Conclusiones probationum omnium, quae in utroque Foro quotidie versantur, 4th ed. 1619; 1st ed., 1584-1588, Conclusio 1122, vol. 3.
50. Averroes. *Ibidem,* i.e., as in note 48: *De Memoria et Reminiscentia,* last chapter (Compendia librorum Aristotelis qui Parva Naturalia vocantur).
51. Plato. *Theaetetus,* cap. 34.
52. Forestus. As in note 41, Liber 10, Observ. 1 in the Scholion, p. 15.
53. Caevalus. Cf. note 33, preface to *Practicae Quaestiones Communes* (probably the same work as that quoted in note 33), Num. 94.
54. Menochius. As in note 16; as above (notes 44, 45, 46), same case (26), Num. 4.
55. Menochius. Ibid., Num. 6.
56. Verallus (Paolo Emilio Verallo, 16th cent.). *Decisiones Aureae Causarum sacri Palatii apostolici,* 1589, decisio 279, Num. 7, pars 3.
57. *Lex Discretis.* Codex, Liber 6, tit. 22: qui testamenta facere possunt, vel non (the text says wrongly: de testamentis, that is: tit. 23) lex 10. para. 1 Sin autem.
58. As in note 57, gloss there on the word "raro."
59. Andreas Laurentius (Andre Du Laurens, 1558-1609). *Historia Anatomica Humani Corporis,* Liber 11, cap. 13: De aure interna, quae verum auditus est organum Controversiae, quaestio 11, De mira aurium & palati, linguae ac laryngis sympathia (1600, p. 430). (In the 1st ed., 1593, *Opera anatomica . . . .* it is Liber 4, cap. 18, q. 26, pp. 745-46.)
60. Hieronymus Fabricius (Girolamo Fabrici d'Acquapendente, 1533-1619). *De aure, Auditus Organo,* pars 1: De dissectione et historia auris, cap. 4: De Membrana Tympano appellata (1600, pp. 4-5, p. 142 in ed. of 1614).
61. Vallesius (Francisco Valles Covarrubias, 1524-1592). *Liber de sacra philosophia sive de iis quae scripta sunt physice in libris sanctis,* 1558, cap. 3.
62. Bartolus. Cf. note 13. *Tractatus de Testimoniis,* Num. 93, *Opera,* 1552, vol. 2, p. 177.
63. Bartolus. *Ibid.,* Num. 97.

64. Cujacius (Jacques de Cujas, 1522-1590). *Notationes ad Justiniani libros IV Institutionum,* Liber 2, tit. 10: de Testamentis ordinandis, vol. 1 of his *Opera* of 1577. Or p. 96 in vol. 1 of his *Opera omnia* of 1658: Notae in Librum 2. Institutionum Justiniani. De testamentis ordinandis, cap. 10, para. 6.
65. Vantius (Sebastiano Vanti, 16. Cent.) *Tractatus de nullitatibus processuum ac sententiarum . . .* 1554. Tit. de nullitatibus ex defectu inhabilitatis Num. 25.
66. Farinacius (Prospero Farinacci, 1544-1618). *Praxis et Theorica Criminalis,* 1597-1610, pars 2, vol. 1, q. 98.
67. See note 63.
68. *Lex Discretis.* Cf. note 57.
69. *Lex Qui in Potestate,* Digesta, Liber. 28, tit. 1: (de Testamentis &) qui testamenta facere possunt, et quemadmodum testamenta fiant, lex 6.
70. As in note 69, para. I, surdus.
71. Decius. Cf. note 11. *In legem Discretis* (quoted in notes 69 and 57), Num. 1.
72. Nepos a Montalbano (Nepos de Montauban, 13th cent.). *Tractatus exceptionum qui dicitur, liber fugitivus,* 1512, artic. 20, Num. 10.
73. Baldus (Baldo degli Ubaldi, 1319 or 1327-1400). *In lege prima,* in 2 col. Codex, Liber 1, tit. 2: de Sacrosantis Ecclesiis et de rebus et privilegii earum, in repetitionibus (i.e., in his Repetiones).
74. Abbas (Panormitanus or Niccolo de Tedeschi, 1389-1466). In cap. cum apud. Num. 6, de sponsalibus(?).
75. Jason (Jason Mainus, 1435-1519). *In legem Mutum,* Digesta, Liber 29, tit. 2. De adquirenda vel omittenda haereditate, lex 5, Num. 4.
76. Brunellus (Jean Bruneau or Brunel, 14??-15??). *Tractatus de matrimoniis & sponsalibus,* 1521, conclus. 14, Num. 6.
77. Ibid. Num. 8.
78. Galenus. Liber 6, de locis affectis, cap. 5; VIII, 419-20, Kuehn.
79. Mascardus. As in note 49, conclusio 1358, Num. 24, vol. 3.
80. *Lex qui id quod. Digesta,* Liber 39, tit. 5. De donationius, lex 33.
81. As in note 80, para 2, mutus.
82. Maranta (Roberto Maranta, 14??-1530). *Singularia et iuris notabilia* (1616), on the word Mutus.
83. Valescus (Valesco de Taranta, 13??-14??). *Philonium* (begun 1418), lib. 2, cap. 50. De nocumentis aurium: et primo de surditate. Clarificatio. Fol. 69ro, ed. of "1401" (1501); fol. 44ro ed. of 1521; fol. 87ro ed. of 1535; 1st print-ed., 1478.

AMBROISE PARE, THE COUNTESS MARGARET, MULTIPLE BIRTHS, AND HYDATIDIFORM MOLE

L. J. RATHER, M.D.

Department of Pathology
Stanford University Medical Center
Stanford, Calif.

IN the 2d (Paris, 1579) edition of Paré's *Oeuvres* may be found the story of Countess Margaret of Cracow, who is reported to have given birth to 36 live infants on January 20, 1269. Paré cites the Polish historian Martin Cromerus as his source:

> Martinus Cromerus au liure 9 de l'histoire de Poulongne escrit qu'en la prouince de Cracouie, Marguerite, dame fort vertueuse & de grande & ancienne maison, femme d'vn Conte dit Virboslaüs accoucha le xx iour de Ianuier 1269. d'vne ventree de trente six enfans vifs.[1]

The story, with identical dates and numbers, appears also in the 4th (Paris, 1585), 10th (Lyons, 1641), 11th (Lyons, 1652), and 12th (Lyons, 1664) French editions of Paré's *Oeuvres*, and in the definitive 19th century edition by J. F. Malgaigne (Paris, 1840-1841).[2] The 3d Dutch edition (Amsterdam, 1615), reprinted from the 2d Dutch edition (Leiden, 1604), reprinted in turn from the 1st Dutch edition (Dordrecht, 1592), which is a translation made from the 4th French edition (Paris, 1585), also gives the date as January 20, 1269 and the number of children as 36.[3] In contrast, the 1st Latin edition (Paris, 1582), which is a translation of the 2d French edition (Paris, 1579), together with the succeeding Latin editions (Frankfurt/M, 1594, 1612), give the date as January 20, *1296* and the number of children as 36. But the first English translation of Paré (London, 1634) and the two subsequently reprinted editions (London, 1649, 1678) give the date as January 20, 1296, and the number of children as *35*.[4] The English editions derive from the Latin edition of 1582 and represent, according to Janet Doe, "a translation not only of a translation but of a poor translation."[5] Thus the following combinations of dates and numbers in respect to Countess Margaret of Cracow: Jan. 20, 1269, and 36 children (French and Dutch editions), January 20, 1296, and 36 children (Latin editions) Jan. 20, 1296, and 35 children (English editions).

But the Countess of Cracow appears not to be the only Countess Margaret reported by Paré to have delivered an extraordinary number of infants at one time. Edward R. Schumann, in the course of a discussion of hydatidiform mole, writes that—

> Ambroise Paré details the case of Countess Margaret of Flanders, who brought forth at one birth 365 infants, of whom 182 were solemnly baptized John, 182 Elizabeth, and the odd one after much ecclesiastical debate was adjudged an hermaphrodite and accordingly buried without baptism.[6]

Schumann gave no bibliographical reference to Paré. He did mention a passage from the diary of Samuel Pepys that noted a visit to Lausdune (Holland) "where the children were born." Pepys, however, says nothing of the ecclesiastical debate on the odd hermaphrodite.[7]

The story of Countess Margaret of Flanders and her 365 children is *not* in the 2d and 4th French editions of Paré, or the Dutch, Latin, and English editions, or in Malgaigne's definitive 19th century edition. The 10th French edition (Lyons, 1641), published 51 years after Paré's death, mentions her by title only and says nothing of the ecclesiastical debate over the odd hermaphrodite or the burial without baptism:

> Mais de toutes ces portées ou enfantemens, il n'y en a point qui approche de la merueille de la Contesse de Flanders, laquelle par vne iuste permission & vengeance de Dieu, conceu & accoucha d'vne seule portée, ainsi que plusieurs Historiens nous ont laissé par ecrit, de trois cent soixante et cinq enfans autant qu' il y a de iours en l'an.[8]

The 11th and 12th editions (Lyons, 1641, 1664) follow suit, with minor changes.[9]

Schumann's source obviously was not Paré, including the Lyons editions. Nor could it have been Gould and Pyle, although their account has some of the missing features. Gould and Pyle offer both Countesses Margaret on the same page:

> Martin Cromerus, a Polish historian quoted by Paré, who has done some good statistical research on this subject, says that Margaret, of a noble and ancient family near Cracovia, the wife

> of Count Virboslaus, brought forth 36 living children on January 20, 1296. The celebrated case of Countess Margaret daughter of Florent IV, Earl of Holland, and spouse of Count Hermann of Henneberg, was supposed to have occured just before this, on Good Friday, 1278. She was at this time forty-two years of age, and at one birth brought forward 365 infants, 182 males, 182 females, and 1 hermaphrodite. They were all baptized in two large brazen dishes by the Bishop of Treras, the males being called John, the females Elizabeth. During the last century the basins were still on exhibit in the village church of Losdun . . . the affliction was ascribed to the curse of a poor woman who, holding twins in her arms, approached the Countess for aid. She was not only denied alms, but was insulted by being told that her twins were by different fathers, whereupon the poor woman prayed God to send the Countess as many children as there were days in the year.[10]

Gould and Pyle cite a 5th French edition of 1595 as their source for the story of Countess Margaret of Cracow in Paré.[11] The 5th edition actually appeared in 1598.[12] They give the combination (January 20, 1296, and 36 children) found only in the Latin editions of Paré. As to the source of the story of Countess Margaret of Flanders, Gould and Pyle are silent.

Dr. Charles McLennan of Stanford directed my attention to J. Whitridge William's textbook as a possible source for Schumann's version of the story of Countess Margaret of Flanders. Williams added to the confusion by introducing a third countess, this one from the Rhine region. With respect to reports of multiple births he wrote that—

> . . . many such are to be found in the older literature the most remarkable being the Rhine legend, according to which the Countess Hagenau was delivered of 365 embryos at a single labor—manifestly an hydatidiform mole.[13]

Williams gives no source for the "Rhine legend." A later edition of his textbook, edited by N. J. Eastman, makes no reference to the Rhine legend and equates the two countesses:

> Miraculous litter size has been imputed to man, the most extravagant recorded being the haughty Countess of Hagenau. Mauriceau discusses the events in his textbook of 1668. "But I esteem it either a miracle or a fable what is related of the Lady

> Margaret, Countess of Holland, who in the year 1313 was brought to bed of 365 children at one and the same time."[14]

It will be seen that Gould and Pyle date Countess Margaret of Holland's delivery of 365 infants on Good Friday, 1278. Eastman, ostensibly citing from the first edition of Mauriceau's textbook (1668), gives the date as 1313. Although Mauriceau did in fact date the event in 1313 he gave the number of children as *363*:

> But I consider a miracle or a fable the history or tale of that Lady Maragret, Countess of Holland, who gave birth to three hundred and sixty three children at one and the same time in the year 1313. This happened to her (so they say) due to the curse of a poor woman who asked her for alms, pointing out the poverty for which her children, whom she had with her, were the cause, to which the Lady replied that if she was now suffering the inconvenience, she had had the pleasure of making them.[15]

In the second edition (1675) of his book Mauriceau gave the number of children as *365* and the date as *1276*. A partial explanation of Countess Margaret's harshness was added:

> . . . that Lady Margaret, Countess of Holland, who gave birth to three hundred and sixty five children at one and the same time in the year 1276, all of whom were baptized and died on the same day as their mother; this happened (so they say) due to the curse of a poor woman who wished that she would have as many of them as there were days in the year, because while asking her for alms and pointing to her own poverty and that of her two children, twins, whom she bore in her arms, the Lady replied to her that if she was now suffering the inconvenience she had had the pleasure of making them, reproaching her also that she could not have conceived these two children from one man.[16]

Eastman's citation corresponds with neither of these two editions of Mauriceau. Gould and Pyle's date for the event (1278) does not correspond with either of the two dates in Mauriceau. As already mentioned, Gould and Pyle gave no source for their account. Neither did Mauriceau in the first edition, but in the second he ascribed it to Schenck von Grafenberg (a contemporary of Paré). In Schenck's late

16th century collection of medical observations both of the dates used by Mauriceau are to be found, together with some additional dates and Countesses Margaret, as well as a Countess Matilda. Schenck also cites Cromerus on the Countess of Cracow, giving the number of children as 36 but the date as January 20, *1270*:

> In the region of Cracow a certain honorable matron, Margaret, wife of Count Virboslaus, brought forth in one birth on the twentieth day of January 1270 thirty six living children. *Cromerus lib. 9.*
>
> Margaret of Florent, daughter of the Count of Holland [*Margarita Florentij Comitis Hollandiae filia*] sharply rebuked a woman who carried twins in her arms and was begging for aid, averring that she could not have borne the two at one birth unless she also had had relations with two men. The beggar woman prayed fervently to God that as a sign of her chastity the pregnant Countess would give birth to as many children as there were days in the year. The prayers were answered, and in the precise time of gestation in the year 1276 on the day before the Sabbath [Friday] Margaret, in her 42nd year, gave birth to 364 infants, partly males, partly females. They were baptized together in a basin, the male being named John and the females Elizabeth, and together with their mother died shortly afterwards, with an historical epitaph. Lodovico Vives, Erasmus of Rotterdam, and Lodovico Guicciardini in the *Topographia Flandriae*, commemorate them. In the year 1313, during the rule of Henry VII, Margaret, Countess of Holstein [*Margarita Comitissa Holsteinij*] brought forth at one birth as many infants as there are days in the year, three hundred and sixty four, all of ripe age and of human form: all too were baptized alive. *Annales Brunsvicensium Albertus Cranzius in Vandalia, Ernestus Brotussus lib. 4. Cap. 4 Historiae Principium Anhaltinensium. Fulg. lib. 1. cap. 6.* In the year 1322 (as Masseus notes) when the leprous infected the fountains throughout Italy [?], Margaret Countess of Holland [*Margarita Comes Hollandiae*] declared adulterous those women who had borne twins, and through the curse of a certain beggar woman whom she had sharply assailed brought forth 365 at one birth, all living and the size of a thumb, which candidates for the sacred font death snatched away, one by one *Gemma*

> *lib. 1. cap. 6. Cosmocrit.* In the same place may be found what happened in the year 1310 after the Virgin Birth, when Henry of Luxemburg ruled in Germany. At this time Margaret, Countess of Holland [?] [*Margarita Olandae Comes*] brought forth three hundred and sixty living children at one birth, all baptized illuminated in character. *Author Baptista Fulgosus. Mizaldus centur. 8. Memorabil.* Margaret, Countess of Holstein [*Margarita Holstenia Comitissa*] equalled with offspring at one birth the number of days in the year. *Zwingerus Comm. Tabula ad lib. Hipp. de nat. pueri.* The *Historia Chronica* and a tomb in Holland with an epitaph testify of the birth of three hundred and sixty live children by Margaret, daughter of the illustrious Florent, Count of Holland [*Margaretae, illustris Florentij Comitis Hollandiae filiae*]. *Ioan Boscius thesi 109. Concordiae Medicorum et Phisicorum de humano concepto, &c.*
>
> Matilda, Countesss of Henneberg, daughter of Florent IV, Count of Passau [?] [*Machtildis Comitissa ab Henneberg, filia Florentij* IV *Bathavini Comitis*], sister of William King of Rome under the Emperor Frederic II, brought forth at the same time fifteen hundred and fourteen children, who were purified with holy water in a wash basin by her uncle, Otho, Bishop of Utrecht [*Trajectensi*] and died shortly thereafter. *Aventinus lib. 7. Analium*[17]

It is unlikely that these different versions can be reconciled. There is little doubt but that the odd hermaphrodite who rounded off the number to 365 was a later embellishment. The ecclesiastical debate and the burial of the hermaphrodite unbaptized were probably added still later. We may be certain, too, that Ambroise Paré reported only the story of Countess Margaret of Cracow and her delivery of 36 live infants, as recorded by Cromerus. The editions of Paré's *Oeuvres* published at Lyons, beginning with the 10th in 1641, did indeed mention a Countess of Flanders. But the Lyons editions were characterized by Malgaigne in the 19th century as "shameful counterfeits," and Janet Doe finds that they contain "indefensible alterations" and are "abominable" and "detestable."[18]

A closing comment on hydatidiform mole itself is perhaps in order. There is no adequate description of this lesion in Paré's *Oeuvres*. True, he describes a *mole* of the uterus, but as a mass so tough that it could hardly be cut with a knife.[19] Paré's contemporary, Francois Valleriola, however, described the lesion very nicely, likening it to a cluster of membranous watery vesicles or a mass of fish eggs: *membranaceum globum totum aquosis bullis, instar ovorum piscium . . . bullae rotundae, tumidae, pellucidae.*[20]

NOTES AND REFERENCES

1. *Les Oevvres d'Ambroise Paré* . . . 2d ed., Paris, 1579, *liv. 24, ch. 5.* In the 4th ed. Paris 1585, the passage appears in *liv. 25, ch. 5.* There was no 3d French ed., according to Janet Doe (*A Bibliography of the Works of Ambroise Paré: Premier Chirurgien and Conseiller du Roy,* Chicago 1937, p. 121). The 5th French edition of Paris 1598 was the last to be revised by Paré, but the text was altered by Paré's editors after his death in 1590 (Doe, *op. cit.,* p. 128).
2. *Les Oevvres D'Ambroise Paré* . . . 10th ed., Lyons, 1641, *liv. 25, ch. 5.* In the 11th (Lyons 1652) and 12th (Lyons 1664) the same passage appears. In J. F. Malgaigne's *Oeuvres Completes D'Ambroise Paré Revues Et Collationées Sur Toutes Les Editions, Avec Les Variantes* . . . 3 vols., Paris 1840-41, the passage may be found in *liv. 19, ch. 5.* Malgaigne based his edition mainly on that of 1598 (Cf. Doe, *op. cit.,* p. 151).
3. *De Chirurgie, ende alle de Opera, ofte* Wercken *van Mr. Ambrosius Pare* . . . Amsterdam 1615, *Boeck 25, cap. 5.* The title and opening pages are missing from the copy at Stanford. It was identified by Janet Doe (personal communication to Lane Library, May 15, 1934).
4. The Works of that famous Chirurgion Ambrose Parey translated out of Latine and compared with the French by Th. Johnson . . . London 1634, *lib. 25, ch. 3* (the first English translation, according to Doe, *op. cit.,* p. 167). The same passage, with identical dates and figures, occurs in the London eds. of 1649 and 1678, in the latter in Bk. 25, ch. III. The ed. of 1634 has recently been published in facsimile by Milford House, Inc., New York (1968). The Latin translation of Paré's *Oeuvres* was first published in 1582, in Paris. Doe writes that the translator "took great liberties with the French text: using the second editon of 1579, he altered, inserted, subtracted even whole chapters, where it suited him" (*op. cit.,* p. 158). In the three editions (Paris, 1582, Frankf./M., 1594 and 1612) of the Latin translation that I have examined the passage in question appears in *lib. 24, cap. 3* (instead of *liv. 24, ch. 5* as in the Paris edition of 1579) with the number of children given as 36 and the date as of Jan. 20, 1296. The English translator (see above) shifted the passage to *lib. 25, ch. 3.*
5. Doe, J., *op. cit.,* p. 170.
6. Schumann, E. R.: In: *Obstetrics and Gynecology,* Hale, A., ed. Curtis, Philadelphia and London 1933, vol. 2, p. 954. Schumann's version of the story was repeated with minor changes ("clerical debate" instead of "ecclesiastical debate," and "buried in unconsecrated ground" instead of "burial unbaptized") by Clayton T. Beecham in *Obstetrics and Gynecology,* by J. Robert Willson, Clayton T. Beecham, and Elsie Reid Carrington, 2d. ed., St. Louis, 1963 (personal communication from Dr. Beecham, Sept. 1, 1970).
7. Schumann cites vol. 1, p. 38 of the Wheatley edition of Pepys diary, but the correct page is 138 (*Diary of Samuel Pepys. ed.* with additions by Henry B. Wheatley, F.S.A., N.Y., 1892, reprinted 1900, vol. 1, pt. 1, p. 138).
8. Paré, 10th ed., *op. cit., liv. 25, ch. 5.*
9. Paré, 11th ed., *op. cit.* and 12th ed., *op. cit.* contain the same passage with minor

typographical alterations. For the readings in the 11th and 12th eds. I am indebted to Professor Otto Guttentag of the University of California.

10. Gould, G. M. and Pyle, W. L.: *Anomalies and Curiosities of Medicine.* Philadelphia, 1897, p. 147.
11. Ibid., p. 925.
12. Doe, *op. cit.,* p. 123.
13. Williams, J. W.: *Obstetrics.* N.Y. and London, 1904, p. 326.
14. Eastman, N. J.: *Williams Obstetrics,* 10th ed. N.Y., 1950, p. 609.
15. Mauriceau, F. *Traité des maladies des femmes grosses.* Paris, 1668, p. 94.
16. Ibid., 2d ed. Paris, 1675, p. 101. The 7th ed., Paris, 1740, has the same date and number.
17. *Observationum medicarvm rarvm . . . Ion. Schenckii A Grafenberg. Freiburg/* Br., 1584-1597, bk. 4, *de partu,* pp. 361-63.
18. Doe, *op. cit.* pp. 137, 142.
19. Paré, *op. cit.,* 2d ed., *liv. 23. ch, XLI,*
20. *Francisci Valleriolae Doctoris Medici Obseruationum Medicinalium,* 2d ed. Lyons 1588, *lib.* I, *obs.* x. Cited from the edition of 1573 by R. Kossmann, Zur Geschichte der Traubenmole, *Arch. f. Gyn. 62:*153-69, 1900.

THE SEARCHERS*

THOMAS R. FORBES, Ph.D.

Department of Anatomy
Yale University School of Medicine
New Haven, Conn.

On May 6, 1578, the Lord Mayor of the City of London issued "A precept for avoydinge the infection of the plague." One of the steps to be taken was to

> appoynte two honest and discrete matrons within everye pish [parish] . . . wch shalbe sworne trulye to search and make viewe of the bodye of anye such psons [persons] as shall happen to dye within the same pish, to the entent they maye make true reporte to the clarke of the parish of all such as shall dye of the plague, That the same maye make lyke report and certificate to the wardens of the pish clerke.[1]

The term *searcher* was not new. The *Oxford English Dictionary* cites use of the word before 1500 to designate customs officers, sanitary inspectors, market inspectors, and so on. Searcher, in the sense of one who searches bodies for signs of plague or other causes of death, does not seem to appear in London records before 1578, but searchers are said to have been referred to in Shrewsbury in 1539.[2]

The Lord Mayor of London issued in 1581 an order almost identical to that quoted above.[3] The vestry minutes of the Church of St. Martin-in-the-Fields, London, for September 1593, a plague year, mention the appointment of male searchers for men's bodies and female searchers for the bodies of women.[4] This seems to be the only record of male searchers.[5] The parish records of St. Botolph without Aldgate for March 26, 1594, tell of the activities of searchers,[6] and Shakespeare refers to "the searchers of the town" in *Romeo and Juliet*, written in 1596 or 1597,[7] so the term was by then well established.

Sometimes the women employed by the parish to inspect a body were said to "view" it. For example, orders issued during a minor outbreak of plague in London about 1570 specified that "Two Vewers of

*This research was supported in part by Public Health Service Research Grant 5 RO1 LM 01538-02 from the National Library of Medicine, Bethesda, Md.

dead Bodies, two vewers of Sick suspected, shall be appointed and sworne."[8] The churchwardens' accounts for St. Benet Gracechurch in 1578 speak of payment to "two women to vew the corpse of the same wyfe."[9] In 1592 it was directed in the City of London that "in or for every parishe there shalbe appointed two sober Ancient Woemen to be sworne to be viewers of the boddies of such as shall dye in tyme of Infeccon, and twoe other to be viewers of such as shalbe sicke and suspected of Infeccon."[10]

There was repeated mention of searchers in the seventeenth century.[11] In 1603 the appointment and swearing in of searchers was authorized by Royal Statute.[12] A letter written in December 1630 by the Lord Mayor and Court of Aldermen of the City of London to the Privy Council, reporting various activities in connection with efforts to control the plague, said the searchers "appointed for the vissitted houses are ancient woemen; And reputed to bee both honest and skilful, who are sworne for the faithful discharging of their duties in their seaverall places, which uppon certificate it appeareth, they have carefully performed."[13]

An order in 1665, the year of the Great Plague, from the mayor and aldermen tells us a good deal more about the searchers.

> That there be special care, to appoint Women-Searchers in every Parish, such as are of honest reputation, and of the best sort as can be got in this kind: And these to be sworn to make due search and true report, to the utmost of their knowledge, whether the Persons, whose bodies they are appointed to Search, do die of the Infection, or of what other Diseases, as near as they can. And that the Physicians who shall be appointed for cure and prevention of the Infection, do call before them the said Searchers who are or shall be appointed for the several Parishes under their respective Cares, to the end they may consider whether they are fitly qualified for the employment; and charge them from time to time as they shall see cause, if they appear defective in their duties. That no Searcher during this time of Visitation be permitted to use any publick work or imployment, or keep any shop or stall, or be imployed as a Laundress, or in any other common imployment whatsoever.

The last sentence obviously reflects the fear that a searcher might herself become a carrier of disease. The order continues:

> For better assistance of the Searchers, for as much as there hath been heretofore great abuse in reporting that Disease, to the further spreading of the Infection: It is therefore ordered, that there be chosen and appointed able and discreet Chirurgions, besides those that doe already belong to the Pest-house: amongst whom, the City and Liberties to be quartered as the places lie most apt and convenient: and every of these to have one quarter for his Limit: and the said Chirurgions in every of their Limits to joyn with the Searchers for the view of the body, to the end there may be a true report made of the Disease. And further, that the said Chirurgions shall visit and search such like persons as shall either send for them, or be named and directed unto them, by the examiners of every Parish, and inform themselves of the Disease of the said parties, And for as much as the said Chiurgions are to be sequestred from all other Cures, and kept onely to this Disease of the Infection; It is ordered that every of the said Chirurgions shall have twelve-pence a Body searched by them, to be paid out of the goods of the party searched, if he be able, or otherwise by the Parish.[14]

This 1665 order is of particular interest. The searchers had serious deficiencies, and these had attracted official attention. That the aged women should be selected and supervised by physicians sounds like a good if belated idea, but there seems to be little evidence that this new regulation was implemented. The fact was that the searchers were paid inadequately, were not trained for their responsibilities, and sometimes shirked what was at best an unpleasant job. If they reported a death caused by plague, the house was quarantined and its occupants were placed under other restrictions. So the searchers might be offered, and might accept, a bribe to report another cause for death.[15] An order from the Lord Mayor on July 20, 1590, had noted that "there is great suspicion . . . the weekely certificates . . . of such dye within this Cittie were not truely reported especially those which are supposed to dy of the Plague."[16] John Graunt, founder of the science of vital statistics, in his analysis in 1662 of the London Bills of Mortality expressed little confidence in the reliability of the searchers.[17] They were defended, but not very convincingly, by John Bell, Clerk of the Company of Parish Clerks, in 1665.[18]

Although the "ancient women" were originally appointed to search for signs of plague, gradually they began to report other causes of death as well. In at least one London parish, causes of death were being recorded regularly by 1583. The practice was fairly widespread by 1607.[19]

The searchers took an oath of office.[20] During the Great Plague of 1665 they swore to make careful search of bodies for the cause of death and to report promptly to the constables of the parish and to the bearers who would remove the corpse. "You shall not make report of the cause of anyone's death better or worse than the nature of the disease shall deserve." The searchers had to promise to live together and as far as possible to shun the company of others, including their families, carrying a white wand at all times so that they could be recognized and avoided.[21] A heavy task indeed. Church records show that in 1578 two searchers were paid 4d. each for "viewing the corps" and an equal amount for searching another body.[22] In another parish in September 1617 "two fit aged women" searchers were "to have ij^{d} a peece for everie bodie they shall vew and search to be paid by the governor of the house where such bodie dieth and is vewed, and if they shall not be able to paie the said iiij^{d} then the said money is to be satisfied and paid by the Collector for the poore for the time being."

By 1625 the fee in this parish was 4d. for each searcher.[23] In another parish the weekly salary for one male searcher was 6d. For a second male searcher it was 12d., and for two women searchers it was 18d. each.[24] There is no explanation for the apparent discrimination. In a third parish a searcher was paid £1 for working for two weeks. The parish record also itemizes: "Paid for ij potts of beare for the Chirurgeon and searchers afore they went into the house [of a sick person] . . . ij^{d}."[25] These were all London parishes. In Reading searchers were paid 4s. a week in 1625, a plague year, and 4s. "a moneth after the ceassinge of the plague."[26] By comparison, it has been estimated that at about 1650 a mason earned 16 to 18d. a day and a laborer, 10 to 12d.[27] Since the searchers were forbidden other employment, their incomes must have been very meager and certainly gave no compensation for the risks involved.

The law dealt harshly with errant or uncooperative searchers: "These vewers to reporte to the Constable, he to the Clarke, and he to the Chiefe of Clark; all upon Pain of Imprisonment. A Paine of standing on the Pillorye for false Reports, by the Vewers; a Loss of Pension to such as shall refuse."[28] A few years later, in 1581, the lord mayor of London ordered that "If the viewers through favour or corruption shall give wrong certificate, or shall refuse to serve being thereto appointed, then to punish them by imprisonment in such sorte as may serve for the terror of others." [29] In 1592 it was directed that every woman searcher

> for any corruption or other respecte falsely reportinge, shall stande uppon the Pillory, and beare Corporall payne by the Iudgemente of the Lord Maior and court of Aldermen . . . . That evry woman or other appointed to any service for the infected and refusinge or faylinge to doe that service, shall not have any Pension owt of the hospitall.[30]

The number and variety of these penalties imply continuing problems with the searchers.

There were further difficulties. The searchers reported, it was said, only what they heard. "For the wisest person in the parish would be able to find out very few distempers from a bare inspection of the dead body, and could only bring back such an account, as the family and friends of the deceased would be pleased to give."[31] A correspondent in the *Gentlemen's Magazine* in 1799 complained: "In two parishes, which I could point out, the searchers cannot write; the mistakes they make are numberless, in the spelling christian and surnames, for, they trust to memory till they get home; then, child or neighbour writes what they suppose it to be." Even the "search" was perfunctory: "they only look at the face, enquire the disorder, and receive their fee." In one such case, the deceased had died in suspicious circumstances, and someone notified the coroner. The searcher was questioned at the inquest.

> *Q.* How did you examine this body?
> *A.* In the usual way; by looking at the face and feet.
> *Q.* What, did you not turn up the shroud, and examine the body all over?
> *A.* No, it is not customary, without we have suspicion.
> *Coroner.* Well, then, as you seem to be ignorant of your duty, I must acquaint you that, by law, you must examine strictly: you are appointed by the parish for that purpose; and, if you do not do your duty, I am authorised to commit you to Newgate . . . .[32]

Not all searchers were so negligent. Ann Dunn and Mary Small were called to an inquest and testified in February 1801 to careful examination of the body of a woman whose death, it was suspected, had been violent.[33]

But generally the searchers failed in their duties. A bitter article in *The Penny Cyclopaedia* called for reform, citing the incompetence and occasional drunkenness and dishonesty of the searchers.

> The fee which these official characters [searchers] demand is one shilling, but in some cases *two* public authorities of this description proceed to the inspection, when the family of the defunct is defrauded out of an additional shilling. They not infrequently require more than the ordinary fee; and owing to the circumstances under which they pay their visit, their demands are generally complied with. In some cases they even proceed so far as to claim as a perquisite the articles of dress in which the deceased died. Such are the means at present employed in collecting medical and political statistics in the metropolis of England.[34]

Relief from this situation finally came in 1836 when the Registration Act was passed.[35] It called for the registration of all births, deaths, and marriages in England. This law does not mention the searchers, but when it became effective on July 1, 1837, the office of searcher became obsolete.

Because of the frequent incompetence and unreliability of the searchers, one might be tempted to dismiss them rather briefly as historical curiosities. But this would fail to recognize their importance in relation to the vital statistics of the 16th through early 19th centuries in England. The information passed on by the searchers to the parish clerks for ultimate tabulation in the Bills of Mortality came, for better or for worse, mostly from the searchers, although others could also make mistakes. Thomas Short, 17th century physician, observed, "In all Bills or Tables of Casualties and Diseases, some of the Totals are always lost, either from the Diseases of some being concealed from the searchers, or not returned to the Clerk's-Hall, and overlooked by them, or not fit to be mentioned, as *Fluor albus*, *Lochia*, *Menses nimii*, & c."[36] Even when a searcher conscientiously did her best, her understanding and description of a fatal disease could seldom be anything but that of a layman. Hence, the "causes" of death that appear in the Bills of Mortality and, exceptionally, in parish records, are recorded in lay terms and indeed are, far too often, not diseases but symptoms—"decline," "fever," "dropsy," "convulsions," and the like.[37] But such information is the best we have and, indeed, can tell us a great deal.

REFERENCES

1. *Journals of the London Court of Common Council.* Corporation of London Records Office, vol. 20, May 6, 1578, fol. 407r. Manuscript. Transcripts of Crown copyright records in the Corporation of London Records Office appear by permission of the Controller of Her Majesty's Stationery Office.
2. Creighton, C.: *A History of Epidemics in Britain.* London, Cass, 1965, vol. 1, p. 320.
3. Ibid., p 319.
4. Kitto, J. V., editor: *St. Martin-in-the-Fields.* London, Simpkin Marshall Kent Hamilton, 1901, p. 582.
5. Wilson, F. P.: *The Plague in Shakespeare's London.* Oxford, Clarendon Press, 1927, p. 65, footnote.
6. Forbes, T. R.: *Chronicle from Aldgate.* New Haven, Yale University Press, 1971, p. 160.
7. Act V, scene 2.
8. Strype, J.: *Survey.* London, Innys and Richardson, 1755, vol. 2, p. 536.
9. *A Survey of the Cities of London and Westminster.* Guildhall ms. 1568 [1578], p. 270, fol. 139v. Guildhall Library, London.
10. *Journals of the London Court of Common Council.* Sept. 7, 1592, vol. 23, fol. 129ff.
11. Middleton, T.: Michaelmas Terme. London, T. H. for Meighen, 1630, Act. IV, scene 1; *Memorials of Stepney Parish,* Hill, G. W. and Frere, W. H., editors. Guildford, Billings, 1890-1891, pp. 78, 105; *Reading Records,* Guildings, J. M., editor. London, Parker, 1895, 1896, vol. 2, pp. 241, 244, 285; vol. 3, pp. 64, 372; vol. 4, pp. 201, 202.
12. *The Statutes of the Realm.* (No place or publisher), 1603, 1 Jac. I. c. 31.
13. *Remembrancia.* Corporation of London Records Office, December 7, 1630, item 60. Manuscript.
14. *Orders Conceived and Published by the Lord Mayor and Aldermen of the City of London Concerning the Infection of the Plague.* London, 1665. (No pagination.)
15. Wilson, op. cit., pp. 66, 206-07; Forbes, op. cit., pp. 122-23.
16. *Journals of the London Court of Common Council,* op. cit., vol. 22, fol. 401r.
17. Graunt, J.: *Natural and Political Observations on the Bills of Mortality.* London, 1759, pp. 8-9.
18. Bell, John: *Londons Remembrancer: or, A true Accompt of every particular Weeks Christnings and Mortality In all the Years of Pestilence. . . .* London, Cotes, 1665. For further discussion, see Forbes, op. cit., pp. 96-99.
19. Forbes, op. cit., pp. xix, 50.
20. *Journals of the London Court of Common Council,* loc. cit.
21. Sometimes the rod was red. It was about three feet long and cost 2d. Any person who had been exposed to plague had to carry a red wand if he visited royalty. *Journals of the London Court of Common Council,* op. cit., September 7, 1592, fol. 129; Creighton, op. cit., p. 689; Kitto, loc. cit.; Wilson, op. cit., pp. Extracts from churchwardens' accounts, 19, 179; Strype, op. cit., pp. 536, 565; *Brit. Mag. 4*:146, 1833; Mullett, C. F.: *The Bubonic Plague and England.* Lexington, Ky., University of Kentucky Press, 1956, p. 89.
22. *A Survey of the Cities of London and Westminster,* loc. cit.
23. Hill and Frere, op. cit., pp. 78, 106.
24. Kitto, loc. cit.
25. Westlake, H. F.: *St. Margaret's Westminster.* London, Smith, Elder, 1914, pp. 74, 76.
26. Guildings, op. cit., vol. 2, pp. 241, 244.
27. Burnett, J.: *A History of the Cost of Living.* Harmondsworth, Middlesex, Penguin, 1969, p. 120.
28. Strype, loc. cit.
29. Creighton, op. cit., vol. 1, p. 319.
30. *Journals of the London Court of Common Council,* loc. cit.
31. [Birch, T., editor]: *A Collection of the Yearly Bills of Mortality.* London, Millar, 1759, p. 7.
32. *Gentleman's Mag. 69*:657-58, 1799.
33. *Coroners' Inquisitions.* Corporation of London Records Office. Manuscript (no pagination).
34. *The Penny Cyclopaedia of the Society*

for the Diffusion of Useful Knowledge. London, Knight, 1835, vol. 4, pp. 407-08.

35. *The Statutes of the United Kingdom.* London, His Majesty's Printers, 1836, 6 & 7 Gulielmi IV. c. 86, pp. 526-44.

36. Short, T.: *New Observations, Natural, Moral, Civil, Political, and Medical, on the City, Town, and Country Bills of Mortality.* London, Longman and Millar, 1750, p. 204.

37. Forbes, op. cit., p. 99 ff; Forbes, T. R.: Mortality books for 1774-1793 and 1833-1835 from the Parish of St. Giles, Cripplegate, London. *Bull. N.Y. Acad. Med. 47*:1524-36, 1971; Forbes, T. R.: Sextons' day books for 1685-1687 and 1694-1703 from the Parish of St. Martin-in-the-Fields, London. *Yale J. Biol. Med. 46*:142-50, 1973.

REPORTS OF EXTRAORDINARY FECUNDITY IN EARLY CALIFORNIA

KENNETH THOMPSON, PH.D.

Department of Geography
University of California
Davis, Calif.

JOHN BIDWELL, coleader in 1841 of the first overland wagon train to California, related that his enthusiasm for California was first kindled by a speaker who described the area as a land of "boundless fertility."[1] The reference was, of course, to agricultural fertility and was typical of many such encomiastic descriptions of California at this period. But there were others at this time who spoke of California with reference to another type of fertility—human fertility—in similarly laudatory terms. This paper is concerned with the past belief that the environment of California was somehow conducive to an extraordinary increase of fecundity in women.

Nowadays, of course, concern is mainly with the possible reduction of human fertility. This was not so in the middle of the last century, when large families were esteemed for social, economic, religious, and other reasons. A married woman not "blessed" with progeny was apt to be regarded as more or less pitiable. Even mothers with small families were often regarded as somehow deficient, and "only" children were stereotypically "sickly." Accordingly, any supposed means of enhancing human fertility was of keen popular interest and was the subject of much superstition and folk medicine. It was treated by a great many mysterious patent medicines, and was the concern of orthodox medical attention as well.

California was rightly recognized to have many desirable and attractive features. Indeed, almost all the contemporary references to early California were eulogistic. The fertility of the soil was praised in terms of superlatives and, for a while, the productivity of the mines was extravagantly lauded. But the most frequently praised feature of California's favored environment was its supposedly unique healthfulness. The benign environmental influence was perceived as more than merely passively salubrious; it was widely believed in medical and lay circles that the California climate was actually therapeutic for a number of serious and prevalent diseases, especially pulmonary tuberculosis.[2]

While belief in the preternatural healthfulness of the California environment was first gaining general acceptance (after the 1830s), some stories circulated concerning the extraordinary fecundity of early California residents. Such accounts were adduced as evidence of a singularly salubrious environmental influence, perhaps even as positive proof of such an influence.

One of the first to comment on the reproductive aspects of health conditions in California was Lieutenant Charles Wilkes of the United States Navy. Writing of his 1841 visit to California, Wilkes made the customary declarations on the general salubrity of the region (but also made some customary exceptions in regard to the indigenous inhabitants) and stated that "The health and robustness of the white inhabitants seem remarkable, and must be attributed to the fine climate, as well as to their simple diet." Wilkes went on to declare that "it is by no means uncommon to see families of fourteen or fifteen children." Wilkes documented this assertion by reporting "an instance . . . of a woman near Yerba Buena [now San Francisco], who had twenty-six [children]."[3]

A few years later, in 1846, the Reverend Walter Colton took note of exceptional fecundity in California and, speaking with the authority of a minister, naval officer, and American *alcalde* at Monterey, declared that the "fecundity of the Californians is remarkable." He further asserted that "it is no uncommon sight to find from fourteen to eighteen children at the same table, with their mother at their head." Colton supported these statements with the following cases. "There is a lady of some note in Monterey, who is the mother of twenty-two living children. The youngest is at the breast, and must soon, it is said, relinquish his place to a new-comer, who will, in all probability, be allowed only the same brevity of bliss." Further: "There is a lady in the department below who has twenty-eight children, all living, in fine health, and who may share the 'envied kiss' with others yet to come."

Typical of an age which attributed prime health significance to the physical environment, Colton did not hesitate to explain the fecundity of California residents in terms of climatic influence, thus ". . . it must be attributed in no small degree to the effects of the climate."[4]

About the same time that the Reverend Colton reported the above,

Edwin Bryant, author of an immensely popular book on pre-Gold Rush California, also claimed to be impressed with the prolificity of the non-Indian population of California: "The fecundity of the *people of reason* [i.e., non-Indian] is extreme. It is very rare to find a married couple with less than five or six children, while there are hundreds who have from twelve to fifteen. Very few of them die in their youth, and in reaching the age of puberty are sure to see their grand-children."[5]

The influx of outsiders to California after the discovery of gold led to further spreading of accounts of the phenomenal reproductiveness of Californians. Thus Buffum, one of the Forty-niners, in recounting his experiences in California, remarked: "The women [in California] are queenly, with dark, flashing eyes, and magnificent busts, and are remarkable for their fruitfulness. Families boasting twelve, fifteen, and even twenty-five children, have been frequently met with."[6] Although Buffum does not explicitly attribute this "fruitfulness" to a climatic influence, such an explanation can be inferred from the context of his remarks and the writer's highly favorable views of the California climate which led him to assert that "I doubt much if any country in the world can boast a more equable and salubrious climate."[7]

Even physicians propagated beliefs in an environmental influence in California that caused prolific human reproduction. Thus the German Dr. J. Praslow, writing in 1849, took a highly favorable view of health conditions in California and saw the environment as somehow conducive to human fertility. Referring to California, Praslow wrote that "Women from Spain and the Eastern United States who are barren give birth readily in this area."[8] Shortly afterward, another medical man, Dr. J. Blake, confirmed the above views and emphatically declared that "there can be no doubt but that the climate is conducive to fertility in the female."[9]

The view that the California environment somehow enhanced human fertility was being reiterated even in the 1860s. Thus, in 1863 Hittell, a historian and author of a book on California resources, reported: "It has been remarked that a multitude of instances have occurred of couples who, after having lived childless for ten, fifteen, or twenty years in other countries, before coming to California, in a year after their arrival here have had children."[10]

Again, in 1869, in another descriptive work on California, Brace commented on the belief that the California climate increased the fecundity of *both* man and animals. In his book he pointed out that:

> The impresssion prevails generally in California that the climate favors the prolific power of both animals and human beings; both certainly mature earlier than in the Eastern States. Physicians, however, are inclined to trace the remarkable effect on women, observed here, as much to change of climate as to any peculiar power in it. I have heard of some very large families here—one of twenty-eight children, all of one mother.[11]

What can one make of these accounts of extraordinary fecundity in early California? It should, perhaps, first be noted that the stories are hardly credible; they share elements of hearsay and are not based on personal observation. The vaguely specific reports of huge families are also fairly close together in time and space—a circumstance which further suggests the possibility of hearsay. Should these stories be regarded as merely idle rumors? Probably so. There are, of course, no reliable data on birth rates and infant mortality in early California but there can be no doubt that both were relatively high. If there is any sort of factual basis to the stories it is quite possibly connected with a high mortality rate among mothers—those prodigious families reported may actually have been born to more than one mother.

It is not intended to attach profound significance to these accounts of phenomenal fecundity in early California. After all, in the considerable literature that described this region, references to human fecundity are fairly few. The topic, however, does recur frequently and consistently enough to suggest a moderately persistent notion. Further, it is possible that Victorian diffidence regarding the topic of child-bearing might well have diminished the references to what was undoubtedly a subject of great interest. There is, of course, no way of establishing the currency and acceptance of this belief in the supposed environmental influence on human fecundity. However, the circulation of what now appear to be extravagant stories, such as concern mothers with 28 living children, illustrates, if nothing else, the radical limits reached by early, and in this case seemingly unwitting, California boosterism.

REFERENCES

1. Bidwell, J.: *In California Before the Gold Rush.* Los Angeles, Ritchie, 1948, p. 7.
2. For further discussion of the environmental influence on health conditions see Thompson, K.: Insalubrious California: Perception and reality. *Ann. Ass. Amer. Geog. 59*:50, 1969; Thomp-

son, K.; Irrigation as a menace to health in California. *Geog. Rev. 59:* 195, 1969; Thompson, K.: Climatotherapy in California. *Calif. Hist. Quart. 50:*111, 1971.
3. Wilkes, C.: *Narrative of the United States Exploring Expedition During the Years 1838, 1839, 1840, 1841, 1842.* Philadelphia, Lea & Blanchard, 1845, vol. 5, p. 175.
4. Colton, W.: *Three Years in California.* New York, Barnes, 1850, p. 27.
5. Bryant, E.: *What I Saw in California.* Philadelphia, Appleton, 1848, p. 284.
6. Buffum, E. G.: *Six Months in the Gold Mines.* From a journal of three years' residence in upper and lower California 1847-1848-1849, Caughey, J. W., editor. Los Angeles, Ritchie, 1959, p. 8.
7. Ibid., p. 7.
8. Praslow, J.: *The State of California: A Medico-Geographical Account.* Original edition published in German (Göttingen, 1857). Cordes, F. C., translator. San Francisco, Newbegin, 1939, p. 8.
9. Blake, J.: On the climate and disease of California, *Amer. J. Med. Sci. 24:*63, 1852.
10. Hittell, J. S.: *The Resources of California.* San Francisco, Roman, 1863, p. 368.
11. Brace, C. L.: *The New West, or California in 1867-1868.* New York, Putnam, 1869, pp. 369-70.

FECUNDITY IN EARLY NEW SOUTH WALES: AN EVALUATION OF AUSTRALIAN AND CALIFORNIAN EXPERIENCE

BRYAN GANDEVIA, M.D., F.R.A.C.P.

Associate Professor of Thoracic Medicine
University of New South Wales Department of Medicine
Prince Henry Hospital
Sydney, Australia

FRANK M. FORSTER, M.B., F.R.C.O.G.

Associate, Department of Obstetrics and Gynaecology
Monash University
Melbourne, Australia

DR. Kenneth Thompson's review of reports of extraordinary fecundity in early California[1] prompted us to examine similar observations made in relation to the first settlement in Australia, which was founded at Sydney Cove in the late 18th century. Accounts of enhanced fecundity or fertility* may prove to be a phenomenon common to colonization elsewhere. If so, pertinent differences in the backgrounds of Australian and California settlement might shed further light on the concept, and its genesis might emerge more clearly through an examination of the very earliest stages of settlement, particularly when some statistical data were available.

THE COLONY OF NEW SOUTH WALES AND THE QUALITATIVE EVIDENCE FOR ENHANCED FECUNDITY

The settlement at Sydney, Port Jackson, New South Wales, was established in January 1788 under Governor Arthur Phillip. The founding population consisted of approximately 750 convicts (including 188 females) and 200 civil and military personnel, with 40 wives, all of whom arrived on the First Fleet. There was no relevant contact with the small indigenous population. No change took place in

*Matthews Duncan, in 1868, was the first to clearly distinguish between these terms: fecundity means "the demonstrated capability to bear children," while fertility, which implies fecundity, "also introduces the idea of number of progeny."[2]

This project was supported in part by a grant to one of us (B.G.) from the Australian Research Grants Committee.

the female population—except for transfers to a small subsidiary settlement established at Norfolk Island some 900 miles to the east—until June 1790, when the *Lady Juliana* arrived with about 230 female convicts. Although some were said to be "loaded with the infirmities incident to old age,"[3] more than 90% were in the child-bearing age range of 15 to 45 years. During the next month, the Second Fleet—notorious for its high mortality on the voyage—landed about 750 convicts, of whom 67 were female. Again with the exception of transfers to Norfolk Island, the female population remained relatively static until the latter half of 1791 and early 1792, when the arrival of the Third Fleet and other ships added about 2,000 male and 218 female convicts. Late in 1792 two ships brought an additional 365 convicts, of whom 74 were women. Over the period from 1788 through 1792 only minor fluctuations occurred in the "free" (nonconvict) female population.

The first five years—indeed, in some respects the first 15 years—of the colony were a struggle for mere existence. Crops failed, gardens withered, livestock died or strayed, and vital stores and provisions which arrived from England at infrequent intervals were deficient in quality and quantity. Starvation was a recurring threat: indigenous food—plant, fish, and kangaroo—was limited and irregular in availability, so that the colony's nutritional status, basically dependent on salt meat and flour, was constantly impaired. Once the first high hopes for a new venture had died there were no enthusiastic accounts of the settlement's progress and prospects; only a few, notably Governor Phillip, retained any faith in its future.[4] In these circumstances no assessment of human fecundity could have been biassed by considerations of the fertility of the soil, the productivity of the region, or the multiplication of the imported livestock.

Even by 1812 the colony was not entirely self-supporting; some more arable country had been opened up with difficulty, but the settlers were not to escape into the rich pastoral lands beyond the formidable Blue Mountains for almost another five years. At this stage, a Select Committee of the British House of Commons inquiring into transportation possibly assumed a correlation between the fertility of man and of his environment, stating: "the soil and climate are described to be extremely fine, healthy, and productive."[5] No other reference of this kind has been found in the early literature relating to the colony.

The first authoritative observation on the subject is provided by the surgeon's mate of the *Sirius*, a naval vessel of the First Fleet, in 1791:[6]

> Our births have far exceeded our burials; and what is more remarkable, women who were supposed to be past child-bearing, and others who had not been pregnant for fifteen or sixteen years, have lately become mothers.

We have identified no similar observation in the diaries or correspondence of other doctors in the colony during its formative years, but a nurse-midwife and a good observer, Margaret Catchpole, a convict transported in 1801, noted that "it is a wonderfull Countrey for to have children in—very old women have them that never had won Before."[7]

In 1793 Captain Watkin Tench, an officer of the marines and a perceptive participant in the colony's first four years, amplifying the statement that "no climate, hitherto known, is more generally salubrious," remarked:[8]

> . . . to this cause, I ascribe the great number of births which happened, considering the age, and other circumstances, of many of the mothers. Women, who certainly would never have bred in any other climate, here produced as fine children as ever were born.

Similarly, John Hunter, a much-travelled naval captain of humanitarian outlook who was destined to become the colony's governor, observed:[9]

> I do not think I can give a stronger proof the salubrity of the climate than by observing that I never saw the constitution of the human race or any other animal, more prolific in any part of the world; two children at a birth is no uncommon thing, and elderly women, who have believed themselves long past the period of childbearing, have repeatedly had as fine, healthy, strong children as evere were seen.

Hunter was referring particularly to Norfolk Island, a more fertile place than Port Jackson, with which he was equally well acquainted. Although the prolific bird life and the island's produce saved Hunter and his associates from starvation during a stay of some 12 months beginning in March 1790, it is difficult to substantiate his impression of human fertility from the available data. Only 15 births occurred during the year among 100 women in the settlement and among another 150 women, mostly from the *Lady Juliana*, who were transferred from Sydney for the latter six months. The population of children increased from about 35 to 65 (a dozen or so probably arrived with the women), so that the proportion of children (almost all less than five years of age) to adult females fell from approximately 1:3 to 1:4.[10] After generous allowance for possible errors, these figures reflect an annual birth rate of less than 100 per 1,000 women, which is low by contemporary standards (see below). Possibly a more significant observation is that only one child had died since the island was settled in 1788.

Although not published until 1822, one account of remarkable fecundity dates back to the early years of settlement; it also includes a new hypothesis as to the cause. John Nicol, steward of the *Lady Juliana* in 1790, gives a colorful and detailed description of her voyage to Australia with some 220 of the lady convicts and of the Sydney scene:[11]

> They have an herb in the colony they call Sweet Tea. It is infused and drank like the China tea. . . . There was an old female convict, her hair quite grey with age, her face shrivelled, who was suckling a child she had born in the colony. Every one went to see her, and I among the rest. It was a strange sight, her hair was quite white. Her fecundity was ascribed to the sweet tea. I brought away with me two bags of it, as presents to my friends; but two of our men became very ill of the scurvy, and I allowed them the use of it, which soon cured them, but reduced my store. When we came to China I showed it to my Chinese friends, and they bought it with avidity, and importuned me for it. . . .

The vine *(Smilax glicyphylla)* is described as a "tolerably pleasant succedaneum" for China tea in the book published by the colony's surgeon-general, John White, where its leaves are also illustrated.[12] Denis Considen, one of White's assistants, wrote to Sir Joseph Banks of its antiscorbutic properties[13] and other "medical gentlemen" described it as a "powerful tonic,"[14] but a veil of professional secrecy appears to have been drawn over its efficacy in increasing fertility. Nicol's account has been quoted in full because, if it fails to establish a case for enhancing fertility, it does contain hints that the tea may have had aphrodisiac properties. Perhaps its continued use for a century and a half as "a sort of cure-all amongst the humblest class of inhabitants

. . . particularly favoured by old dames" lends support to this suggestion.[13] However, evidence from all sources uniformly supports the view that no aphrodisiacs were required by the early colonial girls; as an English neswpaper facetiously put it:[15]

> Governor Phillip finds great difficulty in the due appropriation of husbands. At first he allowed six to each wife; but at present the female convicts having very greatly increased, the number allotted to each is not more than three. This necessary regulation . . . has produced much animosity among the fair sex of the settlement.

A not entirely accurate description of the penal colony at Sydney published in François Péron's account of his voyage of discovery from 1800 to 1804 (first published in French in 1807), records that in their new environment the reformed *filles publiques* revealed the greatest fecundity, much greater than was to be expected in the previous state of debauchery.[16] At the same time, the relative infertility of the Sydney soil was acknowledged. In the English edition of 1809, and later in the second French edition of 1824, this isolated observation is considerably expanded:[17]

> The same [moral] revolution, effected by the same means, has taken place amongst the women: and those who were wretched prostitutes, have imperceptibly been brought to a regular mode of life, and now form intelligent and laborious mothers of families. Though it is not merely in the moral character of the women, that these important alterations are discoverable, but also in their physical condition, the results of which are worthy of consideration, both of the legislator and the philosopher.* For example, every body knows that the common women of great capitals, are in general unfruitful; at Petersburgh, and Madrid, at Paris, and London, pregnancy is a sort of phenomenon amongst persons of that description; though we are unable to assign any other cause, than a sort of insusceptibility of conception: the difficulty of researches, as to this subject, has prevented philosophers from determining how far this sterility ought to be attributed to the mode of life of such women; and to what degree it may be modified or altered, by a change of condition and manners. But both these problems are

*In the French edition of 1824 the word *médecin* is used.

> resolved, by what takes place in the singular establishment that we are describing. After residing a year or two at Port Jackson, most of the English prostitutes become remarkably fruitful; and what, in my opinion, clearly proves that the effect arises much less from the climate, than from the change of manners amongst the women, is, that those prostitutes in the colony, who are permitted by the police to continue in their immoral way of life, remain barren the same as in Europe. Hence we may be permitted to deduce the important physiological result, that an excess of sexual intercourse destroys the sensibility of the female organs, to such a degree, as to render them incapable of conception; while, to restore the frame to its pristine activity, nothing is necessary but to renounce those fatal excesses.

The second French edition was "revised, corrected and augmented" by L. de Freycinet, largely from earlier notes made by Péron; it seems likely that the paragraph may be attributed directly to Péron, a former student of medicine as well as a distinguished naturalist and anthropologist.

Thomas Reid, surgeon superintendent of convict transports, accepted the widely held view that excessive venery impaired fertility, but was less impressed with the moral reformation induced by the benevolent penal arm of British justice. Referring, with a characteristic polysyllabic prolixity, to "that deplorable state of habitual dissoluteness aggravated by heinous indulgence in open violation of decency," he states (1822):[18]

> The evil consequences to the colony from this abuse are innumerable. The continual disturbance of social connections, and disregard of moral obligation, are not its only bad effects; the great hope of colonization is defeated: population is undoubtedly checked in its advance by such pernicious practices. This fact is proved by the concurrent testimony of all nations, and various arguments have been urged in illustration. . . . In reply to this it may be said, that the population in New South Wales has increased in a ratio greatly beyond that of any other country. The extraordinary salubrity of the climate, and other circumstances, may have contributed in a great degree to that remarkable increase, which appears unquestionably without parallel even in the periods of American colonization; but were

> female virtue better protected, and cherished with becoming care, there can be not a shadow of doubt, that the population would be much greater than it is even now.

A critical, indeed an arrogant, medical gentleman from the Bengal Medical Society offered some peculiarly precise statistical information acquired on a brief tour undertaken for the sake of his health.[19]

> The effects of the climate of Australasia [which varies from temperate to tropical], it is well known, are to increase . . . the productive powers of animals of all descriptions . . . probably [in man] owing to the abundance of provision, in conjunction with the well known salubrity of the atmosphere. . . . Almost every woman, under 42 years of age, on her arrival in New South Wales, and properly treated [sic], will beget a large family, producing for a considerable period, a child once a year. Females of a higher class are less affected by the climate.

A measure of official corroboration of the birth of children to older women is found in the report of J. T. Bigge, a judge appointed to inquire into the state of the colony of New South Wales:[20]

> The effects of the licentiousness of the women at Parramatta are more visible in their appearance than in their health. I was much struck with this circumstance, at the first muster that I attended at Parramatta in the year 1819, when most of them were accompanied by fine and healthy children, some of whom had been born after their mothers had attained the age of 45.

In the short period here under review, instances of families of the remarkable size recorded in California cannot be anticipated, but the Reverend J. D. Lang mentions a convict couple from the First and Second Fleets who had seven or eight children.[21] As will appear, perhaps the more significant observation is that "all [of the children] . . . had arrived at manhood" for there were "no infantile diseases whatever" in the colony. Measles, whooping cough, chicken pox, scarlet fever, and smallpox were unknown, and tuberculosis, if endemic at all, was of negligible importance.[22]

The Australian evidence to suggest enhanced fecundity cited thus far resembles closely the Californian information, both in character and quality. Before comparing the experiences of the two colonies, and as a result offering a provisional explanation of the situation, we may profitably examine the statistical data available for New South Wales.

Vital Statistics

For the period 1788 to 1792 inclusive, data on births and deaths in Sydney are considered reasonably accurate,[23] even though they are based chiefly on baptismal and burial records. The derived rates quoted below, although of the correct order of magnitude, should be considered as approximations. Some of the problems in determining rates for births and deaths have been examined more fully elsewhere.[24]

The ages are known for 122 of the 188 female convicts of the First Fleet; 114 of these were in the childbearing ages of 15 to 45 years.[25] After allowing for transfers to Norfolk Island, approximately 200 women, convict and free, may be accepted as having the potential for conception between January 1788 and June 1790. During this period of two and one half years there were 85 births, giving an annual birth rate of 170 per 1,000 females per annum. In the next 12 months, by June 1791 (prior to the arrival of the Third Fleet) there were 43 births in an estimated population of 300 women (possibly an overstimate), giving a birth rate of 143 per 1,000 females per annum. Births to the end of 1792 numbered 117 in an estimated at risk female population of about 400, or a rate of 195 per 1,000. In Norfolk Island for almost the full two years of 1790 and 1791 (a longer and more realistic period than that previously examined in relation to Captain Hunter's visit) an annual rate of 110 births per 1,000 females prevailed.[10]

For comparison, Coghlan, in a careful statistical study of the New South Wales birth rate in the second half of the 19th century,[26] calculated that for *married* women in New South Wales under the age of 45 the annual natality rate in 1861 was 341 per 1,000. As males outnumbered females by more than three to one between 1788 and 1792, and as there were 245 births during those years among approximately 200 women, more than 90% of whom were probably of an appropriate age, we may reasonably assume that most of the convict women were "married" (although relatively few were legally so). On this basis the annual natality rates noted above for this early period are certainly not high.

To compare these rates with conventional birth rates, it is reasonale to divide them by a factor of eight, on the assumption that 25% of a standard population with equal sex distribution would be females of child-bearing age; it is obviously inappropriate to express the birth rate in terms of the actual settlement population with its excess of males and artificial age distribution. Acceptance of this approach permits the conclusion that an over-all birth rate of 25 per 1,000 might be guessed as an upper limit during the settlement's first five years. If it changed at all—there are limitations to the available information—the birth rate tended to fall during the next decade.[27] This birth rate seems unequivocally lower than that of 35 per 1,000, generally accepted for England at the end of the 18th century,[28] and which was certainly reached in both England and New South Wales by the middle of the 19th century. Only three sets of twins, the expected number, occurred among the 245 births.

As Thompson implied,[1] an impression of increased fertility would be conveyed to an observer by a high survival rate among the infants. There were only 77 deaths in childhood in New South Wales in the five years from 1788 to 1792, amounting to 31% of the total births; between 1789 and 1791, when epidemic dysentery was absent, the proportion of child deaths to births was only 21%. Deaths of those under one year of age totalled only about 20% of the births.[24] Thus, the infant mortality rate was probably less than half that of 18th century London.[29]

For whatever reason, the ratio of adult women to children fell from 5:1 at the foundation of the colony to 2:1 in 1795 and 1:1 in 1799, in spite of an increase in the female population. In only a little more than a year (1790-1791) the ratio at Norfolk Island fell from 1:4 to 1:2.7.[10] Thus, the proportion of children (most of whom would be under two years of age) rose at the Port Jackson settlement from about 4% of the total population in 1795 to about 17% in 1799. Such a rapid change, irrespective of the absolute figures, would create the impression of remarkable fecundity and fertility; the accompanying fact that an unusually high proportion of the women were of child-bearing age would easily escape notice. A superficial observer, particularly one of moralistic tendency, might also find support for this view in the low marriage rate[30] (about 2% of single women per annum at its lowest level, between 1798 and 1802),[31] the high illegitimacy rate (in the early 1800s two thirds of all children were illegitimate),[32] and an increasing number of orphans and abandoned children.

We have attempted to identify any births to women of relatively advanced age. Seventeen female convicts in the First Fleet were recorded as being 35 years of age or more in 1787, and eight were already over 45 years. Five women, ranging in age from 36 to 40 years, had acquired husbands but had no recorded issue by 1880. If it be accepted that two children (by different fathers) born in 1789 and 1791 were more likely to be those of a Mary Harrison in her middle 20s than a woman of the same name in her late 30s, then only one of the older females had a child after her arrival: Ann Powell at the age of 39 years had a baby by a seaman in March 1791—a year too late to be the white-haired mother to whom Nicol refers. As far as we know, Maria Haynes, who married a marine, became the oldest First Fleet mother when she had her fifth child in the colony at the age of 44. Sarah Mitchell, of the *Lady Juliana*, gave birth to a daughter in 1792 when she was 42 years of age. Although at least three others from this ship married after the age of 40 (one at the age of 68), we have failed to establish that any woman of exceptional age proved unexpectedly fecund.

One other fragment of statistical information deserves mention: the Reverend Samuel Marsden, who took a special interest in sin, recorded that of 395 married women in the colony in 1806, 90 (23%), all formerly convicts, had had no children. The duration of the marriages is not stated, although the context implies a long enough period to merit the observation. During the same period, another record indicates that the average number of children born to convict mothers (married or unmarried) was 2.32, and to married free women 2.64.[33] Sixty years later Coghlan estimated that in New South Wales only 8% of women marrying at the age of 30 were childless after five years of marriage. J. Y. Simpson estimated in 1844 that 11% of Scottish marriages remained sterile after five years,[35] while a decade later Matthews Duncan's figure for marriages in Edinburgh and Glasgow of three years' duration was 15%.[36] In 1861, 19% of Scottish marriages of unstated duration were childless.[37] By any standards, then, the Australian figure is high. Venereal disease, as well as promiscuity, was present in the colony virtually from its inception,[38] and postgonococcal salpingitis, as well as malnutrition, may well have contributed to impaired reproductive capacity. We have found no allusion to abortion prior to 1832, and examination of female mortality reveals no evidence of its use in the early years of the settlement.

Toward a Comparison

If the qualitative evidence offered by Thompson[1] and ourselves is accepted at its face value, a comparison of the information from both sources is instructive. First, as a cause of increased fecundity, or an impression thereof, a high regional productivity or local soil fertility is excluded; the relevant area of Australia was barren and infertile by Californian standards. Second, diet and nutrition cannot be held responsible, for the early years of Australian settlement were years of semistarvation and malnutrition. Third, moral reformation of the women, associated with a reduction in promiscuity and excessive venery —so attractive to our professional ancestors as an explanation of physical and mental ills—cannot account for any increased reproductive return. By comparison with the Australian female convicts (perhaps 20% of whom had been prostitutes), the Californian women were surely ladies of impeccable respectability. In any case, there is little or no evidence that moral reformation was achieved by transportation to Sydney, a point on which Reid and most contemporary observers came nearer to the truth than did the French scientists. An equable climate with a relatively high proportion of sunshine hours and comfortable nocturnal temperatures remains a common factor in California and Sydney, and thus it is the most plausible of the explanations offered by early commentators. Indeed, a generation or two later, Coghlan concluded that a climatic influence was responsible for the demonstrably greater fecundity of Australian-born married women (of all ages) by comparison with English, Scottish, or Irish migrant women.[39] Prior to the decline in the birth rate in the later decades of the 19th century, the Australian-born women were also more fertile.[40]

Conclusion

The statistical data available for the formative years of settlement in Australia suggest that the birth rate was not high by contemporary standards, and no individual cases of childbirth at advanced ages have been identified, in spite of some dogmatic medical and lay reports. There is, therefore, no unequivocal evidence of increased fecundity. If the quantitative testimony of the Reverend Marsden (supported by the impressions of Péron and Reid) on the high proportion of childless marriages be admitted, some enhancement of fertility among the remainder is not excluded. A striking and rapid change in the age distribution of the population is clearly demonstrable; this is attributable largely to a low infant-mortality rate. The swift increase in the number of young children relative to the adult population could scarcely fail to create the impression of heightened female reproductive powers (virility being accepted tacitly as a biological constant by all contemporary authorities). The early settlers in California probably provided a population structure resembling more closely that of the first Australian settlement than that of an old, established community, and so the same phenomenon may well have occurred. In terms of the age structure of the population, there is a further analogy in the middle of the 19th century, when gold discoveries produced an influx of young adults to both California and Australia. In the present context this analogy cannot be carried too far, because in Australia this last mass migration was quickly followed by a well-defined rise in the birth rate —to the remarkable peak of 40 per 1,000 in the early 1860s.[41]

To examine in detail the reasons for the different experiences of 1800 and 1860 is beyond our present scope, but it is relevant to note that the environmental circumstances were wholly different in the later period: the resources of established towns and pastoral industries were available, there was an adequate food supply, and the economic status of the community was better. The later migrants were basically healthier, but infant mortality did rise to more conventional levels as the acute infectious diseases and tuberculosis became endemic.

This comparison serves chiefly to indicate that an impression of enhanced fertility in a developing community may arise for a variety of reasons, and can be evaluated critically only if enough information exists to define both the community and its environment. Statistical explanations alone, however, are rarely altogether satisfying, and a sociological rationale should at least be sought for the first Australian settlement. In the early stages of the settlement the female convicts "lived in a state of total idleness,"[42] and many of the men were scarcely more industrious. In the knowledge that "the chastity of the female part of the settlement had never been . . . rigid,"[43] we were at first inclined to relate any apparent increase in fertility to a combination of leisure, laxity of morals, and perhaps the effects of Botany Bay sweet tea, but these features would seem less likely to explain the Californian experience.

Further research provided a more profound, as well as a more comprehensive, answer to the problem in the work of Peter Cunningham published in 1827. Cunningham, a naval surgeon of wide experience, gained an intimate knowledge of the colony as a settler and of its convict population as an efficient surgeon-superintendent of five ships of convicts. His essays, written with humour and insight, reveal a tolerance and understanding of human waywardness which is uncommon among his contemporaries. In endorsing his concept, we venture to transcribe not only the sentence which is relevant to the present problem but also the ancedotes so aptly illustrative of it:[31]

> The inauspicious issue of the experimental mission of the Twelve Apostles [A footnote states: Twelve *unfortunate girls*, who had been sent out by some religious society, to get either places or husbands in New South Wales. They were so named by the sailors.] some years back has, I fear, operated against future speculations of this kind; a goodly proportion of that chosen band having been found in a *matronly* way (hanging in a sort of sentimental love-trance round the necks of the sympathizing tars) by the reverend inspector who visited them on arrival, to certify as to their *high* state of *moral* improvement. . . . still the situation of these unfortunates must be *now* out of all comparison superior to their former debased condition in England; while the colony cannot but have profited by such an acquisition as twelve young healthy females, destined perhaps to become mothers of virtuous families, and thus to increase the amount of our industrious population. Their sudden prolifickness doubtless arises partly from change of climate producing a corresponding change in constitution, but may chiefly be ascribed to an alteration of *habits*. The same effect we see coming into play among the street-perambulators in England, since it became fashionable to renovate their constitutions by short sentences to wholesome prison diet, and the wholesome discipline of the treadmill. The *fruitful* effects of these measures most of the parishes frequented by such damsels can abundantly testify. The facetious clergyman of a manufacturing village in the North seemed to understand this matter also:—no illegitimate children had been for a long while forthcoming in the parish, till change of times caused a dispersion of the *manufacturing establishment*, when a sudden fecundity ensued. A

worthy elder, shocked at the scandal of such a numerous illegal progeny being all "on the stocks" at once, waited on his pastor to condole upon the subject, and take steps to avert, as he deemed it, the "increasing depravity",—but was checked by his reverend friend pulling him gently by the sleeve, and whispering in his ear, "No, no, James, no, no! instead of viewing such as tokens of *increasing depravity*, I hail them, James, as the first signs of *returning morality*. . . ." So we may say of our female exiled population; pointing to the fine and numerous families which they rear as triumphant proofs of their moral regeneration.

We trust that Cunningham's Law of Increasing Depravity and Returning Morality will be found equally applicable to other colonies where, as another Australian medical traveler observed, "the healthy aspects, blooming cheeks and expressive eyes of the young damsels . . . show that the soil is as well adapted for the development of female beauty as it is universally allowed to be for the growth of grain."[45]

ACKNOWLEDGMENTS

We are indebted to Mrs. Sheila Simpson for her invaluable assistance, and to the trustees of the Mitchell Library, Sydney, Australia, for permission to study material in their custody.

NOTES AND REFERENCES

1. Thompson, K.: Reports of extraordinary fecundity in early California. *Bull. N. Y. Acad. Med. 49*:661, 1973.
2. Duncan, J. M.: *Fecundity, Fertility, Sterility and Allied Topics.* Edinburgh, Black, 1866, p. 3.
3. Collins, D.: *An Account of the English Colony in New South Wales.* London, Codell, 1798, p. 119. Of the 230 women on the *Lady Juliana,* 50 were 19 years of age or less (including six who were less than 15 years) and 36 were 40 or more, including 11 who were more than 50 years of age. On an average, they were younger than the women of the First Fleet.
4. The modern accounts of the early settlement which are most appropriate in the present context are Eldershaw, M. B.: *Phillip of Australia.* Sydney, Angus and Roberson, 1972; Mackaness, G.: *Admiral Arthur Phillip.* Sydney, Angus and Robertson, 1937.
5. *Report from the Select Committee on Transportation.* Ordered by the House of Commons to be printed July 10, 1812, p. 3.
6. Lowes,—: *Historical Records of New South Wales.* Sydney, Govt. Printer, 1893, vol. ii, p. 771.
7. Written by Margaret Catchpole in a letter to her uncle and aunt, January 28, 1807. Mitchell Library, Sydney, Catchpole mss.
8. Tench, W.: *A Complete Account of the Settlement at Port Jackson in New*

South Wales. London, Nicol, 1793, p. 169.

9. Hunter, J.: *An Historical Journal of the Transactions at Port Jackson and Norfolk Island.* London, Stockdale, 1793, p. 138.
10. *Historical Records of Australia.* Commonwealth of Australia, Series I. Sydney, Govt. Printer, 1914, vol. 1, pp. 148, 166, 203-04, 236, 246, and 298-99.
11. Nicol, J.: *The Life and Adventures of John Nicol, Mariner.* Edinburgh, Blackwood, 1822, p. 131. Nicol admittedly thought that "every thing thrives well" in New South Wales, p. 129.
12. White, J.: *Journal of a Voyage to New South Wales.* London, Debrett, 1790, pp. 195 and 230.
13. Campbell, W. S.: The use and abuse of stimulants in the early days of settlement in New South Wales. *J. Roy. Aust. Hist. Soc. 18*:74, 1932.
14. Collins, op. cit., p. 57.
15. *Public Advertiser,* May 1791; quoted by Mackaness, op. cit., p. 259.
16. Péron, F.: *Voyage de découvertes aux Terres Australes . . . [1800-1804]*, 2 vols. Paris, L'Imprimerie Impériale, 1807, vol. 2, p. 402. See also 2d ed., Paris, L'Imprimerie L'Impériale, 1824, pp. 282-83 and Introduction by L. de Freycinet.
17. Péron, F.: *A Voyage of Discovery to the Southern Hemisphere, 1801-1804.* London, Phillips, 1809, p. 277. A preview of this "official" translation from the French which appeared in the *Naval Chronicle* (*22*:389, 477, 1809) lacks the expanded paragraph, so that it seems de Freycinet was given the opportunity to revise the English text or to supply additional material.
18. Reid, T.: *Two Voyages to New South Wales.* London, Longman, 1822, p. 304.
19. Henderson, J.: *Observations on the Colonies of New South Wales and Van Diemen's Land.* Calcutta, Baptist Mission Press, 1832, pp. 21-22.
20. [Bigge, J. T.]: *Report of the Commissioner of Inquiry into the State of New South Wales.* London, Govt. Printer, 1822, p. 71.
21. Lang, J. D.: *An Historical and Statistical Account of New South Wales, both as a Penal Settlement and as a British Colony,* 2 vols. London, Cochrane and McCrone, 1834, vol. 2, p. 33. At a later period (1857), the convict J. F. Mortlock, referring to a family of 10 fine, healthy children, noted that the climate of Tasmania was particularly favorable "to the first cause for which the holy state of matrimony was ordained." *Experiences of a Convict,* Wilkes, G. A. and Mitchell, A. G., editors. Sydney, Sydney University Press, 1965, p. 83.
22. Wentworth, W. C.: *Statistical, Historical and Political Account of the Colony of New South Wales.* London, Cochrane and McCrone, 1834, p. 55; Cunningham, P.: *Two Years in New South Wales,* 2 vols. London, Colburn, 1827, vol. 2, p. 183; Gandevia, B.: The Medico-Historical Significance of Young and Developing Countries, Illustrated by Australian Experience. In: *Modern Methods in the History of Medicine,* Clarke, E., editor. London, Athlone Press, 1971, p. 75; Thomas, B. and Gandevia, B.: Dr. Francis Workman and the history of taking the cure for consumption in the colonies. *Med. J. Aust. 2*:1, 1959.
23. *Report from Select Committee,* op. cit., p. 9.
24. Gandevia, B. and Cobley, J.: Mortality at Sydney Cove, 1788-1792. *Aust. New Zeal. J. Med. 4*:111, 1974; Gandevia, B. and Gandevia, S.: Childhood mortality and its social background in the first settlement at Sydney Cove, 1788-1792. Submitted for publication. The figures used in the present essay are largely derived from these papers, in which the sources are more fully examined.
25. The ages are given by Cobley, J.: *The Crimes of the First Fleet Convicts.* Sydney, Angus and Robertson, 1970.
26. Coghlan, T. A.: *The Decline in the Birth Rate in New South Wales.* Sydney, Govt. Printer, 1903, p. 4. This paper is subtitled "An Essay in Statistics."
27. Dey, P. and Gandevia, B.: *Childhood Mortality and the Birth Rate in New*

South Wales, 1793-1800. In preparation.

28. The evidence is reviewed by McKeown, T. and Brown, R. G.: Medical evidence related to English population changes in the eighteenth century. *Pop. Studies 9:*119, 1955. See also Griffith, G. T.: *Population Problems of the Age of Malthus,* 2d ed. London, Cass. 1969, Introduction; Krause, J. T.: Changes in English fertility and mortality 1781-1850. *Econ. Hist. Rev. 52:*11, 1958. Krause indicates that in the absence of effective birth registration the ratio of children aged 0 to 4 years per 1,000 women of childbearing age is a measure of fertility. Without subscribing to this concept, we estimate through this method a ratio of 500 per 1,000 as a maximum for Sydney in 1793—more than 100 below the English figure for 1821.
29. Still, G. F.: *The History of Paediatrics.* London, Dawsons, 1965, pp. 445 and 379; Rendle-Short, M. and Rendle-Short, J.: *The Father of Child Care: Life of William Cadogan (1711-1797).* Bristol, Wright, 1966, pp. 39 and 28. See also McKeown and Brown, loc. cit.
30. Robson, L. L.: *The Convict Settlers of Australia.* Melbourne, Melbourne University Press, 1965, p. 141.
31. Calculations based on approximate figures from various sources suggest a decline from about 6.3 marriages per 100 unmarried females per annum between 1788 and 1792 to 1.6 in 1798-1802, followed by a rise to 5.3 in 1807-1810.
32. *Report from Select Committee,* op. cit., p. 12.
33. Marsden, S.: Essays concerning New South Wales 1807-1817, with a list of females in the colony. Mitchell Library, Sydney, Marsden papers. See also Sacleir, M.: Sam Marsden's colony: Notes on a manuscript in the Mitchell Library, Sydney. *J. Roy. Aust. Hist. Soc. 52:*94, 1966; and *Historical Records of New South Wales,* op. cit., vol. 6, p. 162.
34. Coghlan, op. cit., p. 18.
35. Simpson, J. Y.: On the alleged infecundity of females born co-twins with males: With some notes on the average proportion of marriage without issue in general society. *Edinburgh Med. Surg. J. 61:*107, 1844.
36. Duncan, op. cit., p. 186.
37. Census of Scotland, 1861: *Population Tables and Report.* Edinburgh, Secretary of State for the Home Department, Scotland, 1861, vol. 2, p. xxxvi.
38. Collins, op. cit., pp. 26, 446, and 596.
39. Coghlan, op. cit., p. 18 ff.
40. Coghlan, op. cit., p. 40 ff.
41. Cumpston, J. H. L.: Public health in Australia: Part III. Developments after 1850. *Med. J. Aust. 1:*679, 1931.
42. Tench, W.: *A Narrative of the Expedition to Botany Bay.* London, Debrett, 1793, p. 132. Major Robert Ross, when commandant of Norfolk Island, explicitly ordered that "for the further encouragement of such male convicts as are desirous to maintain the females, such females shall not be called upon by the public to do any work" except in special circumstances *(Historical Record of New South Wales,* op. cit., p. 447). Ross claimed to have made an effort to foster family life.
43. Collins, op. cit., p. 81.
44. Cunningham, op. cit., vol. 2, pp. 293-95.
45. Wilson, T. B.: *Narrative of a Voyage Round the World.* London, Dawson, 1968 (first published 1835), p. 297.

BENJAMIN WEST'S OSTEOMYELITIS: A TRANSLATION

ADRIAN W. ZORGNIOTTI, M.D.

Associate Professor of Clinical Urology
Principal Lecturer, History of Medicine
New York University School of Medicine
New York, N.Y.

IN the early 1760s, before settling down in England to a glorious career in painting, Benjamin West (1738-1820) visited the eminent painter Anton R. Mengs in Rome. West's biographer states that because of a fever West was advised by a friend to leave the capital.[1] He returned to Leghorn, where he had been received previously by the merchants Jackson and Rutherford, to whom he had letters of introduction. It soon became apparent that he had an infection in the region of the left ankle and that his condition was worsening. West's friends insisted that he consult Angelo Nannoni (1715-1790), the eminent surgeon of the Hospital of Santa Maria Nuova in Florence. This choice turned out to be felicitous, since Nannoni appears to have achieved a cure after four operations. Nannoni's fame was based in part upon his espousal of simple methods for treating wounds and the infections that almost always accompanied them. At a time when oils, balsams, and other liquids were smeared on wounds and ulcers, Nannoni's use of tepid aqueous irrigations and dry dressings gave notably favorable results.[2] Nannoni also distinguished himself as a lithotomist and as a contributor to surgery of the breast.[3]

Among the Florentine surgeon's case reports is that of West.[4] With casual disregard for his patient's privacy—typical of the times—Nannoni recounts in detail his treatment of the painter:

MEMOIR V, OBSERVATION XVI

Mr. West was born in Pennsylvania of an English father. From the tenderest age he showed great inclination for painting. He cultivated this art in all its aspects in his native America with such fervor that, in a short time, he had made such progress that his father, helped by the advice of authoritative persons, resolved to send him to Italy and in particular to Rome. He disembarked at Leghorn where he had introductions to the late Mr. Giorgio Giasson and to Mr. Rodefort. This occurred around 1759. These gentlemen directed him to Rome and to Mr. Mens, a painter of the highest merit.

Mr. West brought from America to Italy a very delicate complexion which corresponded to a very fervid temperament. The inflammable quality of his humors, and particularly of the combustible substance of the oil necessary for the vital flame, had been the cause of his being tormented with rheumatisms and joint pains in America and in Italy. The joints, which were often attacked by pains, swelled in the form of emphysemas. These are tumors arising from rarefied air caused by manifest inflammation or by cold fermentations. Whether fermentation productive of the release of the air, be it hot or cold, these tumors have sometimes been observed to be mixed with water; hence was born the name hydrarthos or hydrops of the joints.

This tumor, called hydrarthos, which does not occur as frequently as does emphysema, has been the subject of protracted study by some who have devoted themselves to this illness without concerning themselves sufficiently with the search for that cause of which the hydrarthos is an effect, and which cause often consists in a manifest and painful inflammation, or hot fermentation. The latter at times gives rise to abscesses which turn into sores that attract from the air new material for the increase of the inflammation destructive of the joint, and often of life, if one does not succeed in halting the progress of that destructive illness by amputation—which is in itself a remedy full of danger.

The joint pains which often afflicted Mr. West were never the result of so great an inflammation as to give rise to suppurations in these same joints. A suppuration appeared on the external part of the left leg but outside the articulation of this part with the foot. This suppuration followed the painful inflammation productive of rheumatisms. These, with their frequency and persistence, were always accompanied by a thinning of the thigh, leg, and foot. During the period of greatest emaciation, in addition to rheumatic pains there appeared pains in the knee and ankle with weakness throughout the extremity. It was in Rome that Mr. West was attacked by this latest inflammatory illness, which was treated in that large city in the best possible manner to halt the cause productive of ills which progress notwithstanding the greatest human attentions, because human knowledge is greatly inferior to the force of that physical cause which promotes and leads to its end that certain change in structure or substance which is called disease.

The inflammation which in Rome arose around the malleoli of Mr. West's leg produced a swelling with some threat of suppuration at some distance from the ankle. Mr. West's friends in Leghorn, having learned of the illness by which he was menaced, recalled him to Leghorn so that he might be treated under their very eyes. An abscess appeared between the external malleolus and the achilles tendon. This was opened, giving rise to a wound with suppuration. After several months that this wound was present without signs of imminent healing it was decided to send the patient to Florence so that I might treat him. At the end of November 1761 I began this treatment in the house of the painter, Ignazio Hugford.*

The sickness entrusted to my care consisted of a wound with a granulating surface lying between the external malleolus and the achilles tendon. Surrounding the wound there was always a swelling which was both emphysematous and spongy.

The nature of the wound and of the swelling extending around the ankle made me question that carious bone could be present. My doubts increased on reflecting upon the quality of the temperament, the rheumatisms, and the joint pains long suffered in America and in Italy. Further reflection on the long time that there existed a wound with spongy swelling around it over the malleolus and the achilles tendon caused an increase in fears that the bone was already carious. The surgeon who had opened the abscess and treated the wound had detected the existence of a space of such depth that he did not deem any operation feasible.

Before taking any decision on this granulating wound which was without signs of hidden or manifest spaces, I allowed several days to pass, after which I touched it with the infernal stone.** By means of this light caustic the proud flesh was destroyed but new granulation was produced. The same thing followed the use of precipitate† and again

*Ignazio Enrico Hugford (1703-1778), painter of historical subjects and portraitist. Although considered a member of the English School, he was born in Pisa and worked and died in Florence.

**Silver nitrate fused into a stick has only recently been replaced by wooden applicators.

†One of several mercury compounds, most probably mercury bichloride (corrosive sublimate).

with mundificative ointment.* In view of all these things I conjectured that a bad fermentation extending even unto the substance of the bone was the cause of fresh granulation tissue. Eight days after the start of digestive medications, I was able to increase the pressure of my touch over the achilles tendon; it was then that I saw for the first time a small amount of pus in the wound. This casual discovery made me certain of the existence of a sinus, which I then found by means of the probe.

The sinus space ran deeply between the achilles tendon and the malleolus. Notwithstanding the attentions given this, even by the surgeon who had discovered it before me, I determined to open it with a cut. As best I could, I made the incision to the very bottom of the space, sparing the achilles tendon. Once the cut was made there began a great and prolonged pain in the leg and foot. I dressed the wound with dry raw lint,† packing it as much as was needed to keep the edges of the wound separated from each other, so that the base of the ill might render itself always more evident. Continuing this treatment with dry raw lint, one could see healthy flesh everywhere except at the center, which always abounded with corrupt tissue. The caustics were acting upon that product of fermentation so evil that its force, productive of that body of granulation tissue, overcame the action of the most powerful caustics, one of which was alum mixed with precipitate. The mixture of these two powders at times produces an inflammatory fermentation so that the hardest sarcomas are destroyed. In our case the caustic alluded to produced great pain and one always found the wound filled with corrupt tissue. As I advanced with the treatment, which consisted of discontinuing and resuming the caustics according to what seemed to me best, unexpectedly there arose an inflammation with suppuration, after which I discovered a sinus space deeper than the first.

It is not prudent to operate on all recent spaces but in this case I did not know if one could hope to see a cure without cutting, therefore I decided upon this course. I postponed this until a day of clear air because, alas, in the treatment of this wound I had observed how much cloudiness and humidity acted in promoting and increasing bad fermentations.

The opening of this new space also between the achilles tendon and

*Mundificative ointment was used to clean up ulcerations. It usually had emollient and digestive properties.

†Raw lint was obtained by unraveling clean linen cloths, taking pains to mix the threads in such a manner as to create a soft ball which was absorbent.

the fibula had to be made with great care. Despite this the wound turned out very painful and bled heavily. In each of the two incisions which were made to reach the bottom of the space a portion of the muscular substance remained involved. Two days after the last operation I uncovered the wound and, examining it deeply, found a piece of dry bone. I raised this with the spatula, detached it, and removed it from the wound. I continued treatment with dry raw lint. This was followed by sanies. These were the effects of fermentation from suppuration of the tissue. This, breaking down into pus, left new spaces which, as the treatment proceeded, were always found between the achilles tendon and the fibula. The part which gave rise to these spaces did not favor the making of incisions with complete freedom. However, to avoid the risk of a fistula which the nature of these same sinus spaces menaced, I became concerned, and took great pains to open these without causing great harm to the achilles tendon.

I made a third incision. Each of these operations opened the way to new fermentations of suppurations, thus giving rise to new sinuses; these last were the worst because of their extent and hidden course, always between the achilles tendon and the fibula.

I performed these operations, aimed at abolishing the spaces which arose after the removal of the dry bone, after having waited a sufficient time to see if in the usual new animalization* following the destructive suppuration one could acquire some hope that it would not be necessary to do everything by means of the violence of the art. To this end I used for a while a dressing of myrrh in wine. There followed the same suppurations which customarily occurred from fermentations caused by the cloudy air.

Thus while I did the dressing twice daily with myrrh in wine, there followed a great change in the air, which from clear and cold, became humid, and even greater inflammation was rekindled. There were signs of great pain, great heat, red color, and throbbing in the site of the wound with, what is more, fever. The myrrh in wine, not having been capable of preventing even the production of bad flesh, was discontinued, and I returned to the use of the caustic composed of alum and

*This term applies to the creation of new tissue from food substances (*Oxford English Dictionary*). See also Hatchett, C.: *Philosophical Trans. Roy. Soc. 90*:401, 1800. "The clot or crassamentum also affords, by repeated washings, a large proportion of albumen and gelatin; after which a substance remains. This substance (called fibrin by chemists) may be regarded as that part of the blood which has undergone the most complete animalization, and from which the muscle fiber and other organs of the body are formed."

precipitate. This time greater fire than ever was kindled, with most severe pain which lasted 24 hours. The very painful action of the caustic did not free the patient from the necessity of a fourth incision no lesser than the others. From this operation, performed on February 2, there began an inflammation with much drainage. This time those sinus spaces, which the keen observer perceives cannot be overcome except by opening, did not arise. I waited until the suppuration promoted by latest cut ended, I then gave attention to observing the outcome of the cavities newly arising between the fibula and achilles tendon. I packed all these spaces with soft lint.* Going forward in this manner, with the help of the good season of spring, every ulcerated cavity abolished itself and scar appeared. This came about best while the air was clear, thus from this observation one must again point out how much clear weather influences the improvement and care of wounds.

Mr. West's leg remained very thin. This did not prevent him from walking freely. To this freedom of motion a state of looseness of the leg cooperated greatly, and without any help from the art a great binding with filling in of the soft parts joined at the articulation of the foot.

Mr. West, triumphant by our surgery, by which he fully recovered his health after a very complicated illness whose treatment was difficult, left Florence for London, where he is admired for his great talents for painting.

---

*Soft lint was made by scraping well-washed cloths, producing a material which resembles the absorbent cotton in use today.

REFERENCES

1. Galt, J.: *Life Studies and works of Benjamin West, Esq.* London, 1820.
2. Nannoni, A. In: *Enciclopedia Italiana di Scienze, Lettere ed Arti.* Rome, Treccani, 1949, vol. 24, p. 200.
3. Fiorillo, L.: *Elogio Istorico del Celeberrimo Prof. di Chirurgia Angelo Nannoni.* Florence, 1790.
4. Nannoni, A.: *Memorie Di Chirurgia (Per Servire Alla Formazione del Secondo Tomo del Trattato Sopra La Semplicita del Medicare I Mali Curabili Coll'Ajuto della Mano).* Siena, 1774, pp. 61-6.

THE DIAGNOSIS OF NEOPLASM IN MATTHEW BAILLIE'S ATLAS OF ANATOMY (1812)

I. WILLIAM GROSSMAN, M.D.

Brattleboro Memorial Hospital
Brattleboro, Vt.

PRESENT-DAY macroscopical diagnoses of neoplasms are substantiated by histopathological examination and by knowledge of the actual or potential biological activities of the neoplasms. How accurate were the macroscopical diagnoses of neoplasms before the doctrine of cellular pathology was developed (1858) and before the biological activities of the various neoplasms were known? A present-day pathologist may attempt to answer this question by comparing macroscopical diagnoses of neoplasms with those which Matthew Baillie (1761-1823) offered in his *Series of Engravings*,* the first systematic descriptive atlas of macroscopic pathological anatomy. This work was intended as a supplement to Baillie's *Morbid Anatomy*.† The atlas‡ consists of 73 plates divided into 10 fascicles; each plate contains one to five figures. Each figure has a concise legend.

Inflammatory lesions of various organs are portrayed and diagnosed correctly. Neoplastic lesions are depicted accurately (Figures 1 to 3) and can be easily diagnosed by a present-day pathologist. The majority of the neoplastic lesions are diagnosed correctly by Baillie. A present-day pathologist would differ with respect to certain lesions diagnosed as schirrhus. This term signified a firm, malignant neoplasm; today such a lesion would most probably be termed gastric leiomyoma (Figure 1), prostatic nodular fibroadhenomatous hyperplasia, uterine leiofibromyoma, and ovarian thecoma. The macroscopical appearance of encapsulation or benign biological behavior of these lesions was not taken

*Baillie, M.: *A Series of Engravings, Accompanied with Explanations, which are Intended to Illustrate the Morbid Anatomy of Some of the Most Important Parts of the Human Body*. London, Bulmer, 1st. ed., 1799; 2d. ed., 1812.

†Idem.: *The Morbid Anatomy of Some of the Most Important Parts of the Human Body*. London, Nichol, 1793.

‡I have used the 1812 edition of the atlas in the William H. Welch Library, Johns Hopkins University School of Medicine, Baltimore, Md.

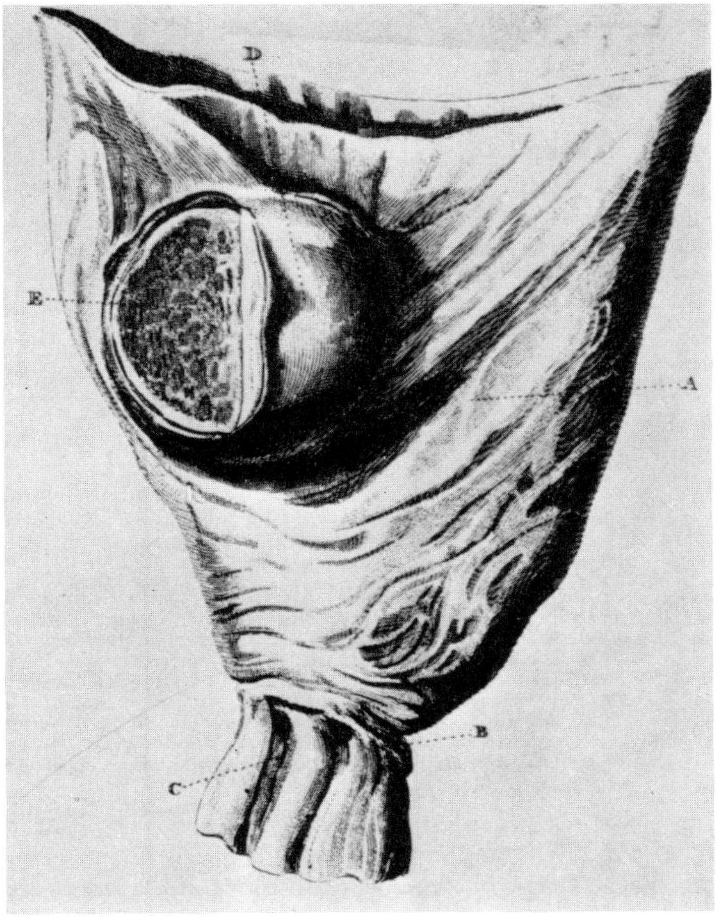

Fig. 1. Segment of stomach with a "circumscribed tumor is covered by the inner membrane of the stomach. In its center there is a small aperture." The lesion most probably represents a submucosal leiomyoma with a peptic ulcer of the overlying mucosa. The cut surface of the lesion shows bundles of apparently smooth muscle interspersed by fibrous tissue. Other lesions that should be considered in the differential diagnosis are submucosal neurofibroma and a metastatic carcinoma (fascicle 3, plate 6, Figure 1).

into account; Baillie apparently characterized these lesions as malignant solely on their consistency.

Baillie did not recognize metastatic neoplasms, although he suspected that the hepatic lesions shown in Figure 2 were malignant. Typical metastatic carcinomas were portrayed in the liver (Figure 2)

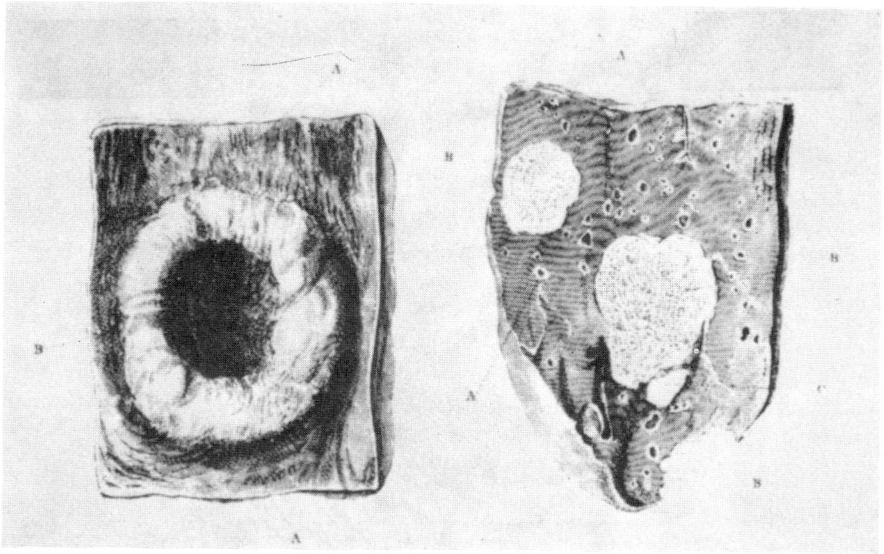

Fig. 2. Segments of liver showing the capsular and cut surfaces with tubercles "firm in its texture . . . generally depressed upon its external surface, and large portions of the liver in the sound state are interposed between the different tubercles. If a judgment were to be formed considering the nature of this tubercle merely from its texture, it would be considered as scirrhous; but in one or two instances I have seen some tubercles of this kind converted into a thick curdy pus, similar to that of a scrofulous gland when some tubercles are formed, the liver is commonly enlarged beyond the natural size." These lesions represent metastatic carcinoma to the liver. The central umbilication of the capsular lesion is characteristic of a metastatic deposit (fascicle 5, plate 3, Figures 2 and 3).

and lungs. The concept of metastasis had to await the discovery of embolism by Virchow (1846) and the knowledge of cellular pathology.[1]

Perhaps the most interesting macroscopical diagnosis in the atlas is that of a polypoid mucosal neoplasm of the bladder in a young child (Figure 3). Baillie interpreted this lesion as benign polypus. On histological examination the tumor, which was preserved in John Hunter's museum, was interpreted 87 years later as a benign rhabdomyoma because of the presence of striated muscle fibers in various stages of the development.[2] This macroscopically and microscopically innocent-appearing neoplasm of the bladder would be diagnosed as a sarcoma botryoides by a present-day pathologist, 159 years after the initial macroscopical diagnosis and 67 years after the initial histological diagnosis, because of present-day knowledge of its potentially malignant biological activity.

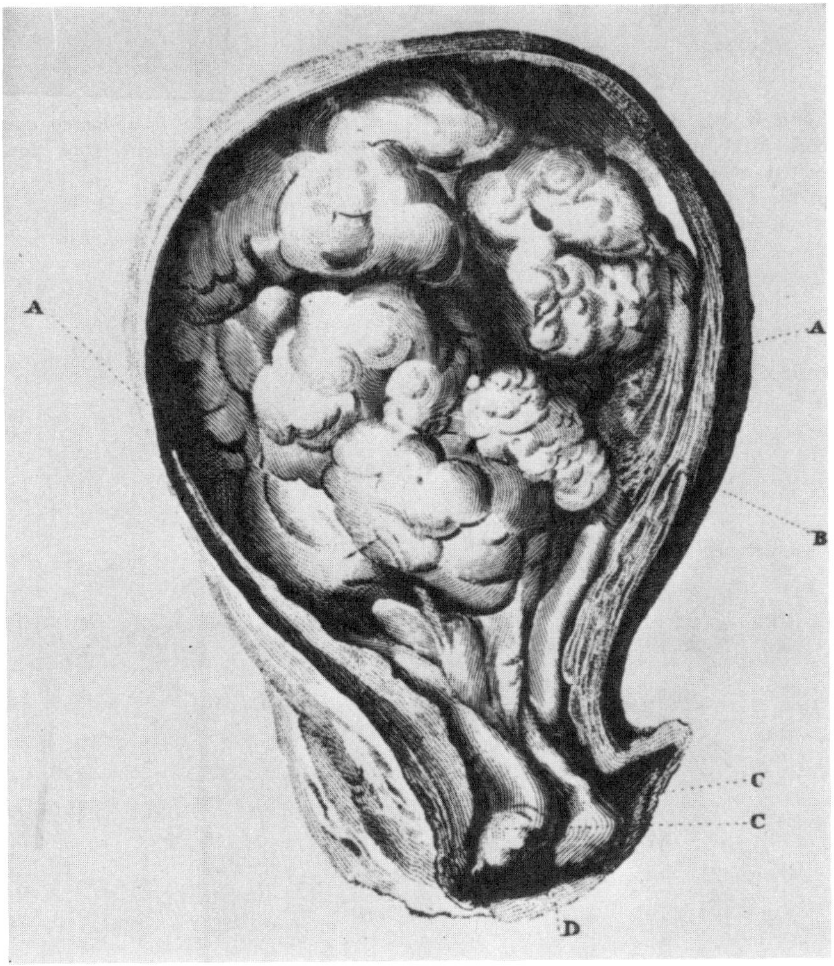

Fig. 3. "Bladder of a child, by which is brought into view a very large polypus, filling up its cavity. The polypus consists of several large projecting irregular masses and two long processes had grown from it, shooting through the urethra as far as its external orifice, and distending very much its canal." The lesion was examined histologically 87 years later, when it was termed a benign rhabdomyoma. This lesion would be diagnosed by a present-day pathologist as sarcoma botryoides, 159 years after the initial macroscopical diagnosis and 62 years after the initial histological diagnosis, because of present day knowlege of its potential malignant biological activity (fascicle 7, plate 4, Figure 2).

The discussion of these three lesions implies that morbid anatomy is not a dead or dying specialty, but a specialty which is continually developing new concepts for the understanding of disease.

REFERENCES

1. Long E. R.: *A History of Pathology.* New York, Dover (enlarged and corrected republication of 1928 ed.), 1965, p. 94.

2. Shattock S. G.: Rhabdomyoma of the urinary bladder. *Proc. Roy. Soc. Med.* *3*:31-41, 1909.

PURKYNE'S FIBERS: THE FIRST REPORT (1839), THE GERMAN VERSION (1845), AND THE ENGLISH VERSION

PROFESSOR VLADISLAV KRUTA

Department of Physiology
Medical Faculty
J. E. Purkyně University
Brno, Czechoslovakia

DURING the last 20 years the fibers of Purkyně have been widely studied because of their unusual physiological properties and their important role in cardiac physiology. The terms Purkyně's (Purkinje's) fibers, Purkyně network, and Purkyně system are among the most frequently used eponyms in medical and biological terminology. Interest in the discovery of the fibers and in the origin of the eponym is therefore not surprising. It has been stated repeatedly that Purkyně first described these structures in 1845 (Aeby 1863, Tawara 1906, Tandler 1913, Tigerstedt 1921, Landois-Rosemann 1923, Hanák 1930, Benninghoff 1930, Rothschuh 1952, Wiggers 1960, W. Coraboeuf 1963); other authors (v. Hessling 1854, Hermann 1932, Franklin 1933, 1949) give 1839 as the year of the discovery. Some commentators (Garrison 1913, Willius and Dry 1948, J. Dobson 1962, Katz and Hellerstein 1964, Burch and De Pasquale 1964), suggest that the dissertation of Purkyně's pupil B. Palicki, *De musculari cordis structura* (Vratislaviae 1839), was the first publication of Purkyně's discovery.

Matousek and Posner (1969) in their recent survey of the history of Purkyně fibers rightly say that these structures are not mentioned in Palicki's dissertation on the course of the muscular cardiac fibers (contractile myocardium) which can be observed in a boiled or fixed heart. However, they are wrong in stating that Purkyně's discovery was first published in 1845. This is obvious from the opening paragraph of the paper, Mikroskopisch-neurologische Beobachtungen (*Müllers Archiv.* p. 281, 1845), which was almost immediately translated into

English by William W. Gull* and published in the *London Medical Gazette*. Gull's translation begins as follows:

> In the summer of the year 1838, whilst making a more extended trial of the value of acetic acid, first introduced by the younger Burdach, for the purpose of rendering very delicate nervous fibers visible, I instituted a set of observations upon the proportion of such elementary fibers in the different tissues. These observations, at the request of several of the Professors of the University of Cracow, were sent to the Annual Report of the Faculty of Medicine,** in which they were printed in the year 1839. It seemed to me, however, that the remarks there contained had not received the publicity which they deserved. A part of them appeared in a small pamphlet by Dr. Benedict Schultz, "*On the Physiology of the Spinal Cord in relation to its Pathological conditions*." Vienna, 1842.† The remainder received but a slight notice. I have therefore thought it might not be superfluous if I again communicated from the Cracow Report these observations to the philosophical world at large.‡ If I have here and there introduced known facts, or negative results, it must be borne in mind, that, in giving an historical sketch of the value of acetic acid in microscopical investigations, I was obliged to mention when its employment was, or was not, successful.

Purkyně repeated his statement in 1858 in the detailed review of his scientific publications in the Czech periodical *Ziva;* he also gave a summary in which he complained again that his Polish paper would have remained hidden, to his own loss and that of science.§ It is astonishing that such a clear statement could have remained unnoticed by so

*Sir William Withey Gull (1816-1890) studied at Guy's Hospital and London University, and graduated in 1847. He was still an undergraduate when he published Purkyně's translations. As lecturer on physiology he remained attached to Guy's Hospital for 20 years. In 1847-1849 Fullerian Professor of Physiology, Royal Institution, he received an honorary degree at Oxford (1868), at Cambridge (1880), and at Edinburgh (1884), and became a baronet in 1872. He was physician extraordinary to the queen, physician to the prince of Wales, etc. Main writings:

The Harveian Oration. London, 1870, 52 pp.

A Collection of the Published Writings of Sir William Withey Gull. Acland, T. D. ed., 2 vols. London, New Sydenham Soc. 1894-1896.

Memoir and Addresses. London, New Sydenham Soc. 1896.

***Rocznik Wydzialu lekarskiego w Uniwersytecie Jagiellonskim, Krakow,* vol. 2, 1839.

†Schulz, B.: *Physiologie des Rückenmarkes mit Berücksichtigung seiner pathologischen Zustände für praktische Ärtze.* Wien, Pfautsch, 1842.

‡. . . to stimulate a wider discussion and further investigation [omitted by the translator].

§*Ziva 6*:41-42, 1858. Reprinted in: *Opera selecta,* Praguae, 1948, pp. 150 and 153.

many distinguished scientists of different nations and at different intervals after the discovery of that peculiar and important structure.

The history of the Polish publication can be reconstructed from the references in the four extant letters of Majer to Purkyně from the year 1839.* On March 29, 1939, Majer and Skobel asked Purkyně to submit a paper on his discovery of nerve fibers in the meninges and certain other organs, or on some other subject, to be published in the *Rocznik Wydziału lekarskiego.* Majer and Skobel wanted more theoretical papers in their periodical, which hitherto had been predominantly clinical; no doubt they felt that a contribution from such an eminent scientist would add to its reputation. On April 12 Majer informed Purkyně of the wish of numerous members of the Cracow Society (Towarzystwo Naukowe), that he should become a member of this learned body, and asked for his acceptance. On June 30 Majer thanked Purkyně for his readiness to send a paper for the *Rocznik,* which Purkyně must have done soon afterward. This is obvious from Majer's letter of September 25th in which he thanked Purkyně for his contributions to the *Rocznik* and told him that he and Professor F. Skobel had translated them. He apologized for the delay in publication. He also sent the diploma of the *Societas Litteraria Antiquissimae Studiorum Universitatis Cracowiensis.* Purkyně's paper was then published in the second issue of the 1839 volume.

Purkyně's contribution to the Cracow annual entitled "New Observations and Research in Matters of Physiology and Microscopical Anatomy" *(Nowe spostrzeżenia i badania w przedmiocie fizyologii i drobnowidzowéj anatomii)* consisted of two papers. The first was on particular subjective skin sensations experienced during a shower bath *(O szczeogólnych, samodzielnych uczuciach w skórez, podczas działania nań kąpieli mglistéj* [*Staub-*] *lub dźdżystéj* [*Regen-Bad*], *Opera omnia* 3, 52-54), and was republished in German in 1854, included with a larger article: *Die Topologie der Sinne im Allgemeinem, nebst einem Beispiel eigenthümlicher Sinne. Empfindungen der Rückenhaut beim Gebrauche des Regenbades* (cf. *Opera omnia* 3, 79-91). The other, entitled Contribution to the Minute Anatomy of Nerves, Especially on Nerves of the Pia Mater and Other Meninges of the Spinal Cord and Brain *(Przyczynek do drobniejszéj Anatomii nerwów, w szczególności o nerwach błony miekkiéj rdzenia pacier-*

*Purkyně's letters to Majer seem to have been lost; cf. Kruta 1970.

zowego i innych blon, tak tu, jak i do mózgu należacych) ends with the description of special threads in the heart. This Polish paper has a different numbering of the paragraphs but is otherwise almost identical with the German version of 1845. The section on the heart is numbered 5 and begins on p. 65. The description of Purkyně fibers is on pages 66 and 67. It is preceded by a paragraph on the occurrence of nerve fibers in the heart. In the German text the section on the heart is number 12; it begins on page 293 and ends on page 295.

There is thus no doubt that Purkyně discovered the special myocardial fibers in 1838-1839 and that the first report of this discovery was published in 1839, not in Palicki's dissertation* but in a paper written by Purkyně himself and published in Cracow.

As the original text by Purkyně was translated into Polish in 1839 by Majer and Skobel, the German text of 1845 is not a translation but the authentic author's text. It may be of interest to quote Purkyně's description in W. Gull's contemporary English translation which, curiously enough, seems to have escaped entirely the notice of English-speaking biologists and cardiologists: **

> On the inner surface of the cavity of a sheep's heart, I first saw with the naked eye, directly under the serous lining, a network of grey, flat, gelatinous fibres,† which were in part continued to the columnae carneae, and into other nervous† bundles whilst other fibres† cross over the fissures between the muscular columns on the walls of the cavity, forming as it were little bridges. By microscopical examination, I found that these fibres† were composed of globules,†† similar to those in the ganglia, closely pressed together, and thus appearing polyhedral. In the interior of each globule‡ two or three granules§ exist, but unlike the nucleus and nucleolus of the globules†† of true ganglia. Each grey fibre† is formed by rows of these globules,‡

*The reference to Palicki seems to appear first in F. H. Garrison's book, a standard and very reliable work, and taken over by the other cited authors.

**It has been recorded recently in J. S. Emmerson's list: *Translations of Medical Classics.* Newcastle upon Tyne, Univ. Library, 1965, p. 64.

†In the German original, *Fäden* = threads, in contrast to *Fasern,* used by Purkyně for nerve fibers.

††In the original, *faserige Bündel,* i.e., fibrous, not nervous.

‡*Körnern* = grains or globules, term used (usually as the diminutive *Körnchen*) by Purkyně for animal cells in contrast to *Zelle,* used for plant cells, formations surrounded by a distinct cell wall.

§I.e., nuclei.

of which there are from five to ten in a transverse section. The fibres are covered with an elastic tissue, which when treated with acetic acid shows transverse marking similar to those of the muscular tissue of the heart. It is difficult to determine whether these are really fibres,* or only markings of the membranous envelope, which, as in the cells of vegetables, surrounds the granular contents. This latter opinion seems to me the most probable, because on a transverse section no free extremities of the fibres* can be seen; at all events they cannot be compared to those nervous filaments which surround the ganglionic globules in the ganglia, although at first sight they have that appearance; nor could I ever succeed in discovering true nervous filaments which would have given to them a distinct ganglionic character.

At present, were I disposed to class this new tissue with cartilaginous formations, yet I do not understand what can be its function, from its softness in comparison to the largely developed muscular mass of the heart; but it seems most probable that it is an arrangement for motion, and that the membranes surrounding the granules are muscular. I found similar granular fibres† in the cow, pig, and horse. On the other hand, I could not discover any in man, the dog, hare, or rabbit. In the hearts of all the ruminants which I have examined I have found, close upon these fibres, and also quite isolated, rounded aggregations of elongated granules inclosed by a delicate membrane. Were they not so constantly present, they might readily be mistaken for the ova of some parasite (pp. 1157-58).

Purkyně's description of the subendocardial fibers remained unnoticed for another seven years, even after the German publication. As Müller's *Archiv* was a leading periodical on anatomy and physiology, the title may have diverted attention. Purkyně's discovery occurred accidentally during his search for terminal nerve fibers in different organs, and his first observations were rather puzzling. Nevertheless, he considered his findings interesting enough to be reported and felt that they would stimulate further investigation.

In his famous *Handbuch der Gewebelehre*, Kölliker (1852) made

**Fasern* = fibers.
†Körner fäden = cellular threads.

the first significant reference to the fibers and thus stimulated further research. The nature and possible function of the fibers were discussed by a dozen distinguished microscopists (Hessling 1854, Siebold 1854, Reichert 1854, Remak 1862, Aeby 1863, Eberth 1866, Obermaier 1866-1867, Lehnert 1868, Frisch 1869, Krause 1876, L. Ranvier 1877, Gegenbauer 1877). These investigators also studied the occurrence of the fibers and details of their morphology before Schmaltz (1886) made the correct inference concerning their functional significance. But discussions and speculations as to whether they were tissues remaining in an early stage of development or whether they had some mechanical function, as Purkyně himself thought, continued for 20 more years. In 1906 Sunao Tawara published the results of his systematic and thorough research, with a detailed and critical review of previous work leading to the well-founded conclusion that Purkyně fibers were nothing else than the terminal extension of the muscular link between atrium and ventricle. Consequently the fibers must have the same function as the atrioventricular bundle.

Tawara's book, because of its systematic histological presentation and interpretation and because of the critical evaluation of the work done by earlier workers, ranks among the great classics of cardiology.

There are errors in scientific literature which seem to be perennial, having been taken over from one paper to the next without verification of the original source. In the case of the Purkyně fibers, the year of their discovery is clearly stated in the second report of 1845, in its English translation, and in Purkyně's 1858 account of his scientific publications. Moreover, both the original Polish and the second German report were reprinted in Purkyně's *Opera Omnia* in 1938 and 1939. None of us is exempt from making such errors. Some errors occur in spite of all possible care, as in the small book on Purkyně edited in 1962 for the centenary of the Czech Medical Society. In the English translation, of which the Czech author (V.K.) was unable to see the proofs, a misprint regarding Purkyně fibers—1829 instead of 1839—remained uncorrected, whilst in the original Czech and four other translations (French, German, Russian, and Spanish) the year 1839 was given correctly. The desire to eradicate a long-established error in the history of this famous discovery and to recall the forgotten early translation of the classical paper justifies the publication of yet another paper on the history of Purkyně fibers.

REFERENCES

Aeby, C.: Ueber die Bedeutung der Purkyně schen Fäden im Herzen. *Z. Rationelle Med. 3:* ser. 17, 195, 1863.

Benninghoff, A.: Blutgefasse und Herz. In: Mollendorff, W. von, *Handbuch der Mikroskopischen Anatomie des Menschen.* Berlin, Springer, 1930, vol. 6, p. 198.

Burch, G. F. and De Pasquale, M. P.: *A History of Electrocardiography.* Chicago, Year Book Med. Publ., 1964.

Coraboeuf, W.: Proprietes du muscle cardiaque. In Kayser, Ch.: *Physiologie, III.* Paris, Flammarion, 1963, p. 254.

Dobson, J.: *Anatomical Eponyms.* Edinburgh & London, 1962.

Eberth, C. J.: Die Elemente der quergestreiften Muskeln. *Virchow's Arch. 37:* 100, 1866.

Franklin, K. J.: *A Short History of Physiology,* 2d. ed. London, 1949.

Frisch, A.: Zur Kenntnis der Purkinje' schen Fäden. *Sitzungsber. Akad. Wiss. Wien,* Abt. B, *60*:341-48, 1969.

Garrison, F. H.: *An Introduction to the History of Medicine.* Philadelphia, Saunders, 1913; 1917; 1921, p. 488.

Gegenbauer, C.: Notiz über das Vorkommen der Purkinje' schen Fäden. *Gegenbauers Morph. Jb. 3*:633, 1877.

Hanak, A.: Ucebnice fysiologie I. Praha, A. Hynek, p. 108, 1930.

Hermann, H.: Le coeur. *Traite de Physiol. norm. et path. 6, Circulation.* Paris, Masson, 1932, p. 150.

Hessling, T.: Histologische Mittheilungen. *Z. wiss. Zool.* 5:189-99, 1854.

Katz, L. N. and Hellerstein, H. K.: Electrocardiography. In: *Circulation of the Blood. Men and ideas.* Fishman, A. P., & Richards, D. W., eds. New York, Oxford Univ. Press, p. 297.

Kölliker, A.: *Handbuch der Gewebelehre des Menschen. Leipzig,* Engelmann, 1852.

Kruta, V.: *Jan Evangelista Purkyně.* Prague, 1962, pp. 13-116.

Kruta, V.: J. E. Purkyně and the Cracow physiologist Josef Majer, *Scripta Med. 43*:217-230, 1970.

Landois-Rosemann: *Lehrbuch der Physiologie des Menschen,* 18th ed. Berlin-Wien, Urban & Schwarzenberg, p. 109.

Lehnert, M.: Uber die Purkinjeschen Fäden. *Arch. f. mikrosk. Anat. 4*:26, 1868.

Matousek, M., and Posner, E.: Purkyně's (Purkinje's) Muscle fibres in the heart. *Brit. Heart J. 31*:718-21, 1969.

Obermeier, O. H. F.: Ueber Struktur und Textur der Purkinjeschen Fäden. *Arch. Anat. Physiol. wiss. Med. 245*:358, 1867.

Palicki, B.: *De Musculari Cordis Structura.* Dissertation, Breslau. Purkyně, J. E., 1964. *Opera omnia,* 6, pp. 265-89, 1839.

Purkinie, J. E.: Nowe spostrzezenia i badania w przedmiocie fizyologii i drobnowidzowej anatomii. *Rocznik Wydzialu lekar. Univ. Jagiel. 2*:44-67, 1839. Reprinted in *Opera omnia,* 3, 1939, pp. 52-63.

Purkinje, J.: Mikroskopisch-neurologische Bechachtungen. *Arch. anat. Physiol. wiss. Med.* p. 281. Reprinted in: *Opera omnia* 2, 1937. Gull, W. W.: Microscopical observations on the nerves. *London Med. Gaz. 1:* 1066-69, 1156-58, 1845.

Purkyně, J. (1858): Podrobne zpravy o mojich starsich i novejsich literarnich, zvlaste prirodnickych pracich. *Ziva 6*:41-42, *Opera selecta,* 151-53.

Ranvier, L. A. (187): *Traite Technique Histologie.* Paris. Savy.

Reichert, K. B.: Bericht über die Fortschritte in der mikroskopischen. Anatomie in Jahre 1854. *Müllers Arch.:* 51-54, 1855.

Remak, R.: Ueber die embryologische Grundlage der Zellenlehre. *Müllers Arch.,* p. 230, 1862.

Rothschuh, K. E.: *Entwicklungsgeschichte physiologischer Probleme in Tabellenform.* Wien, München, 1952.

Schmaltz, R.: Die Purkinje' schen Fäden im Herzen der Haussäugethiere. *Arch. wiss. prakt. Thierheilk. 12*:161, 1886.

Siebold, C. T.: Zusatz von Professor v. Siebold. *Ztschft. wiss. Zool. 5*:199-200, 1854.

Tandler, J.: *Anatomie des Herzens.* Jena, Fischer, 1913, p. 200.

Tigerstedt, R.: *Physiologie des Kreislaufes.* 2. Aufl. 2, Berlin-Leipzig, de Gruyter, 1921, pp. 186-87.

Tawara, Sunao: *Das Reizleitungssystem des Säugetierherzens. Eine anatomisch-histologische Studie über das Atrioventrikularbündel und die Purkinjeschen Fäden.* Jena, Fischer, 1906.

Wiggers, J. C.: Some significant advances in cardiac physiology during the 19th century. *Bull. Hist. Med. 34*:1-15, 1960.

Willius, F. A. and Dry, T. J.: *A History of the Heart and the Circulation.* Philadelphia, Saunders. 1948.

CRAWFORD W. LONG, M.D., A GEORGIA INNOVATOR*

JAMES HARVEY YOUNG, Ph.D.

Professor of History
Emory University
Atlanta, Ga.

THE city in which we are assembled began in 1837 as Terminus, evolved to Marthasville, and became Atlanta in 1845, the same year in which the first physician settled in the town.[1] Several months before the shift from Terminus to Marthasville, in a village some 80 miles to the northeast, another Georgia physician used ether to anesthetize a patient for surgery.

The year was 1842. The village of Jefferson, Ga., lay a short distance east of the Cherokee lands from which the Indians had been forcibly removed four years before and sent westward along the trail of tears. Now the press reported rumors of a vast Indian conspiracy forming in the West, spurred by a dissident Cherokee leader.[2] The nation was in the grip of economic depression. Henry Clay, as a last task before giving up his senatorial seat to his successor, led the Senate in trying to resolve the government's grave fiscal crisis.[3] Not all observers thought Congress was in a sufficiently earnest mood. According to one orator, congressmen, instead of making laws to govern the country, merely played "at the game of president-making."[2] In an Augusta newspaper, a correspondent philosophized on the state of the nation: "Ruin seems to stalk through the country; the low price of all southern and western produce must tend to create a spirit of dissatisfaction that may end in a complete revolution of our political system, provided always that we do not have to fight some foreign power—which, however to be regretted is the only panacea for our present disorders."[4]

War seemed a panacea that might be administered soon. Relations were tense with Britain because of the *Creole* affair.[5] Slaves aboard this coastwise trading vessel had mutinied and taken the ship to Nassau,

*Presented as the Wood Library-Museum of Anesthesiology's Fifth Annual Historical Lecture on October 20, 1971, at the meeting of the American Society of Anesthesiologists in Atlanta, Ga.

where British authorities had freed all the slaves except those who had taken part in the revolt. Even more ominous reports came from the Lone Star Republic. Efforts to influence Mexico to acquiesce in Texan independence had failed. Santa Anna had put his armies on the offensive, predicting that Mexico would "plant her Eagle Standards on the banks of the Sabine."[2] Sam Houston pleaded for volunteers from the United States to help counter the Mexican danger. Such was the news in the Georgia press during the week that Crawford W. Long first used ether.

The story is familiar to you all. Late in 1841, Jefferson's young set learned of the amazing antics brought on by nitrous oxide administered to volunteers by an itinerant showman, one of a host of such performers who had been crisscrossing America for some time. Jefferson's young men besought one of their number, Dr. Long, a 26-year-old bachelor, to make some of the wonder gas for their own private use. Long had no apparatus by which to prepare and preserve the gas. He did, however, have some sulphuric ether which, he said, "would produce equally exhilerating [sic] effects."[6] While in medical school in Philadelphia he had seen a showman use ether, after which Long and other medical students had locked themselves in a room at their boarding house and enjoyed a private ether jag.[7]

Hearing this testimonial from their physician friend, Long's companions were all the more anxious "to witness its effects." Long first gave ether to a member of the group who also had inhaled it on a previous occasion. He took some himself then gave some to all the other young men present. "They were so much pleased with the exhilerating [sic] effects of ether," Long wrote, "that they afterwards inhaled it frequently, and induced others to do so, and its inhalation soon became quite fashionable in this county, and in fact extended from this place through several counties in this part of Georgia."[6]

Nor did observing the ether sniffing remain a male prerogative. Word, of course, leaked to the Jefferson maidens. Preparations were made to admit them to one of the revels in Dr. Long's office. In February 1842 Long wrote to a former member of the Jefferson circle who had moved to nearby Athens and asked him to have some ether sent posthaste. "We have some *girls* in Jefferson," the young physician explained, "who are anxious to see it taken and you know nothing would afford me more pleasure than to take it in their presence & get a few sweet kisses. . . . You will perhaps think the 'darnation['] of such

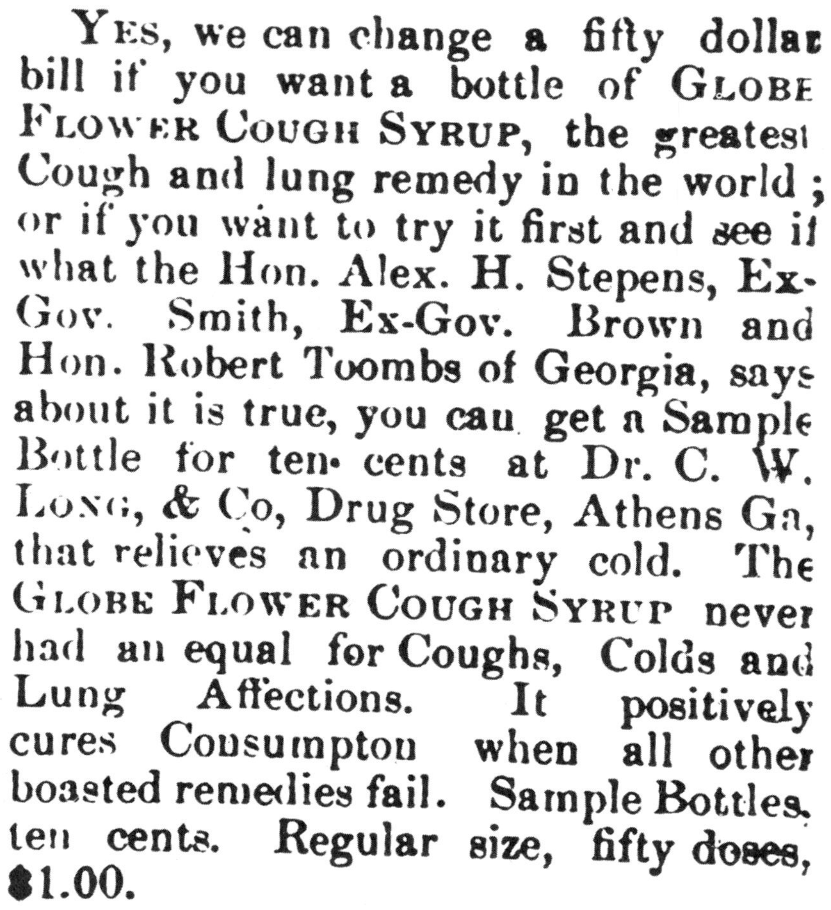

Yes, we can change a fifty dollar bill if you want a bottle of Globe Flower Cough Syrup, the greatest Cough and lung remedy in the world; or if you want to try it first and see if what the Hon. Alex. H. Stepens, Ex-Gov. Smith, Ex-Gov. Brown and Hon. Robert Toombs of Georgia, says about it is true, you can get a Sample Bottle for ten cents at Dr. C. W. Long, & Co, Drug Store, Athens Ga, that relieves an ordinary cold. The Globe Flower Cough Syrup never had an equal for Coughs, Colds and Lung Affections. It positively cures Cousumpton when all other boasted remedies fail. Sample Bottles ten cents. Regular size, fifty doses, $1.00.

Fig. 1. Testimonial by Hon. Alexander H. Stephens and other notables in favor of a cough syrup sold at the drug store of Dr. C. W. Long in Athens, Ga. From the *Southern Banner,* Athens, Ga., August 8, 1878. Reproduced by courtesy of Special Collections Department, the University of Georgia Libraries, Athens, Ga.

troubles, but 'by golly' if you'll attend to it I'll think of you when I am kissing the girls and wish you was present to enjoy some of the pleasure."[8] The event itself turned out to be almost sedate. Warning the girls that they must not hold him responsible for any effects the ether might have on him, Long sniffed the moistened towel, then walked solemnly around the room and kissed each girl in turn.[9]

Contrary to what some writers have asserted, it seems unlikely that among the girls whom Long kissed was Caroline Swain, the young lady 10 years his junior whom he would wed just six months later. For in the first letter Crawford ever wrote to Caroline, who had left Jefferson for a visit to Monroe, Ga., it is apparent that the two had begun to see each other only very recently, had met only a "few times," and then on the most formal basis. Crawford's letter is courtly but ardent, restrained but unquestionable in its amorous intent. Caroline waits a discreet interval and then replies with equal grace and archness, sending him a "watch-paper" she has painted. ". . . we have had but little acquaintance & consequently know but little of each other," she says, yet she makes clear she is fending off the young widower who woos her and tells Crawford she awaits his letters "with impatience" and receives them "with pleasure." The stately waltz continues. Crawford's passion rises. He tells Caroline he has dreamed of kissing her cheek, then apologizes for having written so boldly of this dream. He composes a poem for her, reporting that flowers bloom and birds sing, but he is depressed because "the *girl I love* is now away." Caroline answers immediately. The widower still urges his suit, but Caroline now makes a joke of him. Her growing love for Crawford shines through her formal phrases. She is soon to go to another town and tells Crawford: "if you have not too great a partiality for keeping bachelor's hall I would be pleased to see you." In a postscript Caroline comes even closer to giving her heart away: "I wish to see you very much more than I ever did before, every day *increases*, instead of *diminishes* this desire."[10]

So much for the epistolary beginning of a rapid courtship, the prelude to a life-long love. What relevance do these love letters have to understanding Crawford Long's role in medical history? Intriguingly, this crucial period in Long's personal life and the crucial period in his professional life almost exactly coincide. Crawford's first letter to Caroline is dated March 14, 1842, 16 days before Long, having learned the lesson from his stumbling companions at the office frolics, used ether in operating on one of them. His second letter to Caroline comes three weeks after the operation. In the first letter, Long does not allude to what he might be contemplating, nor in the second does he refer to what he has done. Indeed, he scarcely mentions his medical practice. In his first letter he explains that he must write rather than travel to visit Caroline, because "as you know it is beyond my power to leave home at any time," certainly because his practice keeps him so busy. In his

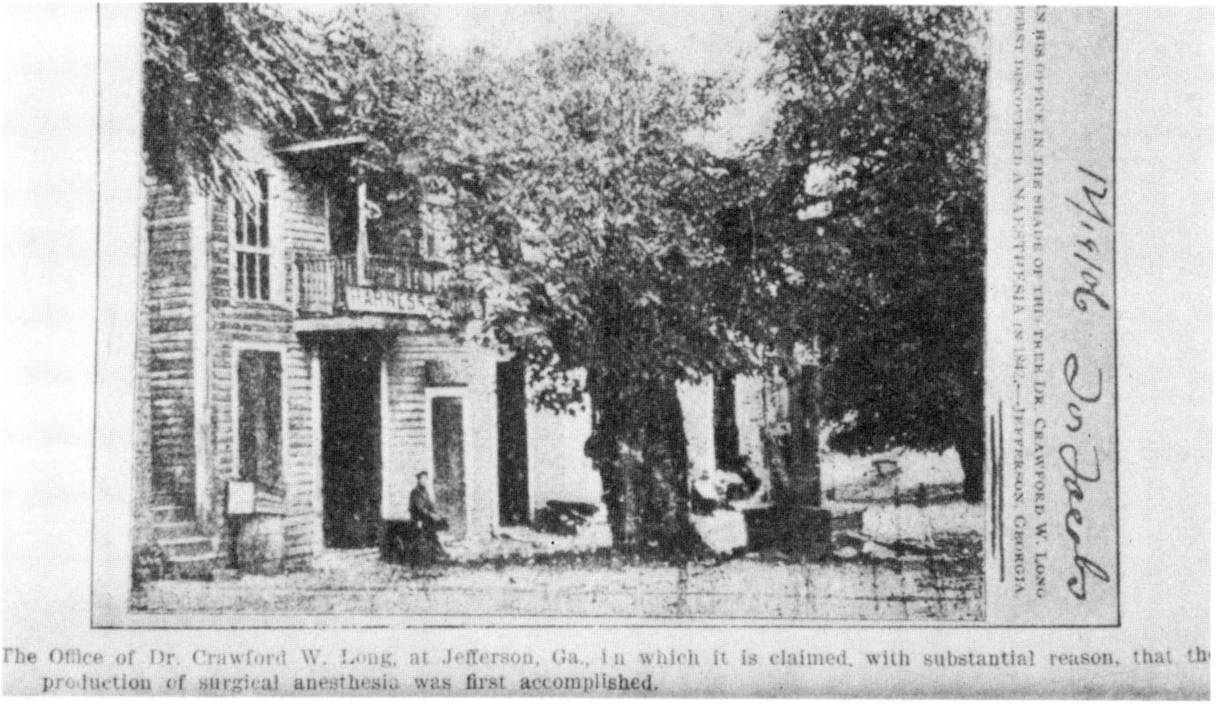

Fig. 2. Long's office in Jefferson, Ga., site of the operation (1842) during which he employed ether to anesthetize James Venable. The office no longer exists. Photograph courtesy of A. W. Calhoun Medical Library, Emory University, Atlanta, Ga. Reproduced by permission of the Parks and Historic Sites Division of the Georgia Department of Natural Resources.

second letter he explains his delay in answering by saying, "I have been absent from my office (unavoidably) every night" since receiving her letter except for one night, and on that night he had begun to compose an answer when "two intruders" came by his office and would not leave until "all the common topics of conversation" had been exhausted. Long was then too tired to continue his epistle. Indeed, he went to bed and promptly had his dream about kissing her cheek. So Long's practice usually kept him busy even at night. Nor do Caroline's letters, except for their salutation, "Dr. Long Sir," make any reference to her ardent correspondent's medical career.

We must recognize that courtship letters, especially in that era of romanticism, conformed to certain conventions. They had a single purpose, and that aim was certainly not to convey the workaday news. Yet one is tempted to wonder if the absence of any comment in Long's letters to Caroline Swain about his employment of ether as an anesthetic may suggest that Long, who certainly did not keep the episode secret, failed at the time to regard his innovation as of momentous significance to surgical history. Might there not have been, even in a love letter, one proud Eureka?

Whether or not Long recognized the full magnitude of his achievement, he certainly did not regard the operation on March 30, 1842, during which he removed the encysted tumor from the back of James Venable's neck while Venable lay anesthetized, as a casual, unique, never-to-be-repeated stunt. Not casual, because Long saw to it that witnesses were present, including the principal of the local academy at which Venable was a student. Not unique, because Long used ether at least five more times before he read in a medical journal about Morton's demonstration in Boston.[6]

Nor were these later operations all merely repetitive. In 1843 Long removed three tumors from a woman's head, the first and third without anesthesia, the second with the aid of ether. In 1845 Long amputated two injured fingers of a slave boy, using anesthesia for one operation but not for the other. Despite the spread of the terrifying rumor that Long was a mad doctor who would put people to sleep and then carve them up, he used ether for operating when the occasion seemed to warrant, which was not often in a country practice in those days.[11] Later Long experimented with ether in his obstetrical practice. His own wife was included among his patients. After the fact, Long ex-

Fig. 3. Marble plaque in Jefferson, Ga., at the site of Long's office, which has been replaced by a museum operated by the Parks and Historic Sites Division of the Georgia Department of Natural Resources. Photograph by the author.

plained his delay in publishing his findings on the grounds of scientific caution.

"At the time I was experimenting with ether," he wrote, "there were physicians 'high in authority,' and of justly distinguished character [especially in Georgia], who were the advocates of mesmerism, and recommended the induction of the *mesmeric state* as adequate to prevent pain in surgical operations. Notwithstanding thus sanctioned, I was an unbeliever in the science, and of the opinion, that if the mesmeric

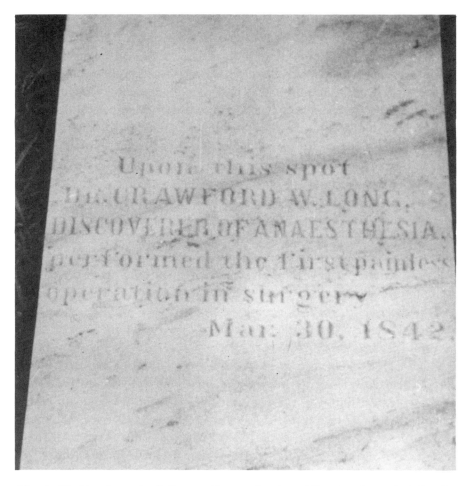

state could be produced at all, it was only on 'those of strong imagination and weak minds,' and was to be ascribed solely to the workings of the patient's imaginations. Entertaining this opinion, I was the more particular in my experiments in etherization."[6]

For this reason and in order to eliminate the possibility that his etherized patients happened to have a high spontaneous resistance to pain, Long performed his experiments on the woman's head and the boy's fingers. Thus, whether or not Long thought scientifically in anticipating publication, he behaved scientifically in following up his discovery.

Nor is this surprising. Long was as well trained as any village doctor in America. His father, a man of substance—plantation owner, miller, owner of railroad stock, clerk of court, state senator—believed in education. He had founded the academy at which Venable later studied. Through his friendship with the president of Franklin College (later the University of Georgia), the senior Long had his son admitted earlier than the stipulated age. Whether or not, as family tradition held, Crawford Long and Alexander H. Stephens actually roomed together, the college careers of the two men overlapped. Upon graduation in 1835, Long returned to Jefferson, ran the academy for a year, read medicine for a while with a local doctor, then rode his horse from Georgia to Kentucky to attend the medical school at Transylvania. Long's father held Henry Clay in high esteem, and Clay entertained Long's son at Ashland. In 1838 Crawford Long transferred to the Medical School of the University of Pennsylvania, from which he was granted his M.D. degree the next year. He had certainly received there the best training the nation offered.[11] One of Long's professors, George B. Wood, an editor of the *United States Dispensatory*, strove through his lectures to improve the quality of American medical publication. He abhorred the reporting of the isolated experiment and he scorned premature announcements. Long's biographers have seen Wood's influence in the Georgia physician's caution in submitting his experiments with ether for publication.[7, 12]

After receiving his degree, Long spent a year and a half "walking the hospitals" in New York City. Not much is known about this significant period. Long's daughter stated that her father specialized in surgery, gained a reputation for his skill, and received counsel that this ability might find a fruitful outlet in the navy.[11] But Long rejected this oppor-

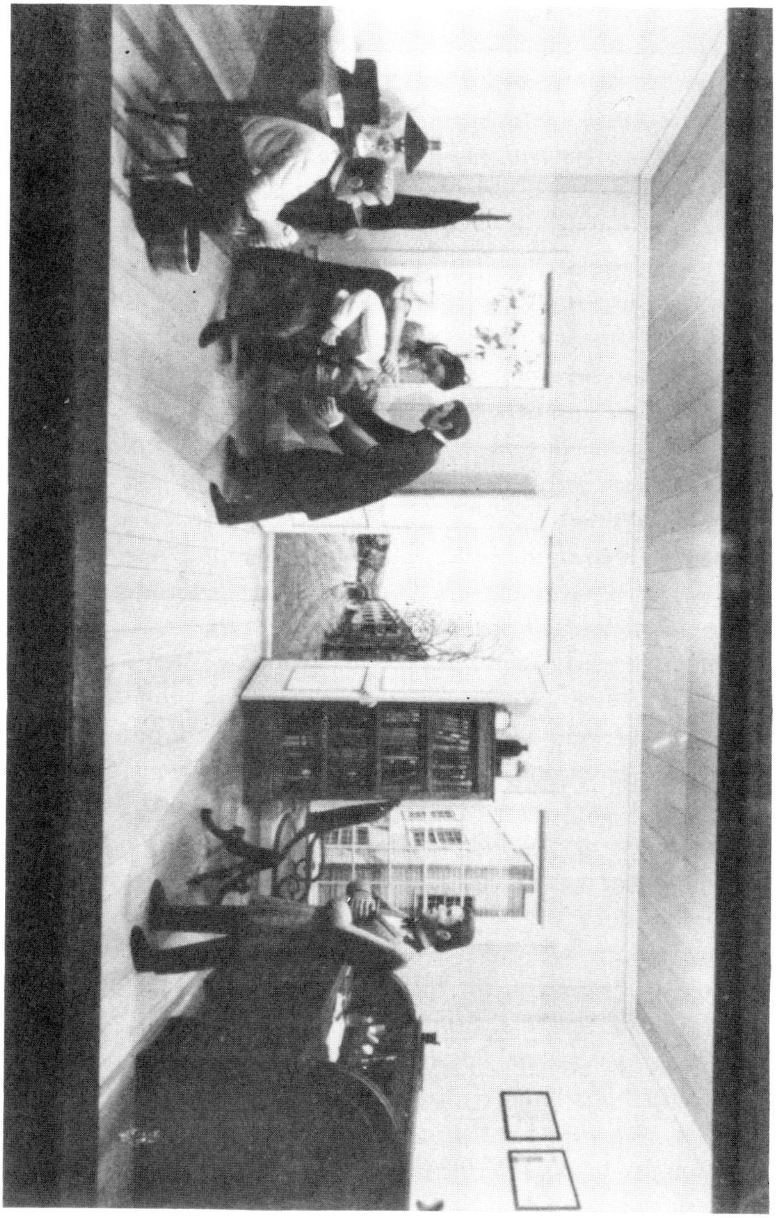

Fig. 4. Diorama in the museum at Jefferson, Ga.; an attempted depiction of the scene of the operation. In his later account Long was chary of details. The diorama version seems unlikely. Photograph courtesy of A. W. Calhoun Medical Library, Emory University, Atlanta, Ga. Reproduced by permission of the Parks and Historic Sites Division of the Georgia Department of Natural Resources.

tunity. Yielding to his father's entreaties, he came home to Jefferson, where he bought the practice of his earlier preceptor. The date was 1841, a year before his rendezvous with Venable.

An unanswerable although pregnant question poses itself: suppose Crawford Long had remained in New York, or had entered the navy, or had returned to Philadelphia, instead of going home to a Georgia country practice, would he have used ether for surgery? Maybe so. In his first paper on the subject he wrote that, when his young companions begged him to make them some nitrous oxide and he countered by suggesting ether, he had told them: ". . . I had inhaled it myself, and considered it as safe as the nitrous oxide gas."[6] No doubt his conviction about the safety of ether rested on his own experience in his Philadelphia boarding house. Whatever the course of his later surgical career, then, at some point, having seen a succession of patients suffering great agony, Long might have remembered ether and sought out its anesthetic properties.

But maybe not. For the received medical wisdom during this period held ether to be extremely dangerous.[12] The shocked reaction of many periodicals to the first report of Morton's experiment testifies to this. It might be argued that an orthodox physician practicing in an urban citadel of orthodoxy might confront barriers to innovation, psychological barriers because of the climate of opinion, and, with respect to surgery, more tangible barriers because hospital surgery was hardly a one-man affair. Had Crawford Long been a city surgeon, then, whatever lessons he had drawn from his medical school ether jag, he might not have put them to use in the operating room. But Long turned his back on urban surgery. As well trained as an American physician could be, he returned to the American frontier, where the heavy hand of medical orthodoxy barely touched his shoulder, and where the pressing exigencies of a far-flung practice for which he alone was responsible fostered innovation. Long's use of ether provides a stellar example of the pragmatic contributions arising from frontier medicine. It is perfectly in character that another such innovator, J. Marion Sims, pioneer operative gynecologist, should later become one of Long's most ardent champions.[13]

And what of that urban medical citadel, Boston, and the famous event that occurred in the surgical amphitheater of the Massachusetts General Hospital on October 16, 1846? To be sure, the highly orthodox

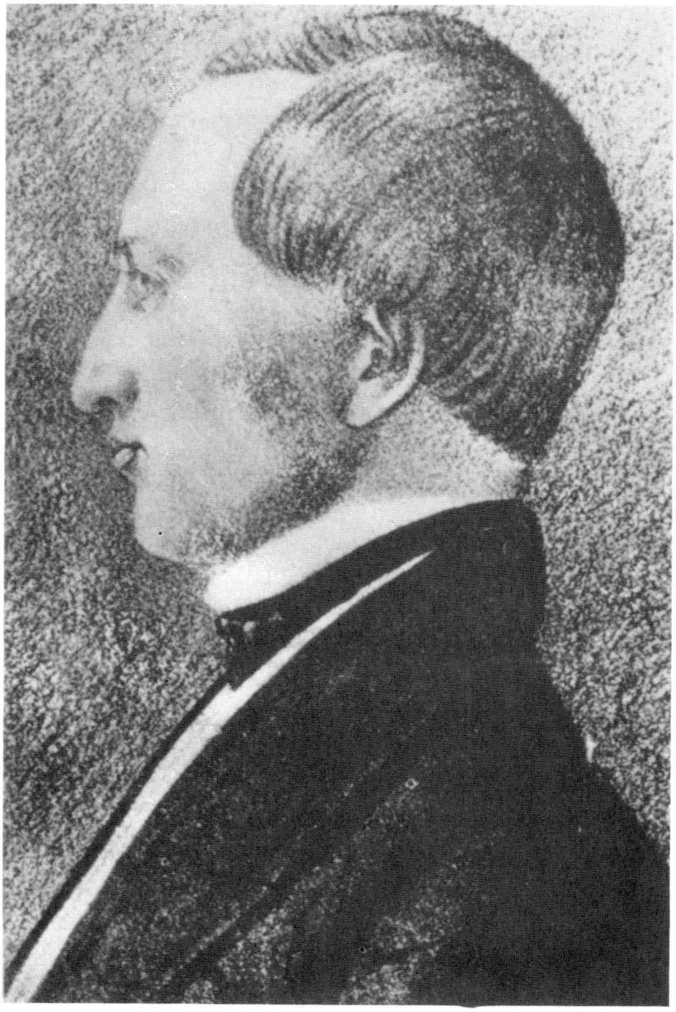

Fig. 5. Crawford W. Long at the age of 26. From a crayon portrait made a few months after his first use of ether as an anesthetic. From Frances Long Taylor: *Crawford W. Long & the Discovery of Ether Anesthesia.* New York, Hoeber, 1928. Photograph by courtesy of Special Collections Department, the University of Georgia Libraries, Athens, Ga.

surgeon, John Collins Warren, performed the operation. But William T. G. Morton administered the Letheon.[14] In the first half of the 19th century, dentistry still stood outside the pale of full respectability as a health profession. In earlier centuries orthodox ethics forbade specialization by the physician, who must accept all comers. The itinerant tooth-puller mingled with the quacks. One such European wanderer advertised his prowess upon entering a new town by pulling a molar with one hand while firing a revolver with the other, his head meanwhile being covered with a sack. Something of this cloud still hung over American dentistry, although pragmatic innovation was bringing major advances. Dentists had a large stake in painlessness, for they hoped to make their patients into steady customers, whereas a surgeon most probably would perform only a single operation on a given patient.[15] Morton was a dentist, and so was Horace Wells. And whatever term might be used to characterize the third member of the Massachusetts triumvirate, the physician-chemist Charles T. Jackson, orthodox is certainly not the word.[9]

Thus Long, a physician with orthodox training who practiced in the free atmosphere of the frontier, and Wells and Morton, members of an as yet scarcely orthodox profession who practiced in urban centers in New England, discovered anesthesia within the same decade. This is the significant generalization, I believe; the tired tussle over priority is not.

Controversy over priority has dominated consideration of the early history of anesthesia from the beginning. Morton, Wells, and Jackson locked horns bitterly, to the ultimate disaster of them all. Profit combined with pride as motives for establishing priority. When Morton could not make his patent on Letheon secure, he sought from Congress a huge sum for his contribution to humanity, a sum that Wells and Jackson and eventually Long wished to share or preempt.[9]

Crawford Long, reading of Morton's administration of ether at the Massachusetts General exhibition, bestirred himself. Long's account book showed that he had charged James Venable two dollars for "Ether and exsecting tumor."[16] But he had not kept contemporary notes. Long finally got around to securing notarized affidavits from Venable and from the witnesses who seven years earlier had watched Long administer the ether and "exsect" the tumor from Venable's neck. Similar documents were acquired from those involved in other of Long's

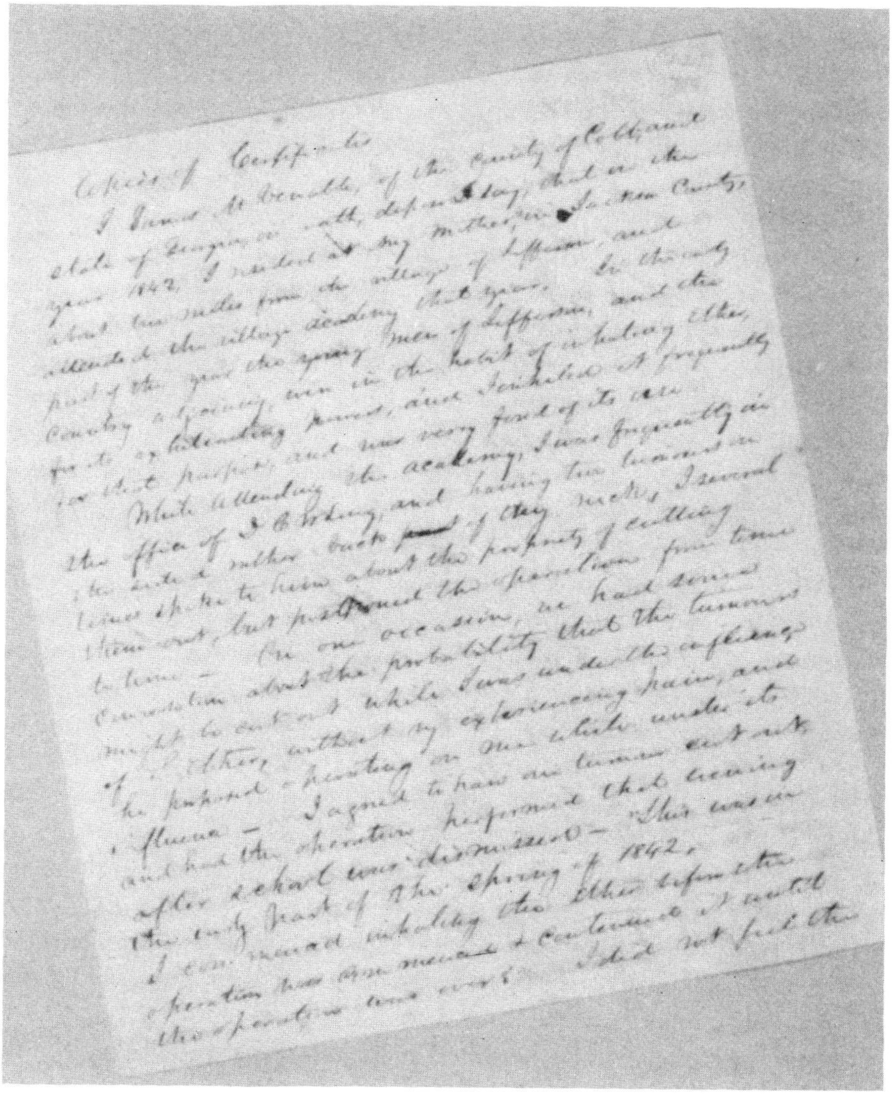

Copy of Certificate

I James M. Venable, of the County of Cobb and State of Georgia on oath, depose & say, that in the year 1842 I resided at my mother's in Jackson County about two miles from the village of Jefferson and attended the village academy that year. In the early part of the year the young men of Jefferson and the country adjoining were in the habit of inhaling ether for its exhilarating powers, and I inhaled it frequently for that purpose and was very fond of its use.

While attending the academy I was frequently in the office of Dr C. W. Long, and having two tumours on the back part of my neck, I several times spoke to him about the propriety of cutting them out, but postponed the operation from time to time. On one occasion we had some conversation about the probability that the tumours might be cut out while I was under the influence of ether without my experiencing pain, and he proposed operating on me while under its influence. I agreed to have one tumour cut out and had the operation performed that evening. This was in the early part of the spring of 1842, after school was dismissed. I commenced inhaling the ether before the operation was commenced & continued it until the operation was over. I did not feel the

Fig. 6. Holograph copy in Long's handwriting of the certificate given him by James Venable, his first ether patient. In 1846, on learning of William T. G. Morton's use of Letheon, Long gathered evidence to establish priority. He secured signed affidavits from patients and from witnesses. The copy in Long's handwriting was later given to the A. W. Calhoun Medical Library by one of Long's daughters. Photograph courtesy of the A. W. Calhoun Medical Library, Emory University, Atlanta, Ga. Reproduced by permission of the Parks and Historical Sites Division of the Georgia Department of Natural Resources.

operations in which ether was used.[6] These documents formed the evidence on which Long based his first published claim, appearing in the *Southern Medical and Surgical Journal* for December 1849, and for his later efforts through a Georgia senator to share in the bounty which Congress was contemplating as a reward for the discoverer of anesthesia. Dr. Long's entrance into the lists further complicated an already confused set of claims. No doubt this factor and the advent of the Civil War caused Congress first to defer, then to abandon, the concept of a monetary grant.

Ethnocentricity has played a major role in many scientific disputes about priority. Unquestionably sectional sentiment helped fire the great ether controversy both before the Civil War and afterward. Morton had champions from north of the Mason-Dixon line, and Long has not lacked Southern defenders, from Marion Sims through Frank K. Boland. One 20th century Georgia governor barred from use in the state's schools a science textbook that gave credit to Morton and neglected Long.[17]

Throughout his long life, marked by no medical pioneering beyond his interest in ether, Crawford Long considered as his greatest treasure the copies penned in his own hand of the certificates he had gathered. By the time of the Civil War Long lived in Athens, where he practiced medicine and ran a drug store. During the summer of 1864 a division of federal cavalry threatened the town. Long quickly prepared to send his family by carriage to a plantation deemed safe from the raiders. Just as the carriage was leaving, Dr. Long hurried from the house with a large jar containing some heirloom watches and a roll of papers. These "are most important," Long said to his oldest daughter, "and under no circumstances must be lost, they are the proofs of my discovery of ether anesthesia." Long besought the girl to bury the jar in a secluded spot until the danger had passed. After much difficulty she did. Later she recovered the treasure. The papers remained Long's prized possession, locked in "a little green traveling trunk" in the attic, which the Long children were cautioned by their mother "never to play with."[11]

All along Long had restudied his documents periodically. He had taken them out to show to Dr. Jackson when that northern claimant came by Athens in 1854 to discuss priority. Even though Jackson, after the conversation, rather swung to Long's side, perhaps to spite Morton, Jackson's visit set at work a suspicion in Long's mind. From a fragment

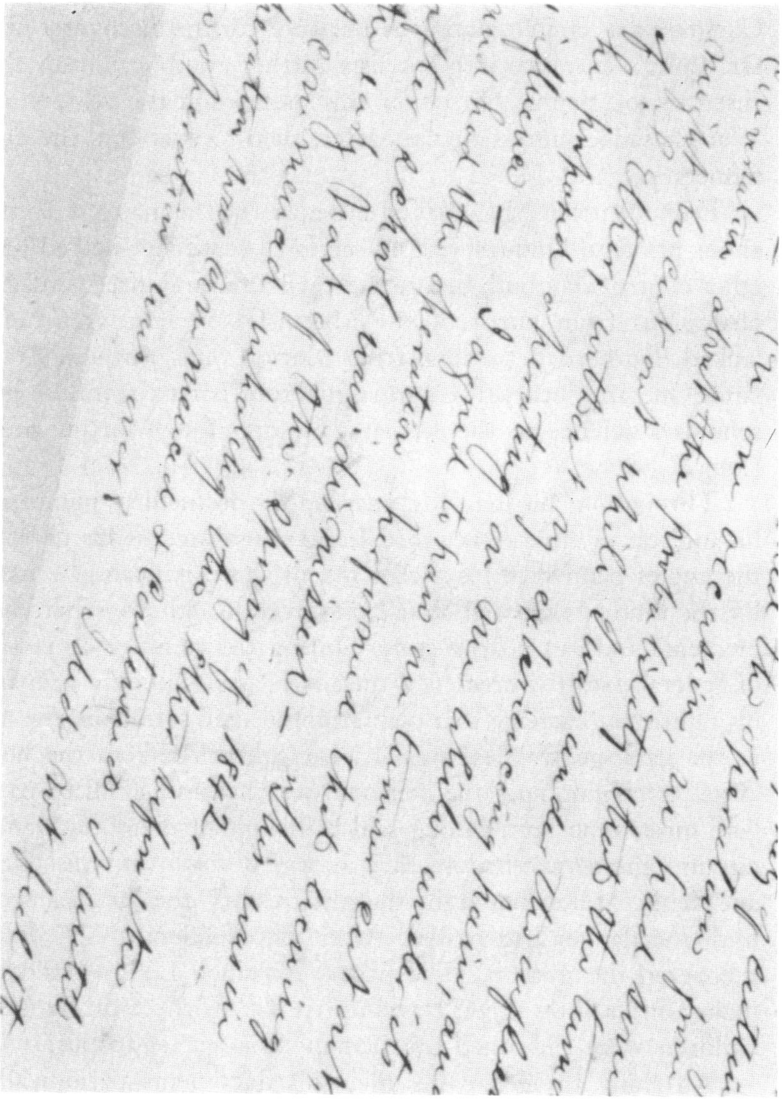

Fig. 7. Detail from Long's holograph copy of Venable's affidavit. The statement reads: ". . . I commenced inhaling the ether before the operation was commenced & continued it until the operation was over. . . ." Photograph courtesy of A. W. Calhoun Medical Library, Emory University, Atlanta, Ga. Reproduced by permission of the Parks and Historic Sites Division of the Georgia Department of Natural Resources.

of a letter in Long's hand, it is apparent that the idea occurred to him that if somebody from Massachusetts could come to Georgia in 1854 why not in 1842 or shortly after, and there hear the talk about Long's use of ether. Indeed, Long remembered, about that time a traveling dentist had come through the county. Could he, Long wondered in retrospect, have been Morton or Wells?[7]

In disputes over priority, this tendency on the part of contestants to suspect the pilfering of their discovery occurs frequently and understandably. Long knew that his use of ether came from his own brain. Surprised by news of another such use at a later time and gradually perceiving dimensions of importance to the discovery not initially sensed, Long would find it as difficult as many other scientists similarly circumstanced not to suspect foul play. The other alternative, independent invention, poses grave threats to self-esteem.

Many latter-day students of the great ether controversy have recognized that both Long and Morton deserve credit, Long for his use of ether for surgery—even though this was not published immediately—and Morton for his public demonstration that enlightened the world. But the partisan polemical nature of much of the commentary has tended to obscure basic aspects of this classic case of multiple discovery.[13] I have alluded to the weight of received opinion, the orthodox view of the danger of ether, as a delaying factor. Yet is this alone enough to explain a delay of more than four decades in the use of *either* ether or nitrous oxide after Sir Humphry Davy's often-quoted broad hint of 1800? "As nitrous oxide in its extensive operation appears capable of destroying physical pain," Sir Humphry wrote, "it may probably be used with advantage during surgical operations in which no great effusion of blood takes place."[14] In addition to this explicit prediction, there was the continuing uncomprehended clue of hundreds of willing exhibitionists bumping painlessly into furniture during theatrical demonstrations of nitrous oxide and ether. The delay, although often noted, has not been assessed fully. Internal medicine possessed more prestige than surgery at the time; doubtless this was a retarding factor.[15] Further detailed study of the period may reveal other medical and social considerations not now recognized as probable hampering forces.

When the decade destined for the multiple discovery came, however, the setting for it was the United States, where orthodoxy rested more lightly than in Europe, and the codiscoverers represented two of the more pragmatic and empirical facets of American medicine, one professional, the other geographical. Wells and Morton practiced dentistry and Crawford Long, the Georgia innovator, a doctor on horseback, exercised his own creative medical judgment on the frontier.

REFERENCES

1. Garrett, F. M.: *Atlanta and Environs.* New York, Lewis, 1954, vol. 1, pp. 150, 189, 216, 224-25.
2. *Georgia Messenger,* Macon, Ga., March 31, 1842.
3. *Southern Whig,* Athens, Ga., April 15, 1842.
4. *Southern Banner,* Athens, Ga., April 8, 1842.
5. *Southern Whig,* Athens, Ga., April 1, 1842.
6. Long, C. W.: An account of the first use of sulphuric ether by inhalation as an anesthetic in surgical operations. *Southern Med. Surg. J. 5*:705-13, 1849.
7. Boland, F. K.: *The First Anesthetic. The Story of Crawford Long.* Athens, Ga., University of Georgia Press, 1950.
8. Incomplete facsimile copy of letter, Long to Robert H. Goodman, February 7, 1842. Crawford W. Long Collection, Special Collections Dept., the University of Georgia Libraries, Athens, Ga. The last sentence of the quotation appears in a handwritten copy of the letter in the Florence Long Scrapbook, *C. W. Long, M.D./1815-1878,* in Special Collections Dept., the University of Georgia Libraries, Athens, Ga.
9. Flexner, J. T.: *Doctors on Horseback. Pioneers of American Medicine.* New York, Viking, 1944, pp. 293-352.
10. Long to Caroline Swain, March 14 and April 20, 1842 and Caroline to Long, April 8, 1842. Box 1, Crawford W. Long Family Papers, Special Collections Dept., the University of Georgia Libraries, Athens, Ga. Caroline to Long, April 25, 1842, Crawford W. Long Memorial Museum, Jefferson, Ga.
11. Taylor, F. L.: *Crawford W. Long & the Discovery of Ether Anesthesia.* New York, Hoeber, 1928.
12. DaCosta, J. C.: Crawford W. Long. In: *Memorial to Dr. Crawford W. Long . . . An Account of the Ceremonies. . . .* Philadelphia, University of Pennsylvania Special Bulletin, April 1912, pp. 8-15.
13. Sims, J. M.: The discovery of anaesthesia. *Va. Med. Monthly 4*:81-100, 1877.
14. Keys, T. E.: *The History of Surgical Anesthesia.* New York, Dover, 1963.
15. Shryock, R. H.: *The Development of Modern Medicine.* New York, Knopf, 1947, pp. 174-76.
16. Long, J. W.: Crawford W. Long. *Trans. Southern Surg. Ass. 37*:312-24, 1924.
17. Unidentified clipping relating to Governor E. D. Rivers (1937-1941). Crawford W. Long Scrapbook compiled by Eugenia Long Harper. Piromis Hulsey Bell Papers, Atlanta Historical Society, Atlanta, Ga.
18. Merton, R. K.: Resistance to the systematic study of multiple discoveries in science. *Arch. Européennes Sociol. 4*:237-82, 1963.

CHEKHOV AMONG THE DOCTORS: THE DOCTOR'S DILEMMA

William B. Ober, M.D.

Attending Pathologist
Beth Israel Hospital

Associate Professor of Pathology
The Mount Sinai School of Medicine of the City University of New York
New York, N. Y.

Gifted with more psychological insight than his biographers and critics, Chekhov appraised his human condition and stated it with his usual concision:

> Self-made intellectuals buy at the price of their youth what gently born writers are endowed with by nature. Go, write a story about a young man, the [grand]son of a serf, the son of a shopkeeper, a choirboy, brought up to respect rank, to kiss the priest's hand, to defer to others' opinions, to offer thanks for every slice of bread, flogged repeatedly, fond of dining with rich relatives, playing the hypocrite before God and man with no other cause than the accepted consciousness of his own unimportance—then tell how this young man presses the slave out of himself one drop at a time, waking up one fine morning to feel that real human blood flows in his veins, not the blood of a slave. . . . (Letter to Suvorin, January 9, 1889,)

Writing this in his 29th year, Chekhov interpreted his quest for identity as an emancipation. His wretched childhood and inferior education are formulaic, but his march to independence began when his father's small retail shop went bankrupt and the family moved to Moscow, leaving the 16-year-old boy to complete his education at the gymnasium at Taganrog, a grubby port on the Sea of Azov. He began to write short sketches, many wryly humorous, for the school paper. By the time he rejoined his family in 1879 to enter the medical school at Moscow, he had mastered the rudiments of the journeyman writer: brevity and speed. His next step toward independence developed when he became the effective head of the household, supporting his mother and younger siblings by writing innumerable sketches and squibs for the lower

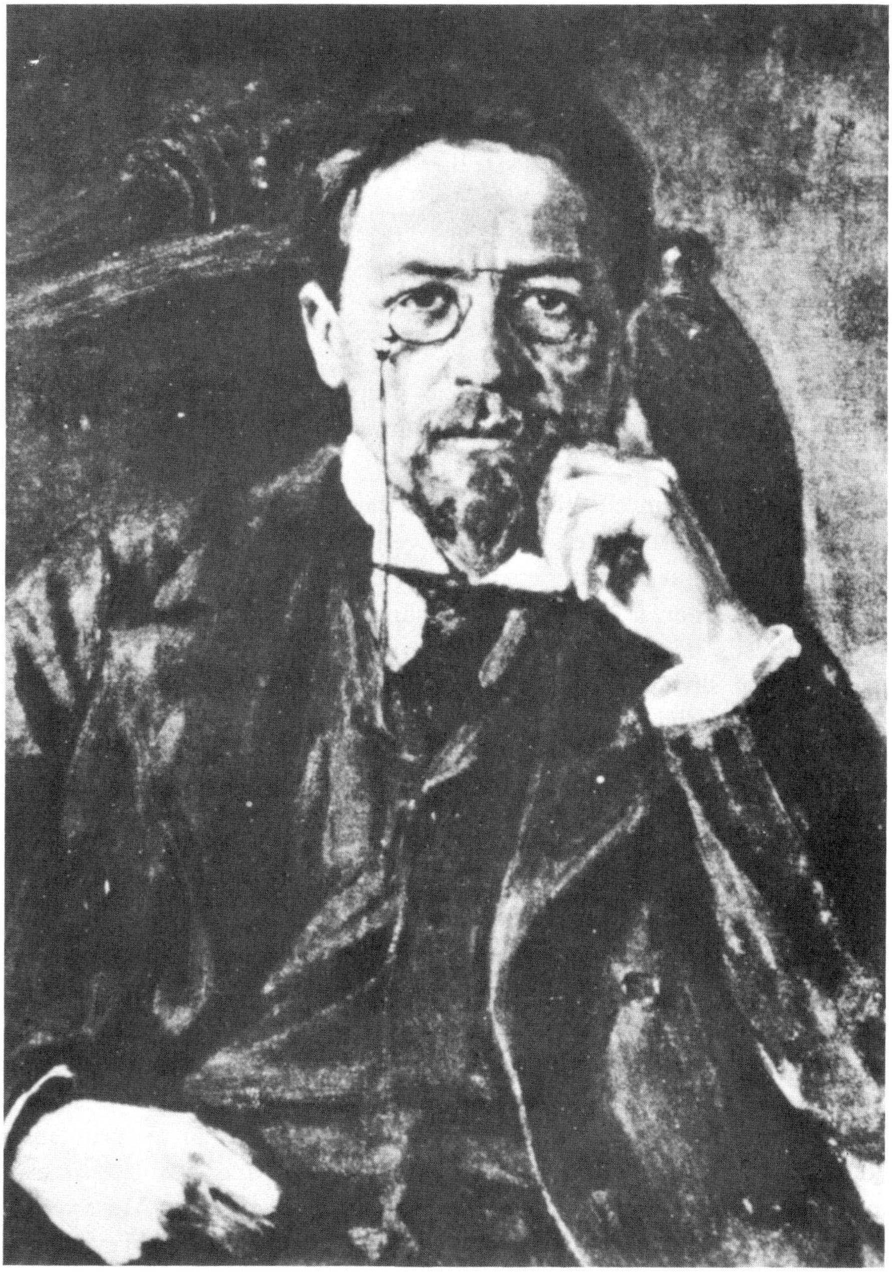

Fig. 1. Portrait of Chekhov by Repin. The three photographs illustrating this article are reproduced by courtesy of the Theatre Collection, New York Public Library, Astor, Lenox, and Tilden Foundations, The Research Libraries, New York, N. Y.

stratum of the Moscow press. He wrote them at top speed, and his unrevised first drafts were "printable."

Chekhov received his medical degree in 1884 and was posted to a *zemstvo* hospital in the country some 30 miles outside of Moscow. He worked there for a year, trying in the meantime to establish a general practice in Moscow and, pressed by circumstances, continued to write in order to make ends meet for his family. All of Chekhov's early pieces were published under the pseudonym of Antosha Chekhonte. It requires little insight to recognize that this was a form of denial; he did not wish his medical colleagues to form an image of him as a writer. But his real name is only thinly veiled, and to it he affixed "*honte*," the French word for shame, whether knowingly or not remaining unknown. However, Chekhov's acquaintances and friends were chiefly drawn from literary and artistic circles. Most of them were struggling or merely scraping by; they were delighted to secure free of charge the services of their young friend, now a qualified physician. Paying patients did not flock to Chekhov, nor did he ever feel his income from medical practice was enough to warrant setting up an office. But his warm, generous nature made it impossible for him to refuse a call, and he continued to live off his literary output. Also, in 1884 he had his first hemoptysis. In retrospect, we know it was tuberculosis, but a single hemoptysis does not make a diagnosis, and Chekhov was quite willing to assume a posture of anosognosia. Repeated episodes of hemoptysis coupled with cough and constitutional symptoms slowly developed and, certainly after 1889, when his brother Nicholas died of tuberculosis, Chekhov was unable to maintain the façade of denial, at least to himself, though he avoided mentioning the disease by name to his family. The inroads of tuberculosis were slow and almost imperceptible; he suffered more conscious pain from hemorrhoids, often aggravated by alternating attacks of diarrhea and constipation. His letters contain more frequent allusions to his rectal problems than to his pulmonary disease, using one level of symptomatic reality to minimize the anxiety engendered by another.

A decisive event in Chekhov's literary career was a letter of praise he received in 1886 from D. A. Grigorovich, then a man of importance in Russian letters. Comments such as "You have a *real* talent, one which places you in the front rank of the coming generation" were coupled with advice to write less prolifically and to concentrate his energies.

It was not easy to cut down production, particularly when money was badly needed, but Chekhov, who had published 129 pieces in 1885 and 112 in 1886, retrenched to 66 in 1887 and only 12 in 1888. Numbers tell only part of the story; Chekhov was able to follow Grigorovich's sound advice because he had established relations with Alexis Suvorin, editor of *Novoe Vremia*, a magazine which not only had prestige but paid high rates. That the magazine's policies were right-wing, anti-libertarian, antiegalitarian and, of course anti-Semitic did not bother Chekhov at the time; he was apolitical. His later breach with Suvorin belongs to another chapter; by that time Chekhov had been exposed to repeated reviews admonishing him for keeping his art separate from life and holding as an example for him Tolstoy's commitment to social causes.

Chekhov's own view of his double life as physician and writer during the period 1886 to 1897, when he finally collapsed with a severe attack of tuberculosis, can be epitomized by two excerpts from his correspondence:

> You advise me not to pursue two hares at a time and to abandon the practice of medicine . . . I feel more contented and more satisfied when I realize that I have two professions, not one. Medicine is my lawful wife and literature my mistress. When I grow weary of one, I pass the night with the other. This may seem disorderly, but it is not dull, and besides, neither of them suffers because of my infidelity. If I did not have my medical work, it would be hard to give my thought and liberty of spirit to literature. (Letter to Suvorin, September 11, 1888.)

It was scarcely two years since Grigorovich's letter had set him to writing seriously. The self-criticism inherent in rewriting first drafts, "rejecting his own thoughts," had shown him explicitly the value of "liberty of spirit," and he had a new sense of his own importance, having adopted a new (and double) persona. The following year he sent an autobiographical sketch for publication in a class album to his classmate, G. I. Rossolimo, one of the few physicians with whom he maintained acquaintanceship:

> My work in medical sciences has undoubtedly had a serious influence on my literary development; it significantly extended the area of my observations, enriched my knowledge, and only one who is himself a physician can understand the true value of

> this for me as a writer; this training has also been a guide, and probably because of my closeness to medicine, I have managed to avoid many mistakes. Familiarity with the natural sciences and scientific method has always kept me on my guard. . . . I do not belong to those literary men who adopt a negative attitude toward science, and I would not want to belong to those who achieve everything by cleverness. (October 11, 1889.)

An added dimension can be given this position statement from a comment of Chekhov's quoted by Ivan Leontiev-Scheglov:

> A simple person looks at the moon and is moved as before something terribly mysterious and unattainable. But an astronomer looks at it with entirely different eyes . . . with him there cannot be any fine illusion! With me, a physician, there are also few illusions. Of course, I'm sorry for this—it somehow desiccates life.

Chekhov's success as a writer stemmed from his ability to adopt a detached clinical attitude, to observe people's conduct, their mixed motives, their compromises with reality—much as a sensible doctor looks at a patient. Consciously, he tried to create artistic unity out of life's disorder by assimilating his view of human behavior into literary expression. His eye was sharp for telling detail, his ear keen for the cadence of everyday speech, even the speech which partly conceals and partly reveals motive, and he had an almost intuitive grasp of character. His biographer Simmons writes, "In his infinite concern to avoid the superfluous . . . he achieved by artistic measure and economy of means a refinement of expression that was truly classical, and an illusion of reality—based on his favorite touchstones of objectivity, truthfulness, originality, boldness, brevity, and simplicity—that seemed quite complete." But, as is usually the case in fiction or drama, it is the *illusion* of reality which is created, and the *seeming* completeness, though it begins with the writer's work, depends in part upon the reader's ability (or willingness) to follow him in his desire and pursuit of the whole.

Literary success and public acclaim—he was awarded the Pushkin Prize in 1889—did not make Chekhov's life complete. Such phrases as "There is a sort of stagnation in my soul" and "For the lonely man, the desert is everywhere" can be lifted from his letters. He had a semiconscious desire to expand his horizons of action, a motive which, coupled with his frustration and loneliness, led to his famous trip to Sakhalin in 1890-1891. For a man who had half-admitted to himself that he had pulmonary tuberculosis, such a trip across the Siberian wastes before the days of the Trans-Siberian railroad was, objectively speaking, sheer folly. And to what end? Chekhov proposed a census of that remote dismal penal colony north of Japan which would be tantamount to a sociological survey (the term had not then been coined) of the life of the exiled felons. Moreover, he proposed to carry out the study without assistants. He prepared for it by reading everything about Sakhalin on which he could lay his hands. He sought help from official quarters but received almost none; the Czar's government was not interested in having the facts of life on its Devil's Island exposed to public view. It took Chekhov three months to get there, and he spent almost four months taking notes, interviewing as many convicts as he could, but it was a period during which he saw nothing but misery and human degradation. Any reasonable fool could have told him he was risking his health, wasting his energy, squandering his talents on a lost cause. But the trip was his catharsis, his private bell for inexplicable needs; possibly he finally resolved his quest for emancipation by comparing his "liberation of spirit" as physician and writer with the lot of the dead souls on Sakhalin. Some sins are not crimes against the state.

On his return he wrote *The Island of Sakhalin*, which was published in 1892, a straightforward piece of reportage describing conditions as he saw them. He had no conviction that such a free-lance study would persuade the government to modify its policies, nor did he ever mount a public campaign for reform, though he continued to correspond with individual convicts whose plight had touched him. Predictably, the book had no effect on penological policy. Viewed in context, Chekhov's mission seems almost a gratuitous act by a man who felt himself superfluous. And, having digested that slice of life, he was satisfied by converting it to a literary experience.

He made one futile gesture to find an audience for his ideas. In 1893 he conceived the notion of submitting *The Island of Sakhalin* as a thesis for the degree of Doctor of Medical Sciences which would have qualified him as a *privatdozent*, permitting him to lecture at the medical school. He enlisted the aid of Rossolimo, then well on his way to distinction as a neuropathologist, writing: "If I were a teacher, I would try to draw my audience as deeply as possible into the area of the subjective feelings of patients, for I think that would prove really useful to the students."

Chekhov's desire to have a foot in academic medicine may have developed from his experiences the previous year when he had returned to active medical work by helping control a cholera epidemic near Melikhovo where he lived, but that could have been only an immediate precipitating cause. A deeper reason was his sensitivity to the emotions he saw being acted out by the people he knew, as well as the implicit recognition, known so well to any man with first hand medical experience, that these emotions are intensified, even uncovered, in the sickbed. Of course, the dean disregarded the petition for the degree, but it can be construed as an example of Chekhov's partly formed ideas on medical psychology (as distinct from clinical psychiatry, which then dealt chiefly with major organic and functional psychoses). It was half a century before the term "psychosomatic medicine" came into vogue, but we can credit Chekhov with having such an idea in embryo and for having derived it himself.

Chekhov's fascination with human conduct and motivation was deep-seated, and upon it depended his ability to create fictional characters who seemed "real" or "natural." Every critic has commented on the vast number of characters from all walks of life who populate Chekhov's pages. Yet Chekhov was not merely attracted to people as a passing parade; he presented their surfaces in order to illuminate their interiors, hence his famous dictum on the style of naturalism in the Russian Art Theatre with which he was closely identified from 1897 to his death in 1904:

> Let everything on the stage be just as complicated and at the same time just as simple as it is in life. People just eat their dinner, just eat their dinner, and all the time their happiness is being established or their lives are being broken up.

Chekhov projected onto his own characters his personal mode of assimilating experience and reacting to it: the perception of reality from inner needs, regardless of external circumstances. Both in his own life and in his fictions the outlook and self-definition of individuals are informed by and result from an internalization of reality.

But one must exercise caution in pursuing Chekhov's psychological insights and analyzing particular stories as if they were designed to illuminate psychological principles. Chekhov's psychology was based on the ideas current in his time, those of the late 19th century. He had no crystal ball to tell him that 20th century psychodynamics would emphasize the unconscious as a motive force, that its *res gestae* would be the ontogeny of individual cases, tracing current problems back to events in childhood and reconstructing elaborations from such starting points. Using the short story and the stage drama as his chosen media, Chekhov limited himself to presenting the "here and now," the situation as it exists in a small segment of time. On at least one occasion he tried to write a novel but found that the extended form was alien to him. Sharp as were his *aperçus* into an immediate situation, he usually lacked the ability to depict its evolution from initiating causes into florid symptoms.

Nor did Chekhov attempt to systematize or develop a set of generalizations from his insights. On many occasions he disavowed the idea that he, as a writer, should either teach or preach. Although, his early years excepted, he was not a miniaturist, he was a particularist. Much like a pointillist painter, he placed his sentences and short paragraphs on paper as if they were small, discrete spots of color on a canvas, creating a picture which became organized as a cognitive entity only when the reader held it at arm's length and examined it from a middle distance. With too close a view his images do not take shape, nor is the relation of one to another decisive; from too great a distance the particularity of the experience being rendered lacks substance, and even its color pales.

In some of Chekhov's short stories the psychological element is typological, for example: Gromov's break with reality in *Ward 6* is readily diagnosable as paranoid schizophrenia with transient, ill-structured ideas of persecution, solipsistic withdrawal, and mental deterioration; in *The Black Monk*, Kovrin experiences visual hallucinations with religious content; in *Grief*, the cab driver Potapov displays the need for catharsis when overwhelmed by the death of his son. But some of the most illuminating examples of psychopathology are to be found among the fictive physicians whom Checkhov created. It is in these, the literary counterparts of members of his chosen profession, that Chekhov most clearly shows his hand. The open question is: To what extent did Chekhov's own limited success in medicine contribute to the projection of doctors in his fictions? How did he internalize the reality of his own status? How did he transform life into letters? Let us examine a few of his doctors and see what light they shed on his dilemma.

Dr. Startsev, the hero of *Ionych* (1898), enters as the rural district medical officer stationed outside a small provincial town. He makes the acquaintance of the Turkin family, the pretentious leaders of the bourgeois intelligentsia, who seem to believe they are running a salon. He falls in love with their daughter Katerina, but she has her heart set on studying the pianoforte at the conservatory, and she trifles with him. Soon after she leaves town, Startsev opens his practice; despite his distaste for the narrow-minded provincial types, he prospers. Katerina returns, having found that her musical talent is inadequate for a career. She would now like to marry Startsev, but his interest in her has flickered out. Chekhov leaves him as a greedy, choleric bachelor whose original ideals have been corroded.

Doubtless Chekhov drew upon his own experiences in provincial towns for the setting, upon his own observations of more than one fellow-physician who succumbed to materialism, and upon any number of pseudointellectuals for the other characters. It is much the same ambience that Sinclair Lewis described in greater detail in *Main Street* and *Babbitt;* both Chekhov and Lewis knew the stifling effect of small towns and hated them. Chekhov's tale is a slice of life, but the picture he draws is too close to the real to be a complete fiction, and his figures are not heroic enough to support the idea of a myth. Underlying the denouement is a theme common to many of Chekhov's stories: namely, that men and women who attempt to develop an intimate relation, whether consummated or not, wind up lonely, frustrated, unhappy, alienated, and defeated. This tells us more about Chekhov than he might wish us to know, but precisely why his Dr. Startsev lacks either the ability to perceive his plight or is unable to escape from it remains uncharted.

A more complex failure is Dr. Ragin in *Ward 6* (1892), the director of a hospital in a small provincial town who gradually withdraws from the task of properly managing his understaffed, poorly equipped hospital, taking refuge in reading philosophy and history, drinking vodka, and eating cucumbers. This doctor rationalizes his maladresse by developing the idea that men must seek peace and satisfaction in themselves, not in the world around them. Though he maintains his internal equipoise, his stance is of little help to the psychotic patients in Ward 6, who are at the mercy of the brutal guard Nikita, who beats them frequently and cheats them of even their few kopecks. Dr. Ragin establishes a quasi-friendship with Gromov, a mildly paranoid schizophrenic on the ward, who contrives to be a philosopher of sorts. Dr. Ragin's inadequacy makes it easy for Dr. Khobotov, his scheming assistant, to force his resignation. Ultimately, after a financially ruinous trip to Moscow with a friend, Dr. Ragin is committed to Ward 6, where Nikita beats him and he dies of a stroke, having lost the comfort of his quietist philosophy, finally aware of the years of physical pain and moral suffering which his withdrawn way of life had inflicted on his defenseless patients.

As Chekhov's fiction goes, it is a long story, even a novella, and here he does have space and scope. Step by step, he shows the gradual nature of Dr. Ragin's withdrawal and his increasingly tenuous grasp of reality. The secondary characters are fleshed out; tension is increased by having first a patient, then a fellow-physician alternate as deuteragonist to the central character. Even as Chekhov leads the reader slowly into the unreal pseudophilosophical world of Dr. Ragin's prolix dialogues with Gromov, he returns him to the level of reality in the scenes with Dr. Khobotov and the intercalated episode of Dr. Ragin's financial ruin. One passage prefigures the existential mode; Dr. Ragin remarks: "My illness is only that in twenty years I've found only one intelligent person in the whole town, and he's a lunatic. There's no illness whatsoever; I simply fell into a bewitched circle from which there's no exit." As the proverb tells us: Life? One can never get out of it alive.

Shorter than *Ward 6* and narrower in scope is *A Dreary Story* (1889), relating the case of Dr. Stepanovich, a professor of medicine, who describes in the third person his failing mental and physicial powers. Insomnia is his chief complaint, but he cannot find a satisfactory cause. The reader is not surprised when the aging professor unwittingly reveals that he is in love with his young ward Katya. Lust and illicit passion are alien to his self-controlled, rational persona; consequently he represses his feelings. The anxiety so engendered manifests itself as insomnia, fear of imminent death, and a congeries of minor psychosomatic symptoms. Much of this story's success depends upon the relatively simple nature of the protagonist's intrapsychic conflict which enables Chekhov to maintain the narrative flow at a single level.

Chekhov's doctors share a lack of self-confidence and purpose; he presents them as incomplete men in an advanced state of copelessness. To generalize that they are projections of himself is a simplistic notion

19 00.

Художественно-Общедоступный Театръ

(Каретный рядъ, „ЭРМИТАЖЪ").

Воскресенье, 8-го Октября:

Дядя Ваня,

сцены изъ деревенской жизни въ 4-хъ дѣйствіяхъ, А. Чехова.

(31-е представленіе).

УЧАСТВУЮЩІЕ:

Серебряковъ, Александръ Владиміровичъ, отставной профессоръ . . . . В. В. Лужскій,
Елена Андреевна, его жена . . . . О. Л. Книпперъ,
Софья Александровна (Соня), его дочь отъ перваго брака . . . . М. П. Лилина,
Войницкая, Марья Васильевна, вдова тайнаго совѣтника, мать первой жены профессора . Е. М. Раевская,
Войницкій, Иванъ Петровичъ, ея сынъ . . . А. Л. Вишневскій,
Астровъ, Михаилъ Львовичъ, врачъ . . . К. С. Станиславскій,
Телѣгинъ, Илья Ильичъ, обѣднѣвшій помѣщикъ . . . . А. Р. Артемъ,
Марина . . . . М. А. Самарова,
Работникъ . . . . М. Г. Григорьевъ.

Дѣйствіе происходитъ въ усадьбѣ Серебрякова.

Режиссеры **К. С. Станиславскій** и **Вл. И. Немировичъ-Данченко.**

Декораціи 1-го дѣйствія художника **В. А. Симова.**

Начало въ 7½ ч. веч., окончаніе около 11½ ч. ночи.

РЕПЕРТУАРЪ.

Понедѣльникъ, 9-го Октября, въ 8-й разъ: **„Снѣгурочка"**, весенняя сказка, А. Н. Островскаго.
Вторникъ, 10-го Октября, въ 31-й разъ: **„Чайка"**, драма А. П. Чехова.

Билеты на всѣ объявленные спектакли можно получать въ кассѣ театра, съ 10 часовъ утра до 10 часовъ вечера.

Цѣны мѣстамъ, со включеніемъ благотворительнаго сбора и за храненіе платья, **на вечерніе спектакли: Верхній ярусъ**—отъ **30** к. до **1** руб. **10** коп.; **Бель-этажъ**—отъ **40** коп. до **1** руб. **80** коп. **Кресла партера**—отъ **85** коп. до **4** руб. **30** коп.; **Ложи**—отъ **5** руб. до **25** руб.. **На утренніе спектакли: Верхній ярусъ**—отъ **20** коп. до **75** коп.; **Бель-этажъ**—отъ **25** коп. до **1** руб. **25** коп.; **Кресла партера**—отъ **40** к. до **2** руб.; **Ложи**—отъ **3** руб. **80** к. до **12** руб.

Главн. режиссеръ К. С. Станиславскій. Завѣд. репертуаромъ Вл. И. Немировичъ-Данченко.

На основаніи ВЫСОЧАЙШЕ утвержденнаго 5 мая 1892 года мнѣнія Государственнаго Совѣта и утвержд. 20 августа 1892 г. правилъ взиманія сбора съ публичныхъ зрѣлищъ и увеселеній, со всѣхъ билетовъ взимается сборъ, оплачиваемый марками, безъ коихъ билеты не дѣйствительны.

Печ. разр. 7 октября 1900 г. Исп. об. Моск. Оберъ-Полиц. Полков. Рудневъ.

Тип. Императорскихъ Московскихъ Театровъ Постав. Двора Его Величества Т-во Скор. А. А. Левенсонъ.

Fig. 2. Playbill of *Uncle Vanya,* Moscow Art Theatre, 1900.

which will not stand under close scrutiny. But Dr. Lvov in *Ivanov* (1888) is young, unmarried, idealistic, and the moral conscience of the play; to that extent he bears a superficial resemblance to his author. However, Lvov stands aghast but impotent as Ivanov cruelly deceives and manipulates his wife, who is dying of tuberculosis. Lvov has a passionate desire to cure humanity's ills but he cannot prevail against Ivanov's cupidity and lechery. Ivanov's wife's distress is made more poignant by Chekhov's casting her as a Jewess who has been rejected by her family for marrying outside her faith and has no recourse. One may speculate that Chekhov was attracted to the theme of intermarriage because in 1886 he was sufficiently in love with a Jewish girl to consider marriage, a scheme which foundered when she would not apostasize and he would not consider civil marriage.

Equally impotent is Dr. Dorn in *The Sea Gull* (1896), an aging bachelor of 55, an engaged bystander to Treplev's love affair with Masha but even more fascinated by Treplev's play. He regrets his limitations: "You know, I've led a varied and discriminating life. I'm satisfied, but if it had ever been my lot to experience the exaltation that comes to artists in their moments of creation, I should have despised this earthly shell . . . and I'd have soared to the heights, leaving the world behind." Alas for his lofty *Anspruchsniveau:* when Treplev commits suicide, the doctor and would-be artist is immobilized; confronted by the suffering of his friends, he can say only, "What can I do, what can I do?"

Another aging, disillusioned doctor is Dr. Astrov in *Uncle Vanya* (written 1890, produced 1898). More interested in forestry than medicine, he comments, "Only God knows what our real vocation is": a fair statement of Chekhov's own plight. Astrov imagines that his reforestation scheme—even the 1890s had their ecological problems—is the plan of a scientist-artist-creator-savior whose change in nature can effect a change in man, a romantic notion which is insufficient to conceal that he is a burnt-out case. Although he is able to talk Uncle Vanya out of a suicidal gesture, he is not able to convince Elena (or himself) that his affection for her is substantial enough to be considered love. Nothing happens, nothing is consummated. Astrov is reduced to the vague hope "that when we are sleeping in our graves we may be attended by visions, perhaps even pleasant ones."

The last of Chekhov's stage doctors is Ivan Chebutykin, an army doctor, in *Three Sisters* (1900-1901). The play deals with the blighted hopes of the principal characters, and Chebutykin's contribution to the general attitude of despair is to add further negative values. Incompetent as a doctor, mildly alcoholic, unlettered, and socially gauche, he is little more than a stock fool. In reply to Irmy's question about an incident on the boulevard he replies: "What happened? Nothing. Nothing worth talking about. It doesn't matter." The schoolteacher Kulygin attempts to draw the incident out of him, but he replies again: "I don't know. It's all nonsense." To which Kulygin responds: "In a certain seminary a teacher wrote 'nonsense' on a composition, but the pupil, thinking it was Latin, read 'consensus.' " Chebutykin is a grotesque caricature of a man. Instead of marrying the widowed mother of the three sisters (are we supposed to think of them as Fates?), he breaks the woman's clock, a symbolic defloration where none would be required, thereby foreclosing a successful resolution. He abdicates his reponsibilities, even pretending ignorance about the arrangements for the duel in which Tusenbach is fated to die and leave Irina bereft. Pretending to know nothing, he becomes nothing, and is even willing to acknowledge his nonexistence:

> Perhaps we imagine that we exist, but we don't really exist at all. . . . Perhaps I'm not even a man at all, but just imagine I've got hands and feet and a head. Perhaps I don't exist at all and only imagine that I walk and eat and sleep. . . . Oh, if only I didn't exist.

Finally, Chekhov has managed to reduce one of his doctors to existential nothingness.

There is no doctor in Chekhov's last play, *The Cherry Orchard* (1903-1904). Following his severe attack of tuberculosis in 1897, Chekhov gave up any semblance of practicing medicine and confined his waning energies to writing. His chief interest lay in the Moscow Art Theatre, which produced his plays, and through it he met the actress Olga Knipper, who became his wife in 1901. Having disposed of the archetype in Chebutykin, he no longer had any need to create lonely, hollow men out of his fictive physicians.

The most frequent comment about Chekhov's plays is that "Nothing happens." That is, "people just eat their dinner. . . ." At the same time the drama of life continues, and the course of these people's lives is being decided at the same time, but they are unable to influence events

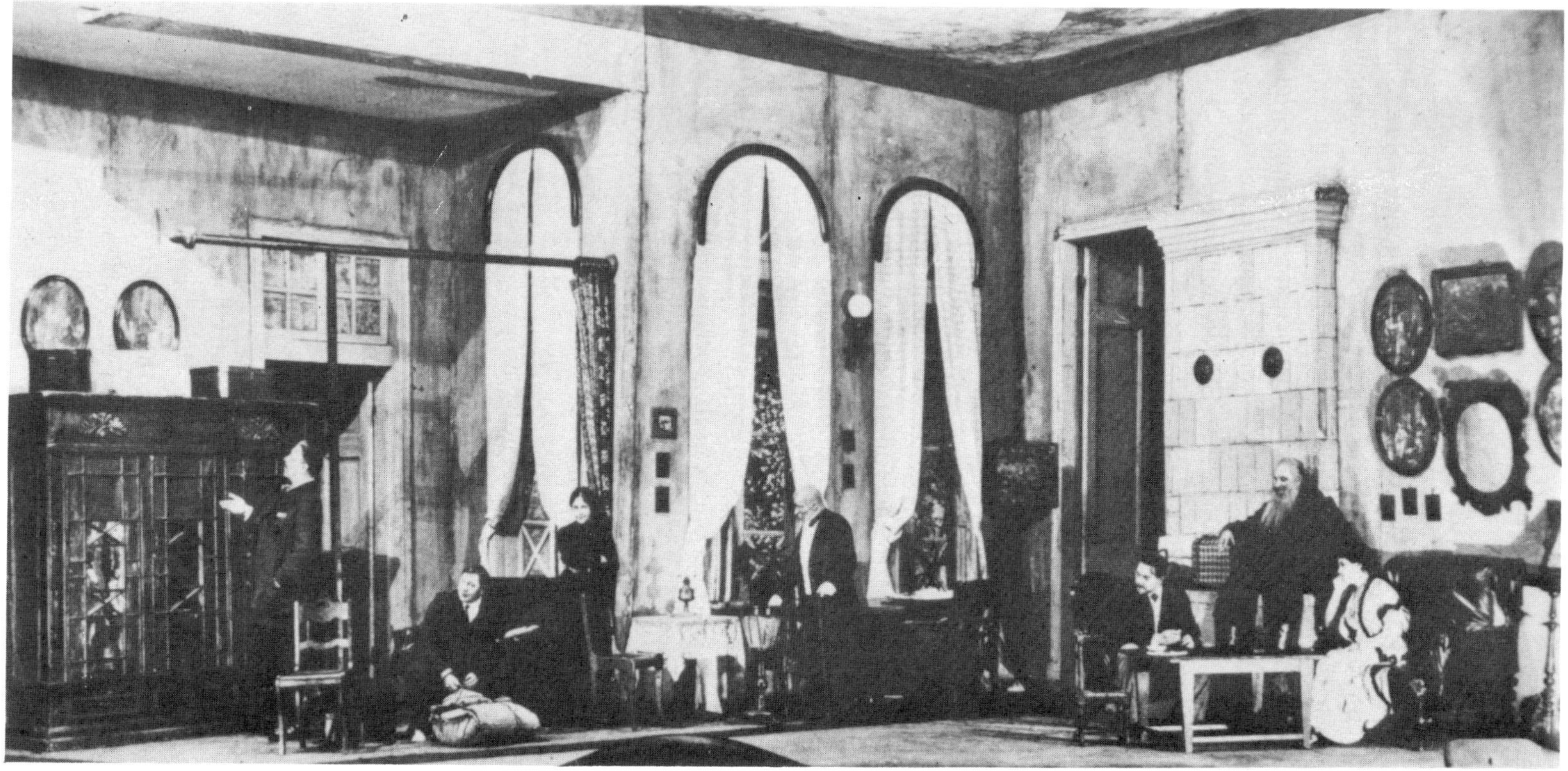

Fig. 3. The set and characters of *The Cherry Orchard* in the Moscow Art Theatre's New York production, 1926.

by insight or will. Even as Chekhov wrote his plays and stories, enjoyed the company of his friends, wrote letters, helped build schools and libraries, courted his wife, and ate his dinner, the tubercle bacillus continued its unremitting work of destruction. The germ which attacked him when he was a young man learning to heal the sick shortened his life, and there is no reason to doubt that for the last seven years of it he knew his time was short. In one sense, the "nothing happens" posture is a defense which implies "nothing is happening to me."

Chekhov died in Germany in 1904. When his doctor wanted to apply an ice bag to his chest, he looked up and said, "One does not put ice upon an empty heart." He then asked for a glass of champagne, drank it, and died. His body was returned to Moscow is a train marked Oysters. Had he been alive to witness it, the bon vivant in him would have commented on the felicity of the final marriage between champagne and oysters, but as it was, "nothing happened," and, as in Werther's sorrows, Charlotte, like a well-bred girl, went on eating bread and butter.

MIGRAINE IN ASTRONOMERS AND "NATURAL PHILOSOPHERS"

IN Charles Hilton Fagge's *Principles and Practice of Medicine*,[1] one of the best medical textbooks ever written, the following remarkable statement occurs in the section on migraine:

> A very curious circumstance in regard to the visual affection is that some of the best and most careful descriptions of it have been written, not by medical men, but by astronomers and natural philosophers. Wollaston, Arago, Sir David Brewster, Sir John Herschel, Sir Charles Wheatstone, Du Bois Reymond, Sir George Airy, and Professor Dufour, of Lausanne, may be mentioned as having been liable to this paroxysmal defect of sight, and as having carefully noted its phenomena; and no similar malady has, within the present century, been the subject of two papers admitted into the 'Philosophical Transactions,' as well as of communications to the 'Philosophical Magazine' and other scientific journals at home and abroad. It may be a question whether persons who are not accustomed to employ the eyes for minute observation would notice the dimness of sight, or regard it as of sufficient importance to be mentioned to their physician. Indeed, when it commences at some distance from the centre of vision, I believe it is sure to be overlooked, unless the patient's attention is specially directed to its occurrence. And this may, perhaps, be the reason why Professor Du Bois Reymond does not mention it in describing this form of headache as he has experienced it himself.

A search for the scientists and the descriptions mentioned by Fagge revealed a plenitude of interesting material.[2] The first author in point of time is William Hyde Wollaston (1766-1828), M.B. 1788, M.D. 1793, the gifted physicist and chemist who discovered palladium and rhodium, invented a method for welding pure platinum, created numerous optical devices, and contributed an early study of the solar spectrum.[3] Since 1800 Wollaston had had occasional attacks of bilateral partial blindness. In 1824 further observation of his hemianopsia led him to the opinion—previously advanced by Sir Isaac Newton[4]—that the optic nerves were semidecussated. Wollaston reported his observations as follows:[5]

It is now more than twenty years since I was first affected with the peculiar state of vision, to which I allude, in consequence of violent exercise I had taken for two or three hours before. I suddenly found that I could see but half the face of a man whom I met; and it was the same with respect to every object I looked at. In attempting to read the name JOHNSON, over a door, I saw only SON; the commencement of the name being wholly obliterated to my view. In this instance the loss of sight was toward my left, and was the same whether I looked with the right eye or the left. This blindness was not so complete as to amount to absolute blackness, but was a shaded darkness without definite outline. The complaint was of short duration, and in about a quarter of an hour might be said to be wholly gone, having receded with a gradual motion from the center of vision obliquely upwards toward the left.

Since this defect arose from over fatigue, a cause common to many other nervous affections, I saw no reason to apprehend any return of it, and it passed away without my drawing any useful inference from it.

It is now about fifteen months since a similar affection occurred again to myself, without my being able to assign any cause whatever, or to connect it with any previous or subsequent indisposition. The blindness was first observed, as before, in looking at the face of a person I met, whose *left* eye was to my sight obliterated. My blindness was in this instance the reverse of the former, being to *my right* (instead of the left) of the spot to which my eyes were directed; so that I have no reason to suppose it in any manner connected with the former affection.

It is of additional interest that Wollaston died in 1828 of brain tumor.

In 1824 François Arago (1786-1853), the astronomer and physicist, published a French translation of Wollaston's paper.[6] To this he subjoined an editorial note[7] in which he stated:

The affection described by M. Wollaston is quite common. I know four persons who are subject to it, and I myself have had three attacks in the last month. The first and second times I could not see things situated to the right of the axis of vision. The third time, on September 27, 1824, objects on the right were, on the contrary, the only ones I could see. For example, having directed my gaze at the right limb of the M of the word BAROMETRE, which

> was written in large characters above an instrument, I could see this stroke perfectly and also the remaining letters ETRE, but I could not see at all either the first upstroke of the M or the BARO. Whichever eye I used, the same phenomenon prevailed. A headache appeared on the right side above the eye about twenty minutes later when the half-blindness ceased. . . .

On February 20, 1865 Sir David Brewster (1781-1868), the famous physicist, eminent for studies of optical phenomena, read before the Royal Society of Edinburgh a paper titled *On Hemiopsy, or Half-Vision.*[8] Brewster wrote:

> . . . Having myself experienced several attacks of hemiopsy, I have been enabled to ascertain the optical condition of the retina when under its influence, and to determine the extent of the affection, and its immediate cause.
>
> In reading the different cases of hemiopsy, we are led to infer that there is vision in one-half of the retina, and blindness in the other. But this is not the case. The blindness, or insensibility to distinct impressions, exists chiefly in a small portion of the retina to the right or left hand of the *foramen centrale*, and extends itself irregularly to other parts of the retina on the same side, in the neighbourhood of which the vision is uninjured. In some cases the upper half of the object is invisible, the part of the retina paralysed being a little below the *foramen centrale*. On some occasions, in absolute darkness, when a faint glow of light was produced by some uniform pressure upon the whole of the retina, I have observed a great number of black spots, corresponding to parts of the retina upon which no pressure was exerted.
>
> In the case of ordinary hemiopsy, as observed by myself, there is neither darkness nor obscurity, the portion of the paper from which the letters disappear being as bright as those upon which they are seen. Now, this is a remarkable condition of the retina. While it is sensible to luminous impressions, it is insensible to the lines and shades of the pictures which it receives of external objects; or, in other words, the retina is in certain parts of it in such a state that the light which falls upon it is irradiated, or passes into the dark lines or shades of the pictures upon it, and obliterates them.

The most valuable of the older descriptions of migraine was com-

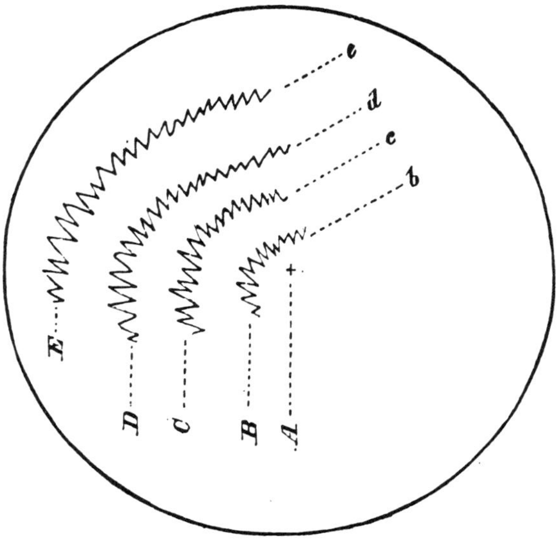

Figure. Disturbance of the visual field in migraine. Drawing by Sir George B. Airy, Astronomer Royal. Reprinted from *London, Edinb., and Dubl. Phil. Mag.,* ser. 4, *30:* 19-21, 1865.

A, the beginning of the disease.

Bb, Cc, Dd, Ee, successive appearances, as the arch gradually enlarges.

posed by Sir George Biddell Airy (1801-92), the Astronomer Royal. Airy wrote as follows:[9]

> I have myself been frequently attacked by it, certainly not fewer than twenty times, probably much oftener; and I am acquainted with two persons who have suffered from it, one of them at least a hundred times. From the information of my friends, and from my own experience, I am able to supply an account of some features of the malady which appear to have escaped the notice of Dr. Wollaston and Sir David Brewster. . . .
>
> I discover the beginning of the attack by a little indistinctness in some object at which I am looking directly; and I believe the locality of this indistinctness upon the retina to be, not the place of entrance of the optic nerve, but the centre of the usual field of vision. Very soon I perceive that the indistinctness is caused by the image being crossed by short lines which change their direction and place. In a little time the disease takes its normal type, and presents successively the appearances shown in the following diagram. [See

Figure.] In drawing this, I have supposed that the principal obscuration of objects is apparently on the left side; by reversing the figure, left to right, the appearances will be given which present themselves when the principal obscuration appears to be on the right side. (In my own experience, I believe it is an even chance whether the obscuration is to the right or to the left.) The bounding circle shows roughly the extent to which the eye is sensible of vision more or less vivid. Only one arch is seen at one time: the arch is small at first, and gradually increases in dimensions.

The zigzags nearly resemble those in the ornaments of a Norman arch, but are somewhat sharper. Those near the letters B,C,D,E are much deeper than those near b,c,d,e. The zigzags do not change their relative arrangement during the dilatation of the arch, but they tremble strongly: the trembling near B,C,D,E is much greater than that near b,c,d,e. There is a slight appearance of scarlet colour on one edge, the external edge, I believe, of the zigzags. As the arch enlarges, vision becomes distinct in the centre of the field. The strongly-trembling extremity of the arch rises at the same time that it passes to the left, and finally passes from the visible field, and the whole phenomenon disappears.

I have never been able to decide with certainty whether the disease really affects both eyes. The first impression on the mind is that only one eye is affected (in the instance depicted above, the left eye). There is general obscurity on one side; but the tremor and boiling are so oppressive, that, if produced only in one, they may nearly extinguish the corresponding vision in the other.

The duration of this ocular derangement with me is usually from twenty to thirty minutes, but with one of my friends it sometimes lasts much longer. In general, I feel no further inconvenience from it; but with my friends, it is followed by oppressive head-ache. . . .

Those who lay stress on psychic predispositions will read with interest the description of Sir George Airy that appears at the beginning of his autobiography.[10]

The ruling feature of his [Sir George Airy's] character was undoubtedly Order. From the time that he went up to Cambridge to the end of his life his system of order was strictly maintained. He wrote his autobiography up to date soon after he had taken his degree, and made his first will as soon as he had any money to leave.

> His accounts were perfectly kept by double entry throughout his life, and he valued extremely the order of book-keeping: this facility of keeping accounts was very useful to him. He seems not to have destroyed a document of any kind whatever: counterfoils of old cheque-books, notes for tradesmen, circulars, bills, and correspondence of all sorts were carefully preserved in the most complete order from the time that he went to Cambridge; and a huge mass they formed. To a high appreciation of order he attributed in a great degree his command of mathematics, and sometimes spoke of mathematics as nothing more than a system of order carried to a considable extent. In everything he was methodical and orderly, and he had the greatest dread of disorder creeping into the routine work of the Observatory, even in the smallest matters.

Elsewhere in his autobiography[11] Airy states that during the meetings of the British Association that were held in Cambridge in June 1833 he had Sir David Brewster and Mr. [John] Herschel as his guests and breakfasted with them daily. We may wonder whether these three migrainous astronomers discussed their common affliction.

S.J.

NOTES AND REFERENCES

1. Fagge, C. H. *The Principles and Practice of Medicine,* Pye-Smith, P. H., ed.; 2d ed. London, Churchill, 1888, vol. 1, p. 781.
2. Emil Du Bois-Reymond, having observed his own case of hemicrania, considered the ailment to be a disturbance of the sympathetic nervous system. See his "Zur Kenntniss der Hemikrania," *Arch. f. Anat. Physiol. u. Wissensch. Med.,* 1860, pp. 461-68.
3. Hartog, P. J. and Lees, C. H. William Hyde Wollaston. In: *Dictionary of National Biography,* vol. 21. London, Oxford Univ. Press, 1921-1922, pp. 782-87.
4. Newton, I. *Opticks* (London, 1730). Reprinted from 4th ed. [London, 1730]. London, Bell, 1931, pp. 346-47.
5. Wollaston, W. H. On Semi-Decussation of the Optic Nerves. *Phil. Trans. 114:* 222-31, 1824.
6. Wollaston, W. H. De la semi-décussation das nerfs optiques. *Ann. de Chimie et de Physique 27:*102-09, 1824.
7. *Ann. de Chimie et de Physique 27:*109-10, 1824.
8. Brewster, D. On Hemiopsy, or Half-Vision, *London, Edinb., and Dublin Phil. Mag.,* ser. 4, *29:*503-07, 1865. Reprinted in *Trans. Roy. Soc. Edinb. 24:* 15-18, 1867.
9. Airy, G. B. The Astronomer Royal on Hemiopsy. *London, Edinb. and Dubl. Phil. Mag.,* ser. 4, *30:*19-21, 1865.
10. Airy, W., ed. *Autobiography of Sir George Biddell Airy.* Cambridge Univ. Press, 1896, p. 2.
11. *Ibid.,* pp. 99-100.

BRAZIL'S LONG FIGHT AGAINST EPIDEMIC DISEASE, 1849-1917, WITH SPECIAL EMPHASIS ON YELLOW FEVER*

DONALD B. COOPER, Ph.D.

Professor, Department of History
The Ohio State University
Columbus, Ohio

"ONE comes to the tropical or semitropical countries for the first time with an idea that they are hotbeds of all disease and veritable pest holes."[1] This statement was made by Dr. W.J.S. Stewart, a United States naval surgeon stationed in Rio de Janeiro in 1904. At the time, few residents of temperate zones would have argued the point with Dr. Stewart and many would have singled out Brazil as one of the world's worst offenders in matters of public health. There is much historical evidence to support such a view; so much so, in fact, that one is surprised to discover that until about 1850 Brazil was widely known for her remarkably salubrious climate. The following statement, written by an English naval physician in 1830, is rather typical of opinions expressed before 1850 on the state of health in South America, including Brazil.

> The inhabitants of the shores of this vast continent [of South America], whether permanent or occasional, enjoy a high and a singularly uniform degree of health.
>
> . . . Epidemic diseases are scarcely known; with widespreading and destructive force they are totally unknown. The [yellow] fever which frequently makes such havoc in the West Indies never makes its appearance here. . . . The people of this continent . . . are not free from febrile disease, but they suffer little from it; and it may be safely asserted that from severe sweeping epidemics of all kinds they are exempt. Even the malignant cholera . . . has not as yet, it is believed, touched South America.[2]

Another English naval physician wrote that before the introduction of yellow fever "the east coast of South America, from Pernambuco

---

*Presented as part of the Macy Conference on the History of Medicine and Medical Education in Latin America held in Antigua, Guatemala, October 11, 1971.

southward to the River Plate, was for Europeans one of the most healthy regions in the whole world, whether they resided permanently on shore, cruised in vessels along the coast, or lay at anchor in the different ports." [3]

Many Brazilians shared the popular view that the intense heat of the equator somehow provided an invisible but effective barrier against the southward spread of great epidemics. Such shallow optimism was obliterated, however, by the double disaster of epidemic yellow fever in 1849-1850 and Asiatic cholera in 1855-1856. Once present in Brazil, these two diseases together claimed upward of a quarter of a million lives over a period of 50 years.[4] Nor was this all. In the last third of the 19th century smallpox—present since the 16th century—suddenly flared up, the toll from malaria steadily increased, beri-beri was commonly reported after the 1870s, and bubonic plague struck Santos in 1899. In just half a century Brazil's reputation had moved full circle.

In the present paper it will not be possible to examine carefully the history of all these diseases, and so, after touching briefly on cholera, I shall focus in some depth on yellow fever. These were the two epidemic diseases that clearly caused the greatest public concern in Brazil, even though both tuberculosis and infant mortality accounted for a greater loss of life. In 1892 the editor of *The Rio News* wrote that "the bare thought of an epidemic of cholera, or [yellow] fever, seems to set a community wild, and to drive out every particle of commonsense and humanity that it ever possessed. . . . " [5]

Let us turn first to cholera. This disease took a larger toll of human life in Brazil than yellow fever, even though it appeared later and was brought under control earlier. The extraordinary epidemic of 1855-1856 caused more deaths in Brazil than have been officially attributed to yellow fever in all years combined. Dr. Estevao Calvacanti Albuquerque, citing official government documents (*relatórios*), reported 130,940 deaths from Asiatic cholera in all of Brazil during 1855-1856; most of these occurred in the northeastern provinces.[6] In later years, however, a report prepared by members of the faculty of Medicine of Rio de Janeiro indicated that "the epidemic of 1855-1856 caused a mortality of more than 160,000 persons. . . ." [7] It seems likely that the larger figure is more accurate, since reports from remote rural areas often took several years to assemble.

The massive outbreak of cholera had been predicted by Dr. Francisco de Paula Cândido, who discovered several cases of the disease in 1854 among sailors arriving from European ports. The first case definitely known to have originated in Brazil was reported from the city of Belém on May 26, 1855. Dr. Cândido wrote that the epidemic attacked mainly persons from the lower classes, such as "soldiers, sailors, and slaves." [8]

By June 21 the cholera had spread to the city of Salvador, capital of the province of Bahia. Dr. Albuquerque wrote that the crisis that ensued was perhaps the worst the city had ever encountered.

> The idea spread of contagion and inevitable death, the most sacred laws were violated, the city was left without physicians, the authorities abandoned their posts; relatives and friends abandoned the unfortunate patients who died unattended; hundreds of cadavers rotted unburied inside houses; consternation was general; emigration became tumultuous, all was confusion, all was horror.
>
> [Furthermore, in the neighboring town of Santo Amaro] . . . The authorities fled, the doctors followed them; the son abandoned the father, the father the son, the daughter the mother, the husband the wife; thus the most sacred and human obligations were forgotten.[9]

By mid-July cholera had appeared in the city of Rio de Janeiro, where the official response was better organized than it had been in the more primitive Northeast. Medical posts and infirmaries were organized in all parts of the city and no charge was made to the indigent for either medicine or hospitalization. Dr. Albuquerque wrote that "the public charity was without limits; even the aristocracy showed itself charitable!!!" Even so, nearly 5,000 persons died of cholera in the imperial capital alone from July 1855 to April 1856.[10]

Physicians were at a loss to know what to prescribe, since the true nature of the disease was unknown and it was, of course, a new malady for Brazil. Dr. Pio Aducci complained that nothing seemed to work with cholera. "In the cure of this disease, the calefacients do not always bring warmth, the refrigerants do not cool . . . the anti-spasmodics do not calm, the stimulants do not excite, and the counter-stimulants do not abate." [11] Dr. Domingos Rodrigues Seixas wrote that "tobacco has been recommended as effective in the cure of cholera. . . . It is always without any harmful effect for the system." [12] He also urged the use of purgatives but condemned the practice, widespread at the time, of employing leeches. Dr. Manoel Ladislão Aranha Dantas, for example, prescribed the application of "fifteen bloodsucking leeches to the anus" [13] of one patient whose life unfortunately was not spared even by this heroic measure. In the realm of preventive medicine Dr. Seixas offered the almost standard advice that one should avoid milk, butter, fish of any kind, acidic fruits, and cold drinks, and added a special caution that "one should not undertake excessive intellectual labors." [14]

The greatest economic consequence of the great cholera epidemic of 1855-1856 was the loss of thousands of agricultural workers, particularly slaves. Dom Pedro II reported in his "Speech from the Throne" in 1856 that "our agriculture has suffered a considerable loss of laborers, and successively it becomes even more urgent [for] the acquisition of [European] colonists who are industrious and of good morals." [15] Had it not been for cholera 1855 would have been one of the most prosperous years ever experienced by the Brazilian economy.

Never again was there a cholera outbreak in Brazil as serious as that first great epidemic, although important outbreaks occurred between 1867 and 1870—especially among troops fighting in the Paraguayan War,[16]—in 1887 in Mato Grasso,[17] and in 1894-1895 in the Paraíba Valley and in Minas Gerais.[18] The threat of cholera was seldom absent during the second half of the 19th century.

At this point we turn our attention to yellow fever. The first recorded outbreak of this disease in Brazil occurred in the province of Pernambuco in the Northeast between 1685 and 1694.[19] For reasons unknown, the disease then seemingly disappeared in Brazil until the city of Salvador was attacked in the fall of 1849. Some 3,000 deaths were reported in Salvador [20] and within a year the fever had radiated to most of the larger urban centers along the coast; Recife, Natal, and Belém in the north, and Santos and Rio de Janeiro in the south were all attacked.

Since yellow fever had never been reported previously in Salvador, it was widely assumed that the disease had been accidentally imported from abroad. The lack of any certain evidence on this point did not prevent elements of the local press from singling out the American brig *Brazil* as the offending party. This ship had arrived in Salvador on September 30, 1849, after earlier stops at New Orleans and Havana—cities in which yellow fever had long been reported. Two crew members had died of the disease en route, and others died shortly after their arrival in Brazil. Once underway, the epidemic spread rapidly among the ships in the harbor, throughout the city, and for some 20 leagues along the beach, where "it decimated a large part of the inhabitants of the province." [21] One doctor estimated that 80,000 persons suffered an attack in Salvador,[22] and another estimated 3,000 actually died from yellow fever in that city.[23] One victim was the American consul in Salvador, Thomas Torner.[24]

Many persons refused to believe that at long last yellow fever had returned to Brazil. The Minister of Empire, the Viscount of Monte Alegre, in a series of well publicized pronouncements insisted that the invading malady was malaria (*sezão*). But the diagnosis of yellow fever was confirmed by Dr. John L. Paterson (1820-1882), the Scotch physician to the British colony in Salvador. Dr. Paterson, Dr. Otto Wucherer (1820-1873), a German, and Dr. José Francisco da Silva Lima (1826-1910), a Portuguese—the most distinguished trio of medical researchers in 19th century Brazil—(all of whom agreed on the diagnosis) were criticized as being "meddlesome foreigners." [25] Dr. José Maria de Noronha Feital later reported a similar reluctance in Rio de Janeiro to face the fact of a yellow fever epidemic. For making such a statement before the Imperial Academy of Medicine he was called a "terrorist" by one of his colleagues. Feital said, "The disease was already with us, and neither the physicians nor the authorities wanted to believe it. The fear of telling the truth was such that nobody wished that I utter the words—yellow fever!" [26]

In Rio de Janeiro the first confirmed case of yellow fever was that of a sailor from the military steamship *Dom Pedro II*, who was admitted to the maritime hospital of Santa Isabel on December 29, 1849.[27] The first confirmed case on shore came on January 7, 1850. Initially the fever spread slowly among seamen in their lodgings on shore. As late as February there were very few cases among the general population, although the fever raged epidemically aboard foreign ships in port. The *London Medical Gazette* reported that several ships lost their entire complement of officers and men.[28] (Some of these ships carried passengers who were bound for the gold fields of California, many of whom had no doubt chosen the long and dangerous passage around Cape Horn by way of Brazil in order to avoid the still more dangerous yellow fever zone in the isthmus of Central America and Panama.)

Observers were puzzled by the shipboard cases since on occasion no communication with land had taken place and most ships remained 40 to 50 yards offshore. In the middle of March there was a sudden spurt in which "nearly all of the population of the city found itself affected." [29] To coordinate the fight against the epidemic, a Central Commission for Public Health was named that included some of the nation's most distinguished physicians, including Cândido Borges Monteiro, José Pereira Rego (1816-1892), later Baron of Lavradio, Roberto Jorge Haddock Lobo, and José Francisco Xavier Siguad (1796-1856), the French physician and author of the classic study *Du climat et des maladies du Brésil.* Neighborhood commissions were organized under supervision of members of the central commission.[30]

Perhaps never before had the city of Rio de Janeiro faced such a grave emergency with so little understanding of the real nature of the problem it faced. Nothing was known about the true cause or mode of transmission of yellow fever, although there were theories aplenty. Treatment of the disease was ineffective if not harmful. Physicians disagreed vehemently as to whether the disease was contagious or not but, in the absence of any certainty on this point, there was reluctance to admit yellow fever patients to the city's regular hospitals, such as the Santa Casa de Misericórdia, Brazil's oldest and best-known medical institution. Consequently, temporary infirmaries had to be established throughout the city or on islands in the bay. No charge was made to the indigent for treatment in these centers but care was minimal at best.[31] For example, the Sisters of Charity, the nursing order that staffed the Santa Casa in 1850, did not provide a single nurse for the yellow fever infirmaries.[32] On occasion sufferers from the disease were removed forcibly to such treatment centers; the police announced a plan of daily inspection of hotels and public houses in an effort to halt the spread of the disease. Another precaution, only indifferently enforced, was a ban on the re-use of funeral accessories, such as coffins, pillows, and drapes.[33]

The members of at least three colonies of foreigners in Rio de Janeiro—the Portuguese, the British, and the French—all sponsored beneficient societies that maintained their own modest hospitals.[34] Still another center of treatment was the Hospital da Veneravel Ordém Terceira de São Francisco da Penitencia, a permanent though private institution that aided many yellow fever victims. During this and later epidemics the Emperor dipped into his personal funds for sizable contributions on behalf of the sick poor.[35]

In large part because of the yellow fever epidemic of 1850, the new medical doctrine of homeopathy won wide public acceptance in Brazil. The homeopaths employed a variety of drugs and minerals, but always in minute doses and with minimal interference with the body's natural processes. To a homeopath "to open the vein in yellow fever is the same as opening the grave for the patient;" they also denounced the use of purges, sudorifics, and massive doses of drugs. The poor in particular favored homeopathy for financial reasons; one could be his own doctor by merely consulting a handbook and buying inexpensive drugs in one of the homeopathic drugstores.

The medical regulars, the allopaths, were uncompromising in their condemnation of "the new barbarians of the medical class," all of whom were denounced as charlatans. Dr. João Francisco Barreiros wrote in 1850:

> There is no place for charlatans like Rio de Janeiro! Expelled, and ridiculed in Europe they come to Brazil, as a safe haven, where charlatanism governs and progresses. In this case it is homeopathy . . . [which has been adopted] by an immense number of individuals who lack any other means of support, and so they take advantage of this. Horse-shoers, tailors, and cobblers drop the horseshoe, scissors and awl and start prescribing globules!!! The *vita brevis, ars longa* Hippocrates is for them a phrase without meaning.[36]

It soon became apparent that the victims of yellow fever did not by any means comprise a cross-section of the general population. Mortality was highest among foreigners, including immigrants, travelers, and seamen, especially those who had come from extratropical or temperate climates. Native-born Brazilians were less affected, and many writers commented on the apparent great resistance of blacks to the disease. With regard to certain of the Europeans, Dr. J. O. McWilliam wrote:

> The mortality among the newly arrived Portuguese was . . . very remarkable. In the literal sense of the word, whole families were swept off by this fever. Next to the Portuguese the Italians suffered the most. Of the company composing the Italian opera, seventeen died; as did also nearly every member of an equestrian company. For a long time not a single image-vender, rag mer-

chant, or umbrella-seller (who are almost without exception Italians) was to be seen in the streets of Rio. In many instances, half the passengers who arrived by vessels from Havre de Grace, nay, sometimes even three-fourths of them, died within three weeks after their arrival.[37]

As for the blacks, numerous physicians agreed with Dr. Manoel de Valladão Pimentel that the number of Negroes in the mortality statistics had been "notably low." [38] Dr. John Wilson Croker Pennell said that he had attended 100 blacks without losing one to the fever. In 1850, according to Dr. Pennell, two thirds of the residents of Rio de Janeiro were either blacks or mulattos.[39]

In figures released at the close of the epidemic the Brazilian government listed 4,160 deaths from yellow fever in Rio in 1850.[40] This figure is certainly too low, but how far short of the mark it may be cannot be determined. Many deaths from yellow fever were attributed to other causes, such as American typhus, bilious fever, or hemorrhagic fever. However, the mortality figures published separately by the two English physicians, Drs. Pennell and J. O. McWilliam, seem to go to the other extreme. Pennell wrote that the official figure was known to be "short of the reality, which was estimated at 13,000 by the most moderate," [41] while McWilliam wrote "it is probable that in Rio [de] Janeiro alone not less than 14,000 or 15,000 persons perished." [42]

The government of Brazil admitted that upward of 100,000 persons had been attacked by the fever in Rio,[43] but the Emperor, Pedro II, in his "Speech from the Throne" of May 1850, deliberately underplayed the entire tragic episode. Never using the frightful words "yellow fever," Pedro matter-of-factly reported that "some cities of our coast . . . have been ravaged in recent months by an epidemic fever. The ravages of the sickness are not in proportion to the terror which it has caused."[44] The terror caused during the next half century could not so easily be ignored, as Pedro himself would have ample opportunity to observe. During 12 of the years between 1852 and 1896 more than 1,500 persons died of yellow fever in Rio de Janeiro and more than 4,000 died there in 1891, 1892, and 1894—the latter being the worst epidemic of the disease ever experienced in one year.[45] Brazil's reputation as a hotbed of tropical pestilence was assured. In fact, as early as October 1853 an Italian medical journal commented that yellow fever "is always found in Brazil." [46]

During the more than 50 years of yellow fever epidemics the effect of the disease on immigration and trade was a lively and important question. Some authorities professed to see no permanent harmful effect. Dr. J. I. Gornet wrote in his thesis of 1853:

> The presence of yellow fever in the cities of America does not cause as much harm as might be thought to the development of commerce and to the various industries. The avid businessman, the bold entrepreneur who takes leave of his country, reckons many times with the probabilities of death, but these become probabilities of fortune for those who have the good luck to escape the danger.[47]

As the years passed and the epidemics continued to come, Brazilians characteristically voiced opinions similar to that of Dr. Fernando Costa Ferraz, who in 1880 wrote that because of yellow fever

> Commerce and industry . . . suffer incalculable damages. Agriculture, counting on the benefits of a torrent of immigration, everyday sees its only rich hope evaporating; through a trick of fate it is condemned to be mongrelized! The fertility of the soil of the empire, the prodigious richness which even the bowels of the earth can't hold back, the variety of climate, all is forgotten before the terror which the yellow fever causes the foreigner.[48]

Many arguments were used in Brazil to convince critics, particularly potential immigrants, that the dangers had been exaggerated or that Rio de Janeiro was hardly unique in its problem of recurring epidemics. Europeans were reminded that both Paris and Brussels, for example, suffered from persistent outbreaks of smallpox and typhoid fever.[49] The journal, *A Immigração*, in an article responding to "various inaccuracies about Brazil," claimed that in Italy in 1886 at least 100,000 persons suffered from pellagra, and that the health of the working class of Europe was in very sad condition. "And the journalists keep screaming about yellow fever!"[50] Nor were the Argentines forgotten. After the *Buenos Aires Standard* editorialized "Better stand before a volley from the volunteers at Palermo than venture to Santos, Rio, or indeed any Brazilian port,"[51] *The Rio News* countered: "But what about Buenos Aires herself, neighbor? Would it not be well to tell Europe how much of influenza, diphtheria, typhoid fever, etc. you are having at home, so that they [sic] may know that by jumping out of the Brazilian frying pan they are getting into the Argentine fire?"[52] Argentina was Brazil's leading South American rival for immigrants.

Dr. João Vicente Torres Homem (1837-1887), the man who is still regarded as Brazil's greatest physician of the Empire period, conceded in 1865 in an essay on climate, that "disease and death are often the consequences of emigration," but that sensible persons who observed certain safeguards could greatly minimize their risk. Torres Homem recommended that before settling in a tropical land such as Brazil all immigrants should first spend several months in some intermediate climatic zone. In making the voyage, the slow-moving sailing vessels were to be preferred to the new-fangled steamers because these tended to reduce the shock to the system caused by a sudden confrontation with tropical heat. Once in Brazil, the new immigrant must be careful to avoid contact with swamps, "night airs," and the direct rays of the sun. One can imagine the intense frustration even sensible persons would have experienced in trying to comply with orders such as these. This may have been the reason why Dr. Torres Homem also recommended a stiff shot of brandy every day at noon. If the brandy did not protect your system against yellow fever at least it made you feel better while waiting to find out if you were going to contract the disease.[53]

Despite efforts made to explain away the epidemics or to reassure immigrants that the risk was not substantial, criticism of Brazil seemed to increase rather than diminish. In 1887 *The Rio News* told potential immigrants that:

> Frankly speaking the empire of Brazil is nothing less than a huge pest-house where smallpox, yellow fever, beri-beri, and various other contagious diseases are constantly in existence. . . . Somehow neither the government nor the people ever learn to take precautions against such plagues. They wait until the enemy has them by the throat and then they beg for mercy.[54]

The Italian physician, Dr. Fillippo Rho, stated in 1886 that the annual death rate in Rio de Janeiro had reached 40.4% and that were it not for the constant flow of immigrants, thousands of them Italians, Rio would suffer a net annual decrease in population.[55] *The Gazeta Medica Italiana-Lombardia* published a notice in 1876 which asserted than one fourth of all victims of the epidemic of 1876 in Rio had been Italians.[56] These figures cannot be confirmed, but there is no doubt about the terrible fate of the Italian crew of the cruiser *Lombardia*. This warship arrived in Guanabara Bay on November 27, 1895, ostensibly on a "good will" mission but actually to back up a large number of Italian financial and diplomatic claims against Brazil. The *Lombardia* arrived with a crew of 249 officers and men, of whom only nine failed to contract the disease; 134 died, including the captain and the ship's physician.[57]

On several occasions the Italian government officially advised its citizens not to go to Brazil, and on at least one occasion the German government did the same. Joaquim da Silva Rocha, author of a history of colonization in Brazil, wrote that the Italians' restrictions adopted in 1889 "caused a considerable decrease in immigration. . . . It suffices to cite the figures for 1888 which reached 133,253 immigrants, while in 1889 it did not exceed 65,246."[58] Communities in Brazil free of the disease naturally used this as a selling point to attract workers. The Companhia Agrícola e Industrial, in a "notice to immigrants" published in 1890, advertised the virtues of the town of Paratí: "So close to the city of Rio de Janeiro and with communication there almost daily, [and yet] the yellow fever and other epidemics never penetrate there!"[59]

Dr. Nuno de Andrade (1851-1922), one of Brazil's best known and most influential doctors, made no effort to minimize the harmful effect of persistent epidemics on the rate of immigration.

> What must be done in order to attract large scale immigration? . . . It is not necessary to reform or modify any institution or create any new laws. These, of course, are very important, but the principal [need] is to combat natural influences because the true cause which impeded immigration is the yellow fever.[60]

Dr. Francisco Simoes Correa feared that if the epidemics were not controlled Brazil would be afflicted with "coolie and African" immigrants, who in the doctor's opinion were "not suitable" for Brazil.[61]

It is impossible to determine how many persons made private decisions to stay out of Brazil because of yellow fever. It is clear that Brazilian officials widely assumed a causal link between the epidemics and the flow of immigrants, although many other factors such as hard times, warfare in Europe, and the existence of slavery in Brazil until 1888, would certainly have affected the rate of immigration. There is no doubt, however, that Brazil's two chief rivals for European immigrants—Argentina and Uruguay—exploited the epidemics to their own advantage.[62] And the Portuguese went right on raising the specter of disease in Brazil long after the outbreaks of yellow fever had ended. As late as 1913—10 years after the last major yellow fever epidemic in Rio de Janeiro—the Lisbon newspaper, *A Capital*, warned Portuguese to keep clear of Brazil. "The land which the emigrant imagines to be a paradise, is in reality a great cemetery, many times of his body, and still more often of his dreams. . . . It is virtually certain that he will be going to a slaughterhouse."[63] Naturally the Brazilian consul in Lisbon denied this outrageous charge; he wondered in print if the Argentines were not really the ones behind it.

In an effort to protect new arrivals from yellow fever, Brazilian government, in cooperation with the various colonization companies that recruited laborers in Europe, began in 1873 to intern immigrants in special camps safely located on high ground beyond the range of the disease. This was one of the most effective measures ever adopted against yellow fever in the 19th century. Of the first 2,068 persons who were moved into the immigrant camps, only one person died of yellow fever.[64] A report in 1875 mentioned that as many as 5,717 were interned at a camp near Vassouras, with some 1,400 persons there at one time.[65] Still the foreigners accounted for most of the deaths. In the epidemic of 1891 in Rio native-born Brazilians accounted for only 249, or 5%, of the 4,454 deaths.[66] It appears that the process of internation ended sometime before 1890.

Between 1889 and 1892 the National Academy of Medicine, the Brazilian Society of Hygiene, and *The Rio News* all advocated that there be imposed a "total" ban of immigration for several years to the ports of Rio and Santos, the two endemic centers of the disease in Brazil.[67] Dr. André Rebouças, the famous engineer and one of Brazil's most distinguished black citizens in the period of the empire, urged still more drastic actions. He compared Rio and Santos to the mythical Augean Stables and urged their abandonment as being unfit for human habitation. "It seems, then, it would be good sense to create new seaports, constructed from the beginning under hygienic conditions, on high and dry ground, perfectly drained . . . with plentiful potable water, with wide streets, avenues and boulevards, and with abundant *squares* or tree-lined plazas." [68]

The serious suggestion of such drastic measures by responsible engineers seems more understandable in light of the enormous economic cost of recurrent epidemics of yellow fever. The following quotation from *The Rio News* of 1889 —admittedly quite long—provides an excellent summary of the over-all economic impact of the epidemics.

> It is a frequent cause of complaint that foreigners should entertain so unfavorable opinions of Brazil, but who is to be blamed? The coast cities are never entirely free from sporadic cases of yellow fever. . . . And as for small-pox, the country is never free from its devastations. . . . If the actual cost in money could be computed there is not a Brazilian who would credit the figures. The large sums spent by the general and provincial governments every year in medical commissions, medicines, and other forms of official relief, are in reality only a small part of the actual cost. Add to these the money expended by private individuals in combatting the disease, the expenses of the refugees, the enhanced cost of food, the destruction of infected clothing, bedding and other property, the losses to merchants, manufacturers, and all the professions and industries which form a part of any well-organized community, and also the wages of laboring people thrown out of employment by the stagnation or suspension of all business, and the aggregate will be something appalling. To this, also, should be added the check to immigration caused by these terrible epidemics of fever and smallpox. . . . In this one respect alone Brazil has suffered immeasurably more that it would have cost to maintain the best sanitary measures in existence.[69]

Not only was European immigration undermined by fears of yellow fever but internal migration was also adversely affected. Dr. J. M. da Silva Coutinho, author of a work on epidemics in the Amazon Valley, said that despite the marvel of steam navigation on the Amazon River the valley had not developed as expected because of the universal conviction of its unhealthfulness. A colonization project planned for the valley in 1857 by the Brazilian government had fallen through after a senator said: "The rivers of Pará are so unhealthful that not even animals can survive along their banks." Silva Coutinho said the basis for such unjust criticism was the general belief that yellow fever prevailed endemically throughout the valley. He was correct in his disclaimer that it was malaria and not yellow fever which then, as now, was the chief danger to residents of the Amazon Valley, but he was perhaps guilty of chauvinistic exaggeration when he went on to claim that the healthfulness of the valley was "in no way inferior to the most favored places on the globe." [70]

Many immigrants who came to Brazil lived for a time in the slum neighborhoods of the big cities, and one such locality in Rio was said to be "for the most part, if not completely . . . inhabited by Spanish and Portuguese of the lowest level." [71] Italians were also very numerous in such communities, as were native-born Brazilians both black and white. A writer in 1896 said that these neighborhoods were "all crowded with men, women, and children of all races and colors pigged together worse than animals." [72] Today we might call such a neighborhood a *favela;* in the 19th century the terms *cortiço* and *estalagem* were commonly used. To many persons of the favored classes the proper name for such a place was simply anathema. One of the many reasons why *cortiços* were held in such dread was the popular view that somehow they served as breeding grounds for epidemics of yellow fever. In 1886, for example, Jorge Mirándola, Jr., was authorized by the Emperor to construct units of low-cost or "proletarian" housing. The Emperor was assured that low-cost housing as an alternative to the *cortiços* would be an excellent means of fighting "one of the real causes of the current epidemic of yellow fever." [73]

The Emperor was further advised by the editor of *The Rio News* that he need only investigate the living conditions of the poor to see "how it is that epidemics are always breaking out and are so difficult to suppress." Most residents of the *cortiços* suffered from an inadequate and monotonous diet, scanty clothing, and irregular employment at best. Most of "these people are huddled together in the smallest and foulest of quarters, living in huts without flooring, and sleeping on mats—sometimes ten to twenty in one small, badly ventilated room."[74]

There was, of course, no certain evidence linking the state of poverty with susceptibility to yellow fever; on the contrary many writers commented on the "aristocratic habits" of the disease since it favored whites over blacks and foreigners over natives. Still, some influential physicians such as Dr. Ataliba de Gomensoro, a member of the prestigious Imperial Academy of Medicine, insisted that the *cortiços* must be eradicated as a public health measure and he included yellow fever as a part of his justification. In answer to his own rhetorical question raised on the floor of the academy, "What must be done about the *cortiços?*" Dr. Gomensoro advised immediate and stern police action. "One must disperse the residents of the infected neighborhoods. . . . [One must] enter in those dirty shacks . . . where dozens of individuals live in air sufficient for only six or eight, and disseminate them, scatter them, and make them breathe unpolluted air." To which Dr. Costa Ferraz replied: "The laws of hygiene are not legislated only for those blessed with good fortune who are able in their own good pleasure to enjoy the delights of our suburbs." It was time, he said, that the government of Brazil stopped acting on the principle that "wisdom exists only at the apex of the social pyramid."[75]

Once a person was unfortunate enough to contract yellow fever he quickly discovered that standards of treatment were as uncertain and controversial as any other aspect of this terrible disease. Every doctor had his own favorite remedies. According to Dr. Sebastiao Barroso, "once a proposition had been advanced, once a diagnosis offered, it had to be sustained come what may."[76] Medical rivalries extended into the community at large as partisans defended their favorite doctors and cures in the pharmacies, social gatherings, street corners, and the press. Nineteenth century Brazilian newspapers and medical journals were filled with the kind of contentious scholarship that Barroso described as "10 per cent substance and 90 per cent insults."[76]

In the realm of therapeutics there was much disagreement regarding the real value of bleedings or quinine in treating yellow fever. (Surprisingly, a few physicians still bled yellow fever patients as recently as the first years of the 20th century.) As for the efficacy of quinine in treating yellow fever, the great Dr. Torres Homem continued to prescribe massive doses of the drug until the time of his death in 1887. The editor of *The Rio News* wrote in 1880 that any person who would learn how to treat yellow fever should

> call upon or communicate with some of the medical geniuses of Rio. Every one has a theory of his own, and a course of treatment different from every one else's, and a patient has only to choose the way he wishes to be cured. We have among many others the following processes: electricity, creosote, cold water, hot water, no water, fumigation, spiritualism, liver pad, and Radway's Ready Relief.[77]

Fortunately for the patient who required hospitalization, the duration of the sickness in yellow fever was brief. Death, if it occurred, usually came on the fourth to sixth day of the illness, and even in convalescence patients rarely needed to be confined longer than 12 days. Following the precedents established in the epidemic of 1850, yellow fever patients continued to be treated in special isolation hospitals or temporary infirmaries. The oldest and largest isolation hospital was the Maritime Hospital of Santa Isabel, located across the bay from Rio in the city of Niteroí. This institution was condemned by doctors, patients, crewmen, and passengers alike in a nearly unanimous chorus. Dr. Antonio Augusto de Azevedo Sodré (1864-1929) wrote of Santa Isabel in 1887: "Abandon hope all who enter here,"[78] and Dr. José Lourenço reported in 1890 that conditions there were so bad that patients avoided it "like the devil fleeing from the cross."[79] Mortality figures at the hospital for the period 1882 to 1889 indicate a death rate of 40%.[80]

The temporary infirmaries which opened shop during the epidemics often reported still higher mortality figures. Dr. José Costa Velho, director of the infirmary of Visitaçao, reported in 1876 the death of 200 of the 412 patients treated there for yellow fever. "As a man this makes me very sad, but as a physician it does not alarm me,"[81] he said. Dr. Costa Velho explained that 75 persons had been admitted moribund. In what must be the worst annual record ever reported by any Brazilian hospital, the infirmary of Nossa Senhora de Saúde (Our Lady of Health), in the one-year period from July 1, 1875 to June 30, 1876, lost 603 of 788 yellow fever patients, and for good measure 133 of 196 smallpox patients—several persons who were recovering from yellow fever died of the smallpox which they contracted at Our Lady of Health.[82]

At this point it seems appropriate to describe briefly the burial practices used in Rio de Janeiro. From 1850 to 1890 burial was a monopoly of the Empreza Funeraria, an adjunct of the Santa Casa de Misericórdia. The Santa Casa was sometimes referred to as "a state within a state," and although this hospital ostensibly was purely a charitable institution, critics charged that its funeral monopoly was one of the most lucrative businesses in town.[83] Some of the profits, however, were used to equip and maintain two infirmaries for yellow fever patients during times of epidemics, of which Our Lady of Health was one.[84] But still the Empreza Funeraria was accused of charging exorbitant prices and cutting corners through the improper reuse of funeral equipment. The Reverend A. S. Hawkesworth, an English minister, wrote that "hospital victims and the poor are not buried in any coffin at all; these are used again and again, while the well-to-do were sent off to the cemetery in style in a funeral *bond*," a plain, open car somewhat like a hearse. Reverend Hawkesworth further related that "the Brazilian coffin is totally different from our Anglo-Saxon one, being made of thin 'match boarding,' . . . the whole [device] covered with tinsel and gaudy cloth; it is at best a 'ramshackly' affair, and resembles nothing so much as a showcase for samples."[85]

The popular dread of yellow fever made it possible for a time to broach in public the sensitive question of cremation, a practice inalterably opposed by the Roman Catholic Church, the established church of Imperial Brazil. Dr. Azevedo Sodré wrote in 1888 that "anyone who speaks about cremation will receive in exchange an excommunication from the lords of the land."[86] This statement seems exaggerated, since in his thesis in 1883 Dr. Carlos Loudares said that some Brazilian soldiers who had died of cholera during the Paraguayan War had been cremated.[87] However, there was still little or no public discussion of cremation until in 1880 a chemist and physician in Rio, Dr. Domingos Freire, made the astonishing claim that he had discovered the specific causative microbe of yellow fever and, further, that these microbes were capable of living indefinitely in the soil of cemeteries where yellow fever victims had been buried. Dr. Freire argued that cremation was the only means of destroying these microbes and he founded a cremation society in Rio de Janeiro.[88] I have found no record of the cremation of yellow fever victims in Brazil, although it was done occasionally in Argentina.[89]

Dr. Freire himself seemed to have lost interest in the matter, since he spent more and more time in his laboratory. In 1887 he announced that he had discovered the specific causative microbe of cancer.[90] His scientific researches were so thorough that almost never did he cite the writings of any other investigator. Freire produced a lengthy bibliography of pseudo-scientific works, written in bad French. Historically, he is chiefly remembered as the first person in any country to attempt to apply microbiological techniques to the study of yellow fever. This is not unimportant. Freire's researches, however overblown and faulty, at least had the merit of moving Brazilian scientific studies into the shadow of the laboratory—removing them from the weird realm of miasmas, "night airs," and effluvia. Perhaps it was just as well that Freire died in 1899; he did not live to see the last remnants of his scientific pretentions destroyed by the Walter Reed commission in Havana in 1900 when it scientifically confirmed the theory of the Cuban physician, Dr. Carlos Juan Finlay (1833-1915), that yellow fever was transmitted through the bite of infected *Aedes aegypti* mosquitos.

In Brazil the findings of the Reed commission were not immediately accepted by all, but one man who never doubted their validity was a young physician, Dr. Osvaldo Gonçalves Cruz (1872-1917),[91] who was the first of his countrymen to study at the Pasteur Institute in Paris. Although only 29 years of age and not well known in his own country, Cruz was appointed Director General of Public Health for Brazil on March 31, 1903. He told the President of Brazil, Francisco Rodrigues Alves, that "the mosquito theory is an accomplished fact, an idea victorious,"[92] and that yellow fever could be eradicated from Rio de Janeiro in three years if the techniques worked out by the Americans in Cuba were applied faithfully in Brazil.

Dr. Cruz said that instead of trying to eliminate the disease through quarantine, which had never worked, one should concentrate on two key points: 1) isolation of yellow fever patients from mosquitoes and 2) eradication of the mosquitoes. These suggestions were implemented as quickly as possible and the campaign was a brilliant success. All but the most prejudiced critics were persuaded. By 1904, after the first real test of the new methods, deaths from yellow fever in Rio de Janeiro were reduced to only 48. Cruz wrote in that year, "never again will we fear epidemics of yellow fever."[93] One of the great milestones in Brazilian history had been passed.

Dr. Joao Baptista Lacerda cogently summed up what this great accomplishment meant to Brazil and Brazilians:

> In no other country of the world have the experiments of Cuba had such a great repercussion as in Brazil. We were exhausted, without courage, and without the will to continue the campaign against yellow fever. In this we employed all the resources which science made available to us; we exhausted our forces in bitter combat against the wrathful disease, and we were always conquered. Abroad we were accused of weakness and ineptness, and the foreigners fled terror-stricken from these

> cursed shores, repeating a black legend of horrors and mortalities that stained the reputation of our country and affronted the honor of its governors. We were already half resigned to an unchangeable fatalism when on the horizon there shone the light of hope coming in intermittent waves from the shores of Cuba.[94]

These brief comments cannot possibly do justice to the great achievements and reputation of Dr. Osvaldo Cruz. He is best known for his fight against yellow fever, but he performed numerous services to science and his country during a short but brilliant career. In 1899 he helped a team of physicians curtail an invasion of bubonic plague in Brazil, although this brought him no great fame. Later he waged a militant although only partly successful campaign against smallpox. He remained as Director General of Public Health until 1909, at which time he resigned to devote full time to the activities of the Instituto Osvaldo Cruz, which was then Brazil's leading medical research center. He continued at this post until his death in 1917 from Bright's disease at the age of 44. He was young in years but bowed down with praise and honors from both the New World and the Old. He had used the enormous prestige he had derived from his victory over yellow fever in Rio de Janeiro to upgrade medical and scientific research and teaching throughout Brazil. Cruz is generally regarded as the greatest figure in the field of public-health administration ever produced in Latin America.

Yellow fever was not eliminated completely in Brazil during the time of Cruz. Foci of the disease remained in such cities as Salvador, Belém, Manaus, Victoria, and even Niteroí for varying periods of time. *Aedes agypti* was completely eradicated in Brazil by 1942 through efforts coordinated by the Rockefeller Foundation, but it has recently been reimported to Belém from the United States, where it has long been common.[95] Unfortunately, the brilliance of Cruz's achievement was such that many Brazilians hastily concluded that most of their health problems had been solved. Nothing could have been further from the truth. Brazilians seemed so dazzled by this one great achievement that less publicized but even more deadly diseases such as tuberculosis, malaria, Chagas' Disease, hookworm, and that old foe smallpox were edged out of public consciousness. Men such as Cruz, Belisário Pena (1868-1939), Emilio Ribas (1862-1925), and Arthur Neiva

(1880-1943) were certainly not blinded by one great victory; they knew that Brazil could not rest on her laurels, but the momentum was not maintained. For example, in the vast interior regions of Brazil, such as the dry *sertão* of the Northeast and the Far West and the trackless green jungles of Amazonia, areas far removed from the crowded coastal cities, hardly a beginning had been made in the realm of public health. In 1918, a year after Cruz's death, Dr. Azevedo Sodré wrote that the *saneamento* (a general uplifting of standards of health) of the vast rural interior region was Brazil's single most urgent problem.[96] In that same year Dr. Miguel Pereira made his famous remark—considered unpatriotic by many Brazilians—that "Brazil is an immense hospital."[97] Pereira in effect chided Brazil for somehow confusing Rio de Janeiro and the coastal zones with the entire country. Important as it was, the victory over yellow fever was only a single battle won in the ever-widening fight against epidemic and endemic diseases. According to Azevedo Sodré, 80% of the rural population of the state of Rio de Janeiro was infested with hookworms, a disease which had aroused virtually no public concern even though, according to Azevedo Sodré, the economic loss from hookworm was twice that which had resulted from 50 years of yellow fever.[98] Cruz had made a great beginning but so much remained to be done.

In conclusion, what was the chief significance of the yellow fever epidemics in Brazil? Most tragic of all was the great loss of human life. The majority of the more than 100,000 persons who died of yellow fever were young adults from Europe, whose services as artisans, laborers, and entrepreneurs were in great demand in a developing country such as Brazil. An American consul in Rio estimated in 1898 that 85% of all the victims had been foreigners.[99] Although precise statistics are not available on this point, it seems certain that thousands of potential immigrants were deterred from settling in Brazil because of the general fear of yellow fever. Most who did settle there decided to locate in the relatively fever-free southern regions, such as the highlands of Sao Paulo, Paraná, and Rio Grande do Sul.

The epidemics of yellow fever were the chief cause of Brazil's dreadful reputation throughout the world as a hothouse of tropical pestilence. It is important to learn, as we have seen in this paper, that this reputation did not derive from the essential tropical condition of the country, about which little could be done, but from an historical situation that could be and was in fact controlled. Similarly, the conquest of diseases such as cholera and yellow fever, along with improved understanding of other so-called tropical diseases, helped to show that "many of the alleged deficiencies of residents of tropical lands, such as lack of energy, vitality, and 'ambition,' ought to be attributed more to the causative effect of disease rather than to inherent racial or climatic factors."[100] After the victory of Osvaldo Cruz, nationalists began to talk less about the dangers of life in the tropics and more of its blessings. José Maria Bello has written that because of Cruz's conquest of yellow fever "all of Brazil seemed to take on new life, with greater confidence and pride in herself."[101]

As we look back over the story of the epidemics of yellow fever and cholera in Brazil we see once again that students of history can gain useful insights and even inspiration from a careful study of the annals of the past; yet each succeeding generation must go forth to fight new battles and win new victories in the ancient struggle between mankind and disease.

Acknowledgment

The author wishes to express his sincere appreciation to the Josiah Macy, Jr., Foundation for courtesies extended during the conference and for permission to publish this paper separately from the forthcoming proceedings of the conference.

Notes and References

1. U.S. Public and Marine-Hospital Service: *Annual Report of the Surgeon-General for the Fiscal Year 1904.* Washington, D.C., Govt. Print. Off., 1904, p. 148.
2. Physician General's Dept.: *Statistical Reports on the Health of the Navy for the years 1830, 1831, 1832, 1833, 1834, 1835, and 1836.* London, Cloes, 1841, p. 39.
3. Physician General's Dept.: *Statistical Report of the Health of the Royal Navy for the year 1856.* London, Cloes, 1858, p. 86.
4. This figure is both tentative and conservative, but it does represent a safe minimum estimate. At this point in my researches I estimate that there were approximately 100,000 deaths from yellow fever in Brazil from 1849 to 1906, and 150,000 deaths from cholera in the second half of the 19th century.
5. *The Rio News,* September 6, 1892, p. 3.
6. Albuquerque, E. C. de: Historia do cholera-morbus nas provincias do Pará, Bahia, Rio de Janeiro e Pernambuco. In: *Do cholera-morbus: sua sede, natureza e tratamento, Sera contagioso?* Thesis, Faculdade de Medicina, Rio de Janero, 1856, p. 37.
7. Faculdade de Medicina, Rio de Janeiro: *Parecer sobre a prophylaxia, natureza e tratamento do cholera morbus.* Rio de Janeiro, 1884, p. 10. (The title page is missing from the copy

used by the author at the library of the Faculdade de Medicina de Universidade Federal do Rio de Janeiro.)

8. Albuquerque, op. cit., p. 26.
9. Ibid., p. 27.
10. Ibid., p. 30.
11. Aducci, P.: *Methodo para preservarse do Cholera-Morbus, applicado aos costumes dos habitantes de Bahia, seguido de um mêio facil e popular, para curar esta doença.* Bahia, 1855, p. 7.
12. Seixas, D. R.: *Do cholera-morbus epidémica de 1855 na provincia de Bahia.* Bahia, Antonio Olavo de França Guerra, 1860, p. 12.
13. Arquivo Nacional do Brasil: "Junta central de Higiene Publica," Sec. IS,[4] Leg. 23, fol. 1.
14. Seixas, op. cit., pp. 262, 264.
15. Empire of Brazil: *Fallas do throno desde o anno de 1823 ate o anno de 1889. . . .* Rio de Janeiro, Imprenta Nacional, 1889, pp. 502, 505.
16. Barretto, R. M.: Historia de cholera no Paraguay. In: *Cholera-Morbus.* Thesis, Faculdade de Medicina do Rio de Janeiro, 1868, pp. 73-84, passim; Benedicto-Ottoni, E. B.: Observações sobre a cholera-morbus de 1867 no Hospital de Marinha da Corte, seguida de breve noticia do cholera-morbus de 1868 no mesmo hospital. *Rev. Inst. Acad. 2*:44, 1868.
17. Anon.: Notre courrier do Rio, La marche du cholera. *Brésil 7*:4, 1887; de Souza Lima, A. J. de: *Discurso proferido na sessão magna anniversaria de Academia Imperial de Medicina no dia 30 de junho de 1887.* Rio de Janeiro, Besnard, 1887, p. 4.
18. Malta, C.: Hygiene em Juiz de Fora: Sua evolução. *Rev. Méd. S. Paulo 4*: 60, 1901.
19. Andrade, G. O. de: *Montebelo, os males e os mascates.* Recife, Universidad Federal de Pernambuco, 1969, *passim.*
20. The yellow and typhus fevers at Rio [de] Janeiro. *London Med. Gaz. 10*: 963, 1850.
21. Rebello, T. de A.: *Discripção [sic] succinta ou breve historia da febre-amarella, que tem reinado epidemicamente na Bahia, desde seu apparecimento em 1849.* Antonio O. da França Guerra, 1859, p. 3.
22. Simões, A.: *Tratamento da febre amarella pela agua chlorada.* Rio de Janeiro, Besnard, 1897, p. 17.
23. *Gaz. Hosp. 1*:35, 1850.
24. Feital, J. M. de N.: *Proposições sobre todas as sciencias que compõem o curso médico e algumas palavras sobre a febre amarella e seu contagio.* Thesis, Faculdade de Medicina de Rio de Janeiro, 1859, p. 22.
25. Amaral, F. C. do: Resposta a observacoes feitas pelo Dr. Luiz Vicente De-Simoni. . . . *Gaz. Hosp. 14*:224, 1851.
26. Noronha Feital, op. cit., p. 27.
27. Ibid., p. 25.
28. The yellow and typhus fevers at Rio [de] Janeiro. *London Med. Gaz. 10*: 963, 1850.
29. Empire of Brazil, Commissão Central de Saúde Pública: *Descripção da febre amarella que no anno de 1850 reinou epidémicamente na Capital do Imperio.* Rio de Janeiro, Imprenta Nacional, 1851, p. 1.
30. Feital, op. cit., p. 29.
31. *Gaz. Hosp. 1*:11, 1850.
32. Ibid., p. 13.
33. Empire of Brazil, Commissão Central de Saúde Pública: op. cit., pp. 10-11.
34. Feital, op. cit., p. 25.
35. *Gaz. Hosp. 1*:34, 1850.
36. Barreiros, J. F.: Relatório do Cirurgiao da 1a Classe da Armada, João Francisco Barreiros . . . sobre a epidemia que grassou nos navios de guerra estacionados ao porto do Rio de Janeiro, em 1849 a 1850. *J. Soc. Sci. Méd. Lisboa 7*:171, 1850.
37. McWilliam, J. O.: Some account of the yellow fever epidemy by which Brazil was invaded in the latter part of the year 1849. *Med. Times 2*:449, 1851.
38. Pimental, M. de V.: *Relatório e observações do Dr. Manoel de Valladão Pimentel sobre o tratamento da febre amarella na grande enfermaria a sua direcção durante aquella epidemia nesta Corte.* Rio de Janeiro, 1850, p. 4.
39. Pennell, [J. W.] C.: *A Short Report*

Upon Yellow Fever as it Appeared in Brazil during the Summer of 1849-50. Rio de Janeiro, Rodrigues e C., 1850, p. 9.

40. Rego, J. P.: *Memória histórica das epidemias de febre amarella e cholera-morbo que tem reinado do Brasil.* Rio de Janeiro, 1873, p. 40.
41. Pennell, op. cit., p. 9.
42. McWilliam, J. O.: *Med. Times 2*:449, 1851.
43. Empire of Brazil: *Relatório apresentado á assemblea geral legislativa na segunda sessão da oitavo legislatura pelo ministro e secretário d'estado de negócios do Imperio, Visconde de Mont'Alegre.* Rio de Janeiro, Typographia Nacional, 1850, p. 12.
44. Empire of Brazil, op. cit. (*Fallas do throno. . . .*), p. 447.
45. Republic of Brazil, Directoria geral de saúde pública (Secção demográphica): *Annuário de estatística demographo-sanitária, 1915-1916.* Rio de Janeiro, Typographia Nacional, 1926, p. 114. The epidemic of 1894 claimed 4,852 lives.
46. *Gaz. Med. Italiana-Lombardia 4*:372, 1853.
47. Gornet, J. I.: *Dissertação sobre a febre amarella.* Rio de Janeiro, Typographia Imperiale constitucional de J. Villeneuve, 1853, p. 12.
48. Costa Ferraz, F. F. da: A febre amarella do novo. *Ann. Brazilienses Med. 31*:308, 1880.
49. Anon.: Lettre de Rio-de-Janeiro, *Brésil 3*:2, 1883; Hygin-Furcy, C.: *L'émigration ouvrière au Brésil actuel (Guide de l'émigrant).* Bruxxelles, 1883, p. 13.
50. *A Imigração* (Org. Soc. Cent. Immig.) *3*:7, 1886.
51. *The Rio News,* April 19, 1892.
52. Ibid., June 28, 1892.
53. Torres Homen, J. V. T.: *Do acclimento (These de concurso).* Rio de Janeiro, Typographia Thevenet, 1865, p. 21.
54. *The Rio News,* June 24, 1887.
55. Rho, F.: Note di geografia medica raccolte durante il viaggio di circumnaviagazione della R. Corvetta "Caracciolo" (1881-82-83-84). *Gior. Med. Eserc. Mar. 34*:149, 1886.
56. *Gaz. Med. Italiana-Lombardia 36*:170, 1876.
57. Belli, M.: L'epidemia sulla "Lombardia" e la profilassi della febbre gialla sulle navi da guerra. *Ann. Med. Nav. 3*:9, 1897. Slightly different figures are given in *The Rio News,* March 17, 1896, p. 8, which indicate a crew of 256 and 127 deaths.
58. Silva Rocha, J. da: *História da colonisação do Brasil,* three vols. Rio de Janeiro, Imprenta Nacional, 1918-19-20, vol. 2, p. 147.
59. Companhia Agrícola e Industrial Fluminense: *Os municípios de Angra dos Reis, Paraty, Mangaratiba e Itaguahy do Estado do Rio de Janeiro, Brasil, Notícia para o immigrante.* Rio de Janeiro, 1890, p. 41.
60. Andrade, N. de: Acclimamento dos europeus nos paizes quentes. In: *Conferencias Populares.* Rio de Janeiro, 1876, pp. 90-91. Andrade's lecture was delivered April 2, 1876. The copy used by author was incomplete, and is located in the library of the Faculdade de Medicina da Universidade Federal do Rio de Janeiro.
61. Corrêa, Júnior, F. S.: *Da febre amarella sob o ponto de vista de sua genese e propagação.* Rio de Janeiro, Imprenta Industrial, 1876, pp. 111-12.
62. The yellow fever epidemic of 1871 in Buenos Aires was worse than any ever experienced in Brazil; the official mortality was 13,615, although *The Standard,* an English-language newspaper published in Buenos Aires, claimed 26,000. See Penna, J.: *Estudio sobre las epidemias de fiebre amarilla en el Río de la Plata.* Buenos Aires, Berra, 1895, pp. iii, iv, 21-76. But after 1871 Buenos Aires was virtually free of yellow fever: i.e., before the great wave of immigration to eastern South America that started in the 1870s.
63. Moreira Telles [A. C.]: *A emigração portugueza para o Brasil.* Lisbon, Livaria Ventura Abrantes, 1913, pp. 3, 11, 13.
64. Empire of Brazil: *Relatório apresen-*

tado á assemblea geral na terceira sessão da décima quinta legislatura pelo Ministro e Secretario d'Estado don Negocios do Imperio, Dr. João Alfredo Corrêa de Olivera. Rio de Janeiro, Typographia Nacional 1874, p. 76.

65. Teixiera Garcia, A.: Considerações sobre a primeira epidemia que assolou a cidade de Vassouras em 1880. *Uni. Méd. 3*:126-27, 1883.

66. Republic of Brazil. Ministerio do Interior: *Relatório apresentado ao Vice-Presidente da República dos Estados Unidos do Brazil pelo Dr. Fernando Lobo Leite Pereira . . . em Abril de 1892.* Rio de Janeiro, Imprenta Nacional, 1892, pp. 78-80.

67. Ibid., pp. 352-53; Sociedade de Hygiene do Brazil: *Relatório apresentado na sessão anniversária de 23 de junho de 1893 pelo secretario geral interino, Dr. Carlos Augusto de Brito e Silva.* Rio de Janeiro, Imprenta Nacional, 1893, p. 7; *The Rio News,* January 28, 1889, p. 2.

68. Rebouças, A.: Portos hygiénicos para immigração. *A Immigração* (Org. Soc. Cent. Immig.) *6*:2, 1889.

69. *The Rio News,* September 16, 1889, p. 2.

70. Silva Coutinho, J. M. da: *As Epidemias no valle do Amasonas* [*sic*]. *Breve notica.* Manaus, Francisco José da Silva Ramos, 1861, p. 2.

71. Arquivo da Divisão da Patrimonio Histórico (Municipal Archives of the City of Rio de Janeiro): Febre Amarella, 1891-99. Letter of Dr. Joaquim Candido de Andrade, 3 de fevereiro de 1894, to Exmô. Senhor Director de Hygiene e Assistencia Pública, fol. 46v.

72. U.S. Public Health and Marine-Hospital Service: *Annual Report of the Supervising Surgeon-General for the Fiscal Year 1896.* Washington, D.C., Govt. Print. Off., 1896, p. 383.

73. Mirándola, Filho, J.: *Hygiene pública e privada: A cooperadora; autorisada por decreto de 17 de outubro de 1885, n. 9509.* Rio de Janeiro, 1886, p. 8.

74. *The Rio News,* September 24, 1883, p. 2.

75. Sessão geral extraordinaria em 27 de janeiro de 1873. *Ann. Brasil Med. 25*: 11, 14, 1873.

76. Barroso, S.: Modalidades clínicas de febre amarella. Fórmas benignas e fórmas graves. Unpublished typescript at library of Institute Oswaldo Cruz, Rio de Janeiro, p. 12 [1922?].

77. *The Rio News,* March 7, 1880, p. 2.

78. A[zevedo] S[odré], [A. A. de]: A febre amarella. *O Brasil-Méd. 3*:17, 1889.

79. Lourenço, J.: *A febre amarella e o regulamento de 3 de fevereiro de 1886.* Rio de Janeiro, Imprenta Nacional, 1886, p. 13.

80. *The Rio News,* February 11, 1889, p. 3.

81. Costa Velho, J. M., Torres Homen, J. V., Menezes Dias da Cruz, F., Alemeida Rego, J. M., and de Souza Lima, A. J. de: *Relatórios das cinco enfermarias creadas pelo governo imperial a cargo da Santa Casa de Misericórdia para tratamento dos doentes de febre amarella em 1876,* p. 74.

82. Pereira das Neves, A. J.: *Relatório e estatística pathólogica do Hospício de Nossa Senhora de Saúde. Anno Compromisso de 1875-1876.* Rio de Janeiro, Imprenta Nacional, 1876, pp. 5, 7.

83. Costa Ferraz, [F.F.da]: da Monopólio sobre os enterros. *Ann. Brasil Med. 31*: 427, 1880.

84. Arquivo Geral do Brasil: Pacotilha Is' 29 (1876), Doc. 102, Letter from Jose Pereira Rego to Minister of Empire, 16 de junho de 1876, fol. 1.

85. Hawkesworth, A. S.: The plague spot of the world—An account of Santos and yellow fever. *Climate: Mag. Med. 2*:186, 1899.

86. *O Brasil-Méd. 3*:16, 1888.

87. Loudares, C. A. de C.: *Da cremação de cadaveres.* Thesis, Faculdade de Medicina de Rio de Janeiro, 1883, p. 61.

88. Ibid.

89. *The Rio News,* February 13, 1900.

90. Brissay, A.: Rapport de l'institute Bactériologique de Rio de Janeiro. *Rev. Med.-Chirurg. Brésil. 1*:267, 1893.

91. This statement was related to me by the late son of Osvaldo Conçalves Cruz, Dr. Walter Cruz.

92. Seabra, J. J.: *Relatório apresentado ao presidente de república dos Estados Unidos do Brasil pelo Dr. J. J. Seabra em março de 1904, Annexo J.* Rio de Janeiro, Imprenta Nacional, 1904, p. 50.
93. Seabra, J. J.: *Relatório apresentado ao Exmô. Senhor Dr. J. J. Seabra pelo Dr. Oswaldo Gonçalves Cruz.* Rio de Janeiro, Imprenta Nacional, 1906, p. 13.
94. Lacerda, J. B.: *Prophylaxia internacional da febre amorella.* Rio de Janeiro Imprenta Nacional, 1904, pp. 82-83.
95. Letter from Dr. Fred L. Soper (former Director of the Rockefeller Foundation in Brazil and former Director of the Pan American Health Organization) to Dr. Eugene P. Campbell, Chief, Agency for International Development, United States A.I.D. Mission to Brazil, April 11, 1968.
96. Azevedo Sodré, A. A. de: *Saneamento do Brazil.* Rio de Janeiro, Besnard, 1918.
97. Andrade, T. de: Um vasto hospital. *O Jornal,* 13 de Julho de 1971, p. 4.
98. Azevedo Sodré, A. A. de, op. cit., pp. 11-14, 24, 44.
99. U.S. Public Health and Marine-Hospital Service: *Annual Report of the Supervising Surgeon-General of the Marine-Hospital Service of the United States for the Fiscal Year 1898.* Washington, D.C., Govt. Print. Off., 1899, p. 581.
100. Cooper, D. B.: Oswaldo Cruz and the impact of yellow fever on Brazilian history. *Bull. Tulane Univ. Med. Fac. 26*:52, 1967.
101. Bello, J. M.: *A History of Modern Brazil, 1889-1964.* Stanford, Stanford University Press, 1966, p. 181.

SOCIAL IMPACT OF DISEASE IN THE LATE NINETEENTH CENTURY

JOHN DUFFY, Ph.D.

Professor of the History of Medicine
Tulane University School of Medicine
New Orleans, La.

THE late 19th century witnessed the bacteriological revolution, without doubt one of the most significant events in the history of medicine. Prior to this, epidemic and endemic dieases were as inextricable and mysterious to man as they had been to his most primitive forebears. A few empirical discoveries, such as vaccination for smallpox, had led to some improvement in conditions of health, but the origin and transmission of diseases were as obscure as ever. Acrimonious debates characterized medical meetings as late as the 1880's as theory vied with theory, and theorist with theorist. The greatest advance in knowledge of infectious diseases until then had come from the general recognition that such diseases flourished in filthy, overcrowded conditions. This development, for which the medical profession deserves only partial credit, resulted in the movement for sanitation, which began reducing the urban death rate well before bacteriology provided health officials with a sound rationale.

Although the movement for public and personal hygiene was firmly established in the second half of the 19th century, and Pasteur, Koch, and their colleagues were unveiling the tangled skein of bacteriology, communicable diseases still remained the leading health problem. The health records of every city show that tuberculosis, diphtheria, scarlet fever, whooping cough, enteric disorders, measles, smallpox, and even malaria were endemic. Infant mortality—largely attributed to such vague causes as summer fever and diarrhea, teething, colic, and convulsions —was a major component of the high total death rate. The loss of so many children, however, was accepted as the inexorable working of fate.

Smallpox, the one disease for which a fairly effective preventive measure was available, should have created no difficulty, yet it continued to flare up in every American city. A series of outbreaks in New York City during the 1870's caused 805 deaths in 1871, 929 in 1872,

484 in 1874, and 1,280 in 1875.[1] During three of these same years the annual death toll from smallpox in New Orleans was more than 500, and Dr. Joseph Jones, president of the Louisiana State Board of Health, later declared that 6,432 residents of New Orleans had died of smallpox in the years from 1863 to 1883. As late as the winter of 1899-1900, three of 12 medical students at Tulane University, infected during a widespread outbreak, died of the disease.[2]

Compared with other communicable infections such as diphtheria, for which little could be done, smallpox was only a minor cause of death. Diphtheria, a fearful disorder with an equally high fatality rate, was a major epidemic disease throughout most of this period. Earlier, during the 1850's and 1860's, it had been merely one of many children's complaints, but its incidence took a startling upturn in the 1870's. From 1866 to 1872 diphtheria deaths in New York averaged about 325 per year. In 1873 the figure jumped to 1,151, increased to more than 1,600 in 1874, and then reached a new high of 2,329 in 1875. From 1800 to 1896 the annual deaths from diphtheria never fell below 1,000; on three occasions the total was well in excess of 2,000. The peak period for diphtheria in New York City came during the 1890's, the years when throat cultures and antitoxin therapy were introduced. New York's problems with diphtheria were in no sense unique.[3] In New Orleans a health official informed a joint meeting of the city's two medical societies in 1887 that diphtheria had long existed there, but never before had it been "so widespread and abundant as now."[4] By this date diphtheria had spread throughout America, ravaging town and country alike. Since many deaths from diphtheria went unrecorded, and the hundreds of infant deaths attributed to croup and other vague causes undoubtedly included some cases of diphtheria, the actual toll was probably larger than the statistics of mortality show.

The most surprising aspect of diphtheria was that it aroused so little concern. One of the few newspaper editorials about it came after an 1873-1874 epidemic which killed 1,344 people in New York City. On this occasion the editor of the *New York Times* declared: "Had a tithe of the number died from anything resembling cholera or yellow fever we should have had a public scare which would have compelled such a cleaning out of tenements, flushing of sewers, and clearing away of street filth as had not been witnessed for many years." [5] Occasional discussions can be found in medical journals and transactions of societies but these centered chiefly around methods of treatment. The casual public reaction to diphtheria contrasts sharply with the attitude of colonists a century or so earlier. When a virulent form of the disease suddenly burst upon Western Europe and the American colonies in the 1730's, it aroused widespread apprehension. By the 1870's, however, diphtheria was a familiar disorder to which the population had become accustomed, and its annual toll among the young had come to be taken as a matter of course. The doctors could do little about it, and the public attitude was one of resignation.

This same fatalistic attitude also characterized the public reaction to scarlet fever, tuberculosis, typhoid, and the other perennial disorders. Dr. Abraham Jacobi, reporting for the Committee on Hygiene of the New York County Medical Society, pointed out that between 1866 and 1890 about 43,000 residents of New York had died of diphtheria and croup and that more than 18,000 had succumbed to scarlet fever. Despite this enormous mortality, the city had made virtually no public provision for the sick. Nine years before, in 1882, he continued, the municipal hospital facilities were so crowded with cases of smallpox, typhus, and typhoid that there had been no room for patients with diphtheria or scarlet fever. Since that time nothing had been done except to open one hospital with 70 beds. Almost in despair, Dr. Jacobi exclaimed: "Seventy beds, and twenty-five hundred cases are permitted to die annually." [6] Dr. Jacobi's statement takes on added significance when one considers that New York City had one of the best health departments in the United States.

In terms of mortality, two diseases, phthisis or consumption (tuberculosis of the lungs), and pneumonia should have caused the greatest outcry. Both, however, were considered "constitutional" diseases, and their very frequence dispelled the fears one might expect to be associated with them. In 1870 tuberculosis of the lungs was responsible for about 4,000 deaths in New York City; this figure rose steadily in the ensuing years until about 1890, when almost 5,500 deaths were reported. Deaths from pneumonia rose even more sharply—from 1,836 in 1870 to 6,487 in 1893. Despite their enormous death toll, these familiar and chronic complaints lacked the drama of the great pestilences, and they went largely unnoticed by the general public.[7]

Although most of these statistics have been drawn from New York and New Orleans, the conditions that they reflect prevailed in all major

American cities. New Orleans and other southern urban areas differed from the North only with respect to malaria and yellow fever. As in the North, tuberculosis and the respiratory diseases were the number one killers, while diphtheria, scarlet fever, smallpox, measles, and other disorders contributed to the general mortality.

Although gradually receding southward, malaria was a major problem in the United States throughout the 19th century. In New York City 457 deaths were attributed to malaria during 1881, and it was 1895 before the city's annual number of deaths from the disease fell below 100.[8] In terms of total mortality, malaria was of little significance to New York and most northern cities, but it was a major factor in the South. In 1888 Dr. Stanford Chaillé surveyed the causes of death in New Orleans and concluded that tuberculosis, malaria, and dysentery were the chief culprits. Bearing out Dr. Chaillé's statement, the records of the New Orleans Charity Hospital for 1883 show that 45% of the 8,000 patients admitted were treated for malaria. But malaria, too, was an old and familiar complaint, and in those areas where it was endemic its recurrence each spring and fall was accepted almost as inevitable as the seasonal cycle itself.[9]

In sharp contrast to this casual acceptance of the diseases mentioned thus far was the public reaction to Asiatic cholera and yellow fever. Although both disorders had reached their peak in the 1850's and henceforth were only a minor cause of morbidity and mortality, they dominated newspaper stories relating to health, preoccupied a good share of the time of the medical profession, and were important factors in promoting public health measures. Had either disease gained a permanent foothold in the United States, it might well have been among the ranking causes of mortality and morbidity, but at the same time it would have become familiar and in the process would have lost its capacity to inspire terror. As it was, outbreaks of cholera in any part of the world or the appearance of a case of cholera or yellow fever in quarantine was enough to arouse the newspapers, medical societies, and civic authorities in every American port.

Of the two diseases, yellow fever had a much longer history in the United States. It first appeared in the late 17th century in Boston and then plagued every American port from Boston southward until the beginning of the 19th century. After a series of major epidemics from 1793 to 1805, the Northeastern section of the United States was virtually free of the disease. Attacks on the South Atlantic and Gulf Coast areas, however, intensified in the first half of the 19th century and reached their peak in the 1850's. The number and intensity of the outbreaks, with one or two exceptions, tapered off sharply after the Civil War, although the disease continued to be a real threat to every southern port.[10]

Yellow fever is a fatal and frightening disease; its attacks on the cities of the Eastern seaboard from 1793 to 1805 left a vivid imprint upon the public mind. Throughout the remainder of the century, memories of this pestilence were constantly revived by grim accounts of the recurrent outbreaks in southern ports. Moreover the disease was endemic in the West Indies, and it was a rare summer when one or more cases were not discovered by northern quarantine officials. In 1856 lax enforcement of quarantine laws resulted in more than 500 cases of yellow fever on Staten Island and the western end of Long Island. The New York City quarantine station was located on Staten Island at this time, and outraged local residents barricaded all entrances to it. When the New York authorities responded in 1857 by buying a new site several miles away, an armed mob vandalized the buildings. The following summer, when additional yellow fever patients were landed, another mob burned the quarantine hospital to the ground. Determined opposition by local citizens at all proposed new sites forced the quarantine officials to buy an old steamer to use as a floating hospital for yellow fever.[11] Although the fever never gained a foothold in Manhattan, every summer New York newspapers carried stories of its ravages in the South, and they rarely failed to editorialize upon its danger whenever cases were reported on incoming vessels.

In southern ports it was not necessary to revive old memories, since most residents had experienced close contact with the disease. In 1866-1867 the fever struck coastal towns from Wilmington and New Bern in North Carolina all the way to Brownsville, Texas. Desultory attacks continued until 1878, when the disease was once again widespread. On this occasion it traveled up the Mississippi Valley as far as St. Louis, Chattanooga, and Louisville. Aside from a major outbreak in Florida during 1888, only scattered cases were reported until 1897-1899 and 1905, when minor epidemics occurred in New Orleans and the surrounding areas. The 1878 outbreak, by far the most severe in the post-war years, resulted in 27,000 cases and over 4,000 deaths in New Orleans and wiped out almost 10% of the populations of Memphis and Vicksburg.[12]

Considering these statistics, it is not to be wondered that rumors of yellow jack or the "saffron scourge," as it was sometimes called in New Orleans, was enough to cause panic. When a reported outbreak of yellow fever in Ocean Springs, Miss., in 1897 led the New Orleans Board of Health to proclaim a quarantine against all Gulf Coast towns, a panic-stricken mob of New Orleans residents vacationing in one of the resorts seized control of a train and brought it to the Louisiana state line. Here the train was held up until the health officials, recognizing the hungry and desperate condition of the passengers, reluctantly permitted them to enter New Orleans. This act of mercy by the Board of Health was assailed bitterly and was a factor in the subsequent resignation of the entire board.[13]

When the disease appeared in New Orleans, the mayor arranged for one of the schools to be used as a temporary yellow fever hospital. The following night an armed mob, objecting to the presence of a hospital in their neighborhood, set fire to the building. When firemen arrived, onlookers cut the hoses, precipitating a fight between the mob and the firemen and policemen. Even as late as 1905 the reaction to the presence of yellow fever was one of profound shock. The president of the local medical society in New Orleans wrote: "When the first knowledge reached our city of the presence of this dread disease in our midst, there was almost a panic—stocks and bonds went begging, a pall seemed to be thrown on all things, a general exodus of those who could afford it took place, and the commercial interests seem paralyzed."[14]

Asiatic cholera, the most feared of all diseases in the 19th century, arrived in the Western World as a by-product of the Industrial Revolution. Because of its short incubation period and rapid course, the disease was restricted to the Far East almost until the advent of steam power and rapid transportation. At the same time, industrialism brought massive urbanization with all its concomitant problems: crowded slums, limited and contaminated water supplies, hopelessly ineffectual methods for eliminating sewage and garbage, and city governments ill-equipped to deal with the explosive growth of population. Thus the Industrial Revolution provided both the rapid transportation necessary for spreading the disease and seed beds where it could flourish in the crowded cities.

Improvements in communication contributed further to enhancing the role played by cholera, for no disease in American history was so widely heralded at its first appearance (1832). The introduction of cheap newspapers and journals had made it possible for the American public to follow the disastrous course of this pestilence as it advanced through Russia, Eastern Europe, and pushed northwestward to the Atlantic. The accounts of its destructive progress built up growing apprehensions which were intensified by urgent warnings from health authorities and medical societies that the filthy state of American communities had already set the stage for explosive outbursts of disease. Cholera struck the United States first in 1832 and returned in 1848-1849. On both occasions it swept through cities and towns within a few weeks, killing thousands. In 1866 and 1873 the disease again threatened, but prompt sanitary measures limited its effect. Without knowing precisely why, health authorities recognized that the infection was spread through the feces of infected persons, and they resorted successfully to disinfecting procedures.[15]

Unlike yellow fever, which periodically demonstrated the reality of its threat, Asiatic cholera was never more than a potential danger in the years which followed the Civil War, yet it received an inordinate amount of attention from newspapers and journals in all sections of the United States. Most of the civic cleanups and sanitary campaigns were sparked by what was considered to be the imminent danger from this disease. It shared with yellow fever the capacity for creating panic and brutalizing decent citizens. Victims of Asiatic cholera were often dumped ashore by crews and passengers of river boats, much to the dismay of local residents, who occasionally left them there to die. When the disease appeared in Pittsburgh in 1849 and the Sisters of Mercy opened their hospital to its victims, meetings were held by indignant neighborhood residents and local newspaper correspondents attacked the sisters bitterly. In nearby Allegeny the same situation held true for the Reverend Passavant when he, too, offered help to cholera patients.[16]

The reaction of Americans to a threatened cholera outbreak in 1873 shows how the apprehensions aroused by earlier epidemics carried over into the postwar years. As the disease began spreading into Europe, the newspapers were filled with cholera stories, and the *New York Times* editorialized on "cholera panics." The editor of a medical journal declared that in the United States cholera was the "all-absorbing topic." Responding to demands from newspapers and medical societies, the New York City Health Department promptly began a major effort to alleviate the worst sanitary conditions within the city.[17]

A few years later, when cholera broke out in Toulon and Marseilles, American newspapers once again carried daily front-page reports of the disease. In July 1884 President Chester Arthur reflected national concern by issuing a proclamation warning state officials to be on guard. Throughout the following winter cholera continued to preoccupy public attention. In January a group of New York businessmen organized the Sanitary Protective Society to mobilize all existing health agencies within the city. As the public clamor for action increased, the city board of health secured a special appropriation of $50,000. When the expected epidemic did not materialize, the board was given permission to retain the fund for future use. The following year Asiatic cholera was reported in Italy, and President S. Grover Cleveland was requested to prohibit all Italian immigration until the danger was over.[18]

The last major cholera scare came in 1892. Once again a state of alarm characterized the entire American seaboard. Daily front page stories reported enormous casualties in Russia and hinted of comparable figures in western European cities. Municipal authorities, collaborating with health officials, initiated massive sanitary campaigns, checked on food and water supplies, and made preparations for the expected assault. In New York the city health department retained its summer corps of 50 physicians on an emergency basis; the St. John's Guild lent its "floating hospital" for the use of cholera cases; J. P. Morgan offered the use of a steamship to house cabin passengers from immigrant vessels during the quarantine period; and the directors of St. Mark's Hospital organized a volunteer medical and nursing corps. On the national scene President Benjamin Harrison responded to the crisis by ordering all immigrant vessels to perform a minimum 20-day quarantine. To facilitate the procedure of quarantine, the state of New York leased buildings on Fire Island for the use of healthy cabin passengers during the quarantine period. On hearing this news, the local board of health promptly deputized all citizens and prepared to resist. An armed mob lined the pier, and it was not until the governor mobilized the National Guard that the mob dispersed and passengers were able to land without being molested.[19]

Since most societies tend to operate on a crisis basis, the diseases which were most effective in precipitating social change were those with the greatest shock value. In this category it is clear that Asiatic cholera and yellow fever stood by themselves, with smallpox a poor third, and the other disorders ranking well behind. The outbreaks of yellow fever which struck the Eastern seaboard from 1793 to 1795 had the immediate effect of bringing into existence temporary boards of health, which had surprisingly wide powers. In New York City, for example, the board of health was given the authority and funds to evacuate large sections of the city and to provide food, housing, and medical care for the poor. A permanent result of these outbreaks was the creation of the office of city inspector, a forerunner of New York's health department. Throughout the century yellow fever scares continued to give impetus to health reform. The outbreaks in the 1850's in New Orleans and the southern states had repercussions in every Eastern port and greatly strengthened the position of reformers fighting for permanent boards of health.

In the Southern states, which bore the brunt of the attacks in the 19th century, yellow fever provided the chief stimulus to health reform. Two major epidemics in Louisiana in 1853 and 1854, the first of which killed almost 9,000 residents of New Orleans and the second another 2,500, were directly responsible for the creation of the Louisiana State Board of Health, the first such agency in the United States.[20] Successive epidemics strengthened this board until 1897, when the consternation aroused by the reappearance of yellow fever after an absence of several years forced the members of the board to resign and led to a reorganization of the state board and the establishment of a separate board of health for New Orleans. In 1878 the disastrous outbreak, which affected almost every major town on the South Atlantic and Gulf coasts and spread far up the Mississippi Valley, aroused the entire nation. In Memphis, a city which had not recovered from the Civil War, the loss of 3,500 residents to yellow fever brought a major social and political upheaval.[21] On the national scene, Congress reacted by passing the first national quarantine act. As the full impact of the 1878 epidemic was felt, health reformers were able to secure from Congress a second measure creating the National Board of Health. Neither of these laws proved effective; the quarantine law was weak, and the National Board of Health, after a stormy existence virtually disappeared in 1883 when Congress eliminated its appropriation. Nonetheless, during its brief lifetime the National Board of Health did help to arouse a public health consciousness, and it paved the way for the creation of the United States Public Health Service a few years later.

Asiatic cholera, because it constituted a threat to all areas, was possibly even more significant than yellow fever. The first two waves of this disorder, 1832-1835 and 1848-1855, struck at the coastal cities and then followed the unexcelled waterways of North America. In their wake they left not only a trail of death and suffering but also a host of temporary health boards. During the first attack on Pittsburgh, for example, a 10-man sanitary board was appointed and given an appropriation of $10,000. The following year the funds were reduced to $6,000 and, as the threat of cholera receded, the board disappeared and the funds for sanitation were virtually eliminated from the municipal budget.[22] The second wave of Asiatic cholera at the mid-century coincided with the emerging sanitary movement and the peak years of yellow fever. The two diseases were largely responsible for the organization of the National Sanitary Conventions which met from 1856 to 1860. These gatherings of state and municipal health officials and representatives of medical societies were the first attempts to devise national quarantine and public health programs, and they helped lay the basis for the subsequent establishment of the American Public Health Association.

The second and third waves of Asiatic cholera played a significant role in the establishment of the Health Department of New York City. More than 5,000 New Yorkers died of cholera during 1849 and several hundred more died of it in 1854. Since sanitationists argued that cholera was the product of crowding, the filth and quarantine faction believed that it was a specific communicable disease which could be kept out of the city, cholera supplied both factions in the health movement with ammunition in their effort to obtain a permanent health agency for the city. In the years following the cholera outbreaks of 1849-1854, campaigns to educate the public gradually gained momentum. Several health bills for New York City were introduced into the state legislature during the early 1860's but they all failed. At this stage the third epidemic wave of Asiatic cholera appeared, and its threat in the winter of 1865-1866 led to the passage of a Metropolitan Board of Health Act for New York City. The first problem confronting the Metropolitan Board was to deal with the imminent danger from cholera. An energetic sanitary campaign combined with rigid isolation, quarantine, and disinfection measures kept the number of cases to a minimum. This 1866 attack on the United States was relatively mild and probably would have had a minor effect on New York City. New Yorkers, remembering the 5,000 deaths a few years earlier, gave full credit to the Metropolitan Board of Health. This auspicious start left a residue of good will which resulted in strong public support for the health department for many years.[23]

Repeated cholera scares continued to remind New York officials and the general public of the need for a strong health department, but it was not until 1892 that the disorder again made a permanent impact on the city. The widespread alarm touched off by cholera in that year has already been mentioned. For several years prior to it Drs. Hermann M. Biggs and T. Mitchell Prudden had been advocating the establishment of a bacteriological laboratory. Capitalizing on the general apprehension, Dr. Biggs won his point with the city Board of Estimate and, in September 1892, New York City established the first laboratory to be used for the routine diagnosis of disease.

Possibly more important than the direct effect of epidemic diseases upon social and political reform was their indirect impact. The middle and upper classes sought to insulate themselves from the deplorable condition of the working class, but for those members who encountered the appalling infant mortality and the ravages of disease among the lower economic groups the experience was often traumatic. Morever, as conditions in the urban slums worsened, the diseases of the poor could not be contained, and public health became a matter of concern for all the people.

Members of the medical profession were among the first to encounter the disease and misery of the poor. It was recognized that clinics and dispensaries catering to the poor were essential to medical training and research, and young physicians and surgeons were thrown into direct contact with the realities of poverty. Not surprisingly, in America physicians were among the leading advocates of public health. More significantly, since the integral relation between poverty and disease was all too obvious, they were also among the leaders of social reform.

During the terrible epidemics of Asiatic cholera and yellow fever volunteer groups of all sorts came in contact with dire poverty, and many individuals seeking to help the deserving poor gradually came to realize that even the undeserving poor were the product of their brutalizing environment. In the South a notable example of the volunteer groups was the Howard Association, named after John Howard, the famous English reformer. Originating in New Orleans during a yellow fever epidemic in 1837, its program gradually spread to other southern cities and towns. The members were young businessmen who volunteered their services during major epidemics. The Howards, as they were called, organized massive relief programs to provide medical care for the sick poor and housing and food for their families. The willingness of these men to volunteer for work with the Howard Association evidences some degree of social conscience, but their intimate contact with poverty created a new awareness of social needs.

As far back as the 16th century it had been argued that a country's population was a major form of wealth. By the mid-19th century demography was emerging as a science, and improvements in the collection of vital statistics began to reveal the high morbidity and mortality rates in urban areas. One of the major arguments used by health and social reformers was the economic cost of sickness and death. Estimating the productivity per adult worker, they calculated the loss of productivity caused by the many deaths and added to it the cost of medical care for the sick. The validity of this argument was demonstrated clearly by the repeated epidemics of yellow fever which effectively closed down southern cities and brought all economic activities to a halt. Throughout the 19th century most physicians and laymen believed that epidemic diseases were either propagated or nurtured in conditions of dirt and overcrowding. This environmental concept led to an assault on the atrocious tenement conditions, nuisance trades, deplorable working conditions, and other abuses.

Late in the century the bacteriological revolution turned the medical profession away from environmentalism and focussed its attention upon pathogenic organisms. The germ theory had the beneficent effect of awakening the upper classes to the realization that bacteria were no respecters of economic or social position and that a man's health was dependent to some extent on the health of his fellowmen. The knowledge that the diseases of the workers who sewed clothes in their filthy tenement homes or who processed food could be spread to decent, clean, and respectable citizens served as a powerful incentive to the reform of public health. Since public health could not be separated from social conditions, the net result was an attack on poverty.

The best evidence that a concern for public health underlay much of the effort for social reform is to be found in the multiplicity of volunteer sanitary associations which sprang up in the late 19th century. In every city private groups worked to establish or improve water and sewerage systems, to clean streets, to provide pure milk for the infant poor, to remedy abuses in municipal hospitals and other institutions, and to establish dispensaries, clinics, and hospitals. Examples of these groups in New York City were the Association for Improving the Condition of the Poor, the New York Sanitary Reform Society, the Ladies Health Protective Association, the St. John's Guild, the Sanitary Protective League, the Sanitary Aid Society, and the New York Society for the Prevention of Contagious Diseases. Of the many voluntary organizations operating in New York during this period, some sought only one immediate objective and disbanded after a brief existence, others created organizations that survived for many years. What they all shared in common was the belief that a healthy population was basic to a sound society.

In glancing back over the 19th century one can safely conclude that the rapid expansion of urban areas provided fertile grounds for communicable diseases, and that these diseases were both a cause and effect of the desperate poverty which characterized so many of the cities. At the same time the frightening sickness and death rates drew attention to the deplorable condition of the poor. Dramatic outbreaks of yellow fever and cholera profoundly stirred public opinion and directly and indirectly contributed to the growth of public health institutions. Meanwhile statistical evidence was developing which showed an even heavier toll from chronic and endemic disorders. The net effect, as shown by even the most cursory reading of late 19th century newspapers, was that public health and sanitary reform became major public issues. And for nearly all social reformers, whether their concern was with infant welfare, tenement conditions, or even political reform, the elimination of sickness and disease became a major aim.

NOTES AND REFERENCES

1. See the *Annual Report of the New York City Health Department, 1871-75* (the title varies, sometimes designated as the *Annual Report of the Board of Health . . . .*).
2. Duffy, J., ed.: *The Rudolph Matas History of Medicine in Louisiana,* (2 vols.) Baton Rouge, 1958, vol. 2, pp. 438, 442-43.
3. *Ann. Rep. N. Y. C. Health Dept.,* 1866-1896.
4. *New Orleans Med. Surg. J. 15*:470-74, 1887-1888.
5. *New York Times,* July 14, 1874.
6. Jacobi, A.: The unsanitary condition of the primary schools of the City of New York. *Sanitarian 28*:331-24, 1892.
7. *Ann. Rep., N. Y. C. Health Dept.,* 1870-1893.
8. Ibid.
9. Chaillé, S. E.: Life and death rates; New Orleans and other cities compared, *New Orleans Med. Surg. J. 16*:85-100, 1888-89. Ibid., *12*:716-17, 1884-85.
10. Duffy, J.: Yellow fever in the continental United States during the nineteenth century, *Bull. N.Y. Acad Med. 54*:687-701, 1968.
11. Duffy, J.: *A History of Public Health in New York City, 1625-1866.* New York, 1968, pp. 101-23, 440-60.
12. Duffy, J.: Yellow fever in the continental United States, pp. 639-96.
13. Duffy, J.: *The Rudolph Matas History of Medicine in Louisiana.* vol. 2, p. 430.
14. Augustin, G.: History of Yellow Fever in New Orleans, 1909, pp. 1061-62.
15. For an excellent account, see Rosenberg, C. E.: *The Cholera Years: the United States in 1832, 1849 and 1866.* Chicago, 1962.
16. Duffy, J.: The impact of Asiatic cholera on Pittsburgh, Wheeling, and Charleston. *Western Penn. Hist. Mag. 58*:199-211, 1964.
17. *Sanitarian 1*:228-29, 1873.
18. This material was taken from chapter 7 of the author's second volume on the public health history of New York City, currently in preparation for publication.
19. Ibid.
20. Duffy. J.: *Sword of Pestilence: The New Orleans Fever Epidemic of 1853.* Baton Rouge, 1966, pp. 139, 167.
21. Ellis, J. H.: Memphis' sanitary revolution, 1880-1890. *Tenn. Hist. Quart. 23*: 59-72, 1964.
22. Duffy, J.: Impact of Asiatic cholera on Pittsburgh, Wheeling, and Charleston, pp. 202-03.
23. Duffy, J.: *History of Public Health in New York City,* pp. 441-46.

DISSECTION AND DISCRIMINATION: THE SOCIAL ORIGINS OF CADAVERS IN AMERICA, 1760-1915

David C. Humphrey, Ph.D.

Department of History and Philosophy
Carnegie-Mellon University
Pittsburgh, Pa.

"In Baltimore the bodies of coloured people exclusively are taken for dissection," remarked Harriet Martineau upon visiting the Maryland port in 1835, "because the whites do not like it, and the coloured people cannot resist."[1] In 1845 six members of the Board of Guardians of the Philadelphia almshouse, seven eighths of whose inmates were whites,[2] implored the board to prevent the robbing of bodies from the almshouse graveyard: "That it occasions dread and anxiety in the minds of some of the inmates of this House, is a well known fact," protested the six. Many paupers were acutely aware that burial at the almshouse was a mockery whenever classes were in session at nearby medical colleges, "and to be buried elsewhere is some times asked as the last and greatest favor." The board rejected the plea, contending that "the colleges must have subjects" and should grave robbers be barred from the almshouse they would plunder church cemeteries and other private burial grounds.[3] Blacks in Baltimore and paupers in Philadelphia found themselves victims of a set of circumstances which affected many other blacks and poor whites in 19th century America: their powerlessness and their marginal social status afforded little protection for their dead in the face of persistent shortages of cadavers needed for medical dissections.

A century and a half ago no state permitted the use of unclaimed bodies for dissection, and no one willed his body to medical science. Many Americans considered dissection a degrading and sacrilegious practice, an act to be inflicted on an outcast as punishment—much like the medieval rite of drawing and quartering a criminal.[4] Those few states which created legal channels for procuring cadavers thus restricted them to executed criminals. Even this solution was pitifully inadequate. Massachusetts executed less than 40 persons between 1800 and

1830—hardly enough to supply Bay State anatomists for one year. So anatomists either abandoned the dissection of humans or stole them. But snatching a body to dissect it only compounded the sin, rendering it so gruesome in the eyes of some Americans that riots occasionally erupted. By the early 19th century most states had made grave robbing a crime.[5, 6] How, then, did anatomists procure cadavers without constantly provoking public outrage? The safest way was to steal the dead of groups who could offer little resistance and whose distress did not arouse the rest of the community. Blacks and white paupers provided attractive targets.

Samuel Clossy, New York City's first professor of anatomy, discovered in the 1760s what Harriet Martineau learned in Baltimore 70 years later: blacks lacked the power to protect their dead. Clossy launched his initial anatomy course by dissecting a white and a black, but he soon found, as he confided to a friend, that he and his students were "so known in the place that we could not venture to meddle with a white subject and a black or Mullato I could not procure. . . ." Obviously, dissecting a white was risky business. Dissecting a black was largely a matter of finding a body. Clossy finally procured another cadaver shortly after completing his course: "a Male Black" who had "belonged to a friend of mine," Clossy noted. He dissected it "for the sake of the Skeleton," which he used in courses the following years.[7]

Body snatching proliferated in post-Revolutionary New York when medical students began dissecting cadavers themselves, instead of just watching their professors. By 1788 rumors crisscrosed the city that few blacks were "permitted to remain in the grave." The city's free and enslaved blacks soon petitioned the New York City Common Council to halt the desecration of their burial grounds by medical students: under "cover of the Night, and in the most wanton sallies of excess," they dig up the bodies of blacks, "mangle their flesh out of a wanton curiosity, and then expose it to Beasts and Birds." The Common Council ignored the appeal. After all, wrote one New Yorker, "the only subjects procured for dissection are the productions of Africa . . ." and executed criminals, "and if those characters are the only subjects of dissection, surely no person can object."[8, 9] Some whites did object, but largely because body snatchers recklessly started to rob the graveyards of such city churches as Trinity Church and Brick Presbyterian Church or, as the *New York Packet* put it: "The interments not only of strangers, and the blacks had been disturbed, but the corpses of some respectable persons were removed."[10] Popular anger at body snatchers and anatomists exploded in a riot that lasted two days. The mob ransacked Columbia Medical School and harassed numerous city physicians. By the time troops restored order several rioters had been killed.

Despite the violent response to grave robbing, New York did not legalize the dissection of unclaimed bodies until 1854, when body snatchers were emptying at least 600 or 700 graves annually in and about New York City.[11] Massachusetts passed a similar law in 1831. No other state passed an anatomy act and left it on the books before the Civil War, notwithstanding the fact that some 85 medical schools had been organized before 1860 and that dissections by students had become a normal part of medical education.[12]

Blacks were not the only victims of the widening gap between the legal supply of cadavers and the demands of medical schools. Body snatchers preyed most frequently on the dead of impoverished and powerless whites. White paupers crowded the country's almshouses, particularly outside the South,[13] and in death filled most of the graves in potter's fields—the name traditionally given in each town to the burial ground for the indigent and the unknown. "Were you ever shot at?" a reporter asked a Louisville, Ky., grave robber in 1878. "Oh no," he replied. "We let private cemeteries alone." This grave robber pilfered nearly all his cadavers from potter's fields.[14] Like the use of blacks, the theft of bodies from cemeteries for paupers started with the inception of formal anatomical instruction in America. William Shippen, Philadelphia's first professor of anatomy, calmed suspicious Philadelphians in the 1760s by assuring them that he confined his dissections to executed criminals, suicides (he had dissected a black suicide the previous year), and an occasional body from potter's field; he "never had one Body from the Church, or any other private Burial Place."[15]

The "prudent line of stealing only the bodies of the poor"—as a leading anatomist described the practice in 1896—led to extensive snatching of bodies before burial as well as after.[16] "Those in charge of morgues, the dead rooms of hospitals, and potter's fields, could tell some startling things about how bodies disappear from those places," asserted a doctor in an 1879 issue of *Penn Monthly* magazine. "The number of bodies that are allowed to go into the potter's fields throughout the country is very small, and the majority of those that reach them are not allowed to rest in them many hours."[17] An anatomist at Chicago Medical College in the 1860s later admitted that he procured cadavers from three sources, all illegal: potter's fields, other cemeteries, and almshouses and prisons (before burial), which required judicious bribery.[18] The demonstrator of anatomy at the University of Michigan explained to the university trustees in 1880 that the "better people" could rest easy. Although his annual legal supply of cadavers often fell short of the 90 to 100 that he needed, he made up the difference with the bodies of the "pauper and friendless dead" from the "county houses and asylums."[19] One authority estimated in 1879 that about 5,000 cadavers were dissected each year in the United States and that "at least a majority" were procured illegally.[20] Doubtless a disproportionate number of immigrants ended up in the illicit cadaver traffic. One eighth of the population in 1880 was foreign born, but immigrants comprised almost one third of the paupers in almshouses.[21]

Nineteenth century newspapers abound in stories that describe the many unsavory aspects of body snatching: midnight raids on graveyards, the corruption of cemetery officials, fake burials with empty coffins, the discovery of dead relatives at medical schools or in crates awaiting shipment. Often the reports disclose the lamentable fate of some prominent citizen, for body snatchers at one time or another stole from all social strata. A "well-known citizen of Cleveland, Ohio," was buried on a Monday and his body turned up Tuesday in the pickle tank of the Cleveland Homeopathic Medical College.[22] In another instance a search party discovered the body of Congressman John Harrison, son of President William Henry Harrison and father of President Benjamin Harrison, at the Medical College of Ohio, in Cincinnati.[23] The newspapers played up such incidents, but they dealt with only a fraction of the illicit body traffic. Rarely did the papers inform their readers of the extensive grave robbing in black burial grounds and potter's fields, or of the bodies that disappeared from hospitals, prisons, almshouses, mental institutions, and morgues, or of the bodies of slaves that owners delivered to anatomists.

However, Philadelphia newspapers occasionally made press out of the ceaseless thieving of bodies from the almshouse graveyard. It was this practice which the Board of Guardians refused to halt in 1845, despite the plea of several board members that anxiety over the prospect of dissection imperiled the health of some inmates. Body snatching at the almshouse had already "prevailed for years" by 1845; 15 years later it was still a thriving enterprise. So customary had it become that some Philadelphians believed that the almshouse was a legal source of supply. Philadelphians in the know nicknamed the guardians the Board of Buzzards.[24, 25]

Bodies also disappeared regularly from several other graveyards in and about Philadelphia and from the city morgue.[26] In 1867 Pennsylvania politicians finally confronted the problem. The legislature empowered officials in Philadelphia and Allegheny counties to supply anatomists with all unclaimed bodies which required burial at public expense. But the eight medical and surgical schools in Philadelphia soon found that unclaimed bodies in the two counties amounted to 400 annually, only about half the number needed. Jefferson Medical College—and probably other medical schools—tried to make up the difference by using bodies snatched from Lebanon Cemetery, a black burial ground in Philadelphia. For some 10 years grave robbers preyed on the cemetery, eventually operating in an organized gang that included professional "resurrectionists," doctors, and the superintendent of the burial ground. In 1882 the *Philadelphia Press* exposed the ring. Philadelphia's black community responded so angrily that city medical leaders and Pennsylvania politicians agreed on a second anatomy law, requiring public officials throughout the state to turn over all unclaimed bodies to a state anatomy board.[27]

Fourteen other states had passed similar anatomy acts by the early 1880s, but a smattering of state laws did not quash body snatching in the United States. In 1913 Alabama and Louisiana still provided no legal way for their medical schools to obtain cadavers, while North Carolina and Tennessee furnished their medical schools only with bodies of deceased criminals. Even the passage of a liberal anatomy act did not necessarily eliminate body snatching, since obstinate officials often refused to cooperate with the laws.[28, 29] In 1893, a decade after Maryland passed an anatomy act, legal channels supplied only 49 cadavers for the 1,200 students at Baltimore's seven medical schools.[30] State laws faltered also because the illicit traffic in cadavers was a far-flung, interstate business. Southern body snatchers, for instance, regularly shipped the bodies of Southern blacks to Northern medical schools. For several years during the 1880s and 1890s a professor of anatomy at one New England medical college received a shipment of 12 Southern blacks twice each academic session,[31] while the bodies of blacks filched in Tennessee furnished the entire supply of anatomical material for another northern medical school in 1911.[32]

Grave robbers still operated in Tennessee in the 1920s, selling bodies to Nashville's four medical schools and sending surplus cadavers to Iowa City.[33] But the passage of anatomy acts eliminated body snatching in most parts of the United States by the second decade of the 20th century. Legalization, however, did not substantially alter the social origins of the supply. It simply assured that cadavers would come entirely—rather than primarily—from America's lowest social strata. According to Massachusetts' leading anatomist at the time, Harvard began to obtain an ample supply of legal cadavers about 1850, "particularly in consequence of the influx of Irish paupers, and the great mortality among them."[34] Johns Hopkins finally acquired an adequate number of cadavers through legal channels in 1898; of the 1,200 cadavers received there during the next six years, two thirds were blacks.[35] Like Boston's Irish in 1850, Baltimore's blacks in 1900 suffered from the effects of grinding poverty, social discrimination, and rampant disease.[36, 37] A 1913 survey of 55 medical schools revealed that a "large majority" relied on almshouses as the "sole or main" source for their cadavers, while several schools depended chiefly on hospitals treating victims of tuberculosis,[38] a disease which ravaged blacks and poor whites and killed more than 150,000 people annually at the turn of the century.[39] By 1910 close to half the paupers in almshouses outside the Southern states were foreign born, mainly Irish and German.[40]

The passage of anatomy acts thus did not signify that Americans had come to regard dissection as a legitimate use of the body after death. In practice, if not always in conception, the anatomy laws confined dissections to a voiceless, widely-scorned segment of society. The procurement, dissection, and disposal of cadavers became for most citizens an invisible process and a distant issue. Legalization did expand the supply of cadavers and, by limiting dissections to unclaimed bodies, substantially reduced the amount of personal suffering caused by the seizure and dissection of recently deceased relatives and friends. But legalization also perpetuated an attitude that had not changed much since the days when judges condemned criminals to dissection after execution: dissection remained a humiliation imposed on social outcasts.

From the perspective of the 1970s, legalization appears to have provided a temporary solution that reflected the social values and economic conditions of a passing age. In recent decades the number of unclaimed bodies has dwindled. Affluence, Social Security and other welfare programs which facilitate the burial of the poor, and humanitarian sympathy have undermined a system that depends on social discrimination and abject poverty to operate effectively. Anatomists have gradually discovered that plugging the legal and administrative leaks in the procurement of unclaimed bodies no longer suffices to combat periodic shortages of cadavers. Fearful of arousing latent antagonism toward dissection, medical leaders hesitated for some time to call on a broad spectrum of Americans to assume voluntarily the responsibility of providing the materials of medical instruction and research. By the 1950s, however, the medical community realized that changing attitudes toward death had substantially reduced the need to hide its work from public view.[41-46] A 1967 survey of 87 medical schools in the United States and Canada disclosed that 16 schools obtained almost their entire supply of cadavers through bequests, while another 47 schools relied on donors for anywhere from 10 to 50% of their anatomical material.[47]

In the 1970s medical schools in the Northeast, the South, and the Middle West once again face a shortage of cadavers, since the steadily rising number of bequests has not yet offset the diminishing supply of unclaimed bodies.[48] Undoubtedly unclaimed bodies will continue to be an important source of cadavers for some years to come, and their number may rise should burial become less common in future years. But in a democratic country where 2 million people die each year, increased voluntarism would appear to offer a more suitable and a more promising solution.

Acknowledgments

I thank the National Endowment for the Humanities, Washington, D.C., and Carnegie-Mellon University, Pittsburgh, Pa., for grants which made possible the preparation of this article.

REFERENCES

1. Martineau, H.: *Retrospect of Western Travel.* London, Saunders & Otley, 1838, vol. 1, p. 140.
2. *A Statistical Inquiry into the Condition of the People of Color of the City and Districts of Philadelphia.* Philadelphia, Society of Friends, 1849, excerpted in Bracey, J. H., Jr., et al., editors: *The Afro-Americans: Selected Documents.* Boston, Allyn & Bacon, 1972, p. 107.
3. Lawrence, C.: *History of the Philadelphia Almshouses and Hospitals. . . .* Philadelphia, 1905, pp. 160-61.
4. Edwards, L. F.: Dr. Frederick C. Waite's correspondence with reference to grave robbery: Part II. *Ohio State Med. J. 54*:600, 602, 1958.
5. Blake, J. B.: The development of American anatomy acts. *J. Med. Educ. 30*:433-34, 1955. Massachusetts also permitted the dissection of persons killed in duels.
6. Waite, F. C.: Grave robbing in New England. *Bull. Med. Libr. Ass. 33*:272-76, 1945.
7. Samuel Clossy to George Cleghorn, received Aug. 1, 1764. In: Saffron, M. H.: *Samuel Clossy, M.D. (1762-1786). . . .* New York, Hafner, 1967, pp. xxx-xxxi.
8. Ladenheim, J. C.: "The Doctors' Mob" of 1788. *J. Hist. Med. 5*:23-36, 1950.
9. Gallagher, T. M.: *The Doctors' Story.* New York, Harcourt, Brace & World, 1967, pp. 48-49, 53.
10. Victor, R. G.: An indictment for grave robbing at the time of the "Doctors' Riot," 1788. *Ann. Med. Hist. 2*:368, 1940.
11. Heaton, C. E.: Body snatching in New York City. *N. Y. J. Med. 43*:1864, 1943.
12. Blake, op. cit., pp. 432, 434-35.
13. Bureau of the Census: *Paupers in Almshouses, 1904.* Washington, D.C., Govt. Print. Off., 1906, pp. 6, 12.
14. *New York Times,* Aug. 16, 1878, p. 2.
15. *Pennsylvania Gazette,* April 12, 1764, Sept. 26, 1765.
16. Dwight, T.: Anatomy laws *versus* body-snatching. *Forum 22*:499, 1896.
17. Sozinsky, T. S.: Grave-robbing and dissection. *Penn Monthly 10*:216-17, 1879.
18. Arey, L. B.: *Northwestern University Medical School, 1859-1959: A Pioneer in Educational Reform.* Evanston and Chicago, Northwestern University Medical School, 1959, p. 128.
19. Kaufman, M. and Hanawalt, L. L.: Body snatching in the Midwest. *Mich. Hist. 55*:35-36, 1971.
20. Sozinsky, op. cit., p. 216.
21. Bureau of the Census, op. cit., p. 6.
22. *New York Times,* Sept. 19, 1878, p. 4.
23. Ibid., May 31, 1878, p. 1.
24. Lawrence, op. cit., pp. 160-61, 207-08, 252-53, 269-71.
25. *New York Times,* Aug. 5, 1879, p. 3.
26. Ibid.
27. Montgomery, H.: A body snatcher sponsors Pennsylvania's anatomy act. *J. Hist. Med. 21*:382-91, 1966.
28. Blake, op. cit., pp. 435-36.
29. Report of the Committee on the Collection and Preservation of Anatomical Material. *Science 3*:78, 1896.
30. Mall, F. P.: Anatomical material—Its collection and its preservation at the Johns Hopkins anatomical laboratory. *Bull. Johns Hopkins Hosp. 16*:38-39, 1905.
31. Waite, op. cit., pp. 283-84.
32. Edwards, op. cit., p. 602.
33. Truax, R.: *The Doctors Warren of Boston: First Family of Surgery.* Boston, Houghton Mifflin, 1968, p. 313.
34. Warren, E.: *The Life of John Collins Warren, M. D. . . .* Boston, Ticknor & Fields, 1860, vol. 1, p. 411.
35. Mall, op. cit., p. 39.
36. Handlin, O.: *Boston's Immigrants: A Study in Acculturation,* revised ed. Cambridge, Mass., Harvard University Press, 1959, pp. 115-18.
37. Paul, W.: The shadow of equality: The Negro in Baltimore, 1864-1911. University of Wisconsin, unpub. Ph.D. diss., 1972, abstracted in *Dissert. Abst. Int. 32*:6349A, 1972.
38. Jenkins, G. B.: The legal status of dissecting. *Anat. Rec. 7*:395, 1913.
39. Bureau of the Census: *Tuberculosis in the United States.* Washington, D.C., Govt. Print. Off., 1908, pp. 18-19, 60.

40. Bureau of the Census: *Paupers in Almshouses, 1910.* Washington, D.C., Govt. Print. Off., 1915, pp. 22, 27-28.
41. Woodburne, R. T. and Gardner, E.: Report of the Round Table Discussion on Procurement of Anatomical Material. Proc. Amer. Ass. Anatomists, 67th Meeting. *Anat. Rec. 120*:158-65, 1954.
42. Special report on the supply of anatomical material. *Bull. Med. Res. 10*: 10-25, 1955.
43. Overholser, M. D., et al: Can Missouri schools continue the teaching of human anatomy effectively? *Mo. Med. 53*:474-76, 1956.
44. Cadaver shortage. *Science 126*:1059, 1957.
45. Woodburne, R. T.: Anatomical material and anatomical procurement, 1954-1959. *Anat. Rec. 136*:1-3, 1960.
46. Baumel, J.: Donation of bodies for medical education. *Nebraska Med. J. 53*:90-92, 1968.
47. Smith, R. D.: A survey of the cadaver supply in the medical schools of the United States and Canada. *J. Med. Educ. 44*:628-29, 1969.
48. Altman, L. K.: Body shortage curbs medical schools. *New York Times,* June 25, 1972, pp. 1, 36.

THE DEATH OF THE ASYLUM?*

ERIC T. CARLSON

Department of Psychiatry
The New York Hospital-Cornell Medical Center
New York, N.Y.

To paraphrase an old regal pronouncement: "The asylum is dead: long live the asylum." At first glance the analogy may appear bizarre, but I expect that my purpose will become clear as the following exposition unfolds. "Asylum" was the name given to the mental hospital in the United States throughout much of the 19th century. Today, with many traditional institutions coming under attack, we read not only of the death of marriage and the family, but even of the demise of God. In a similar vein—and history probably will record this as part of the broader fabric—many are sounding the death knell of the mental hospital.

The present radical-reform philosophy runs as follows: mental illness does not exist. If by any remote chance some similar condition is manifested, a biological or "medical model" has no pertinence: the causation of any such condition lies in the turmoils and deficiencies of society alone. If there is anything to treat, it should be done in the setting of the community. The mental hospital, with its taint of medical orientation, should be used neither for treatment nor for the training of potential therapists. It lacks function or future, and its demise is proclaimed. In order to understand the rise of the asylum and the hopes that it once aroused, it is useful to consider its history, especially as exemplified by the founding of the McLean Asylum near Boston.

As is well known, the colonization of North America had its earliest successes in the southernmost portions through the efforts of Spanish explorers and soldiers of fortune. One of the latter, Bernardino Alvarez, arrived in Mexico in 1537 to begin a career of soldiering, drink-

*An essay review of Nina Fletcher Little: *Early Years of the McLean Hospital.* Boston, Francis A. Countway Library of Medicine, 1972. 176 pages, 40 illustrations. $8.95 (obtainable from the Countway Library, Roxbury, Mass.).

This study was supported in part by National Institutes of Health Grant LM00919 from the National Library of Medicine, Washington, D.C., and aided by the editorial assistance of Jeffrey Wollock.

ing, robbing, and exploring, which led eventually to the accumulation of a large fortune. In his maturity Alvarez found financial security but no peace, until his guilt forced him back to his Catholic religion and to the doing of good deeds. One of these was the establishment of a hospital (1567), named after Saint Hippolitus, the patron of Mexico City. Following earlier precedent, contributions from many quarters helped make this pioneering effort possible. The church gave Alvarez the license to proceed; this then was approved by both the viceroy and the king of Spain. Friends gave the land, and many other persons contributed to construction. The hospital was established not only to serve the insane but also the infirm, both convalescent and chronic, the aged, etc.—a whole spectrum of dependency. It was the first of a chain of hospitals that would extend from coast to coast. The rambling, two-story, red-brick building, which still stands next to its church near the heart of Mexico City, accepted purposefully many psychiatric patients, and thus became the first psychiatric hospital in North America.[1]

This hospital well illustrates its Mediterranean background. Although the origin of hospitals disappears in the obscurity of history, it is known that the Chinese and the Indians constructed such institutions long before the Christian era, and these establishments appear to have flourished under the teachings of Buddha. The earliest Christian hospital dates from the period of Constantine (after 335 A.D.); Islam produced its first at Baghdad at the close of the eighth century. As Islamic culture spread westward along both shores of the Mediterranean Sea, the rediscovered and embellished Greek medical writings were introduced into Italy and Spain. Along with this cultural flow came the introduction, in Spain, of the first mental hospitals. The first psychiatric hospital in the Western world was founded in Valencia in 1410. Started through the leadership of a Catholic priest inspired by his sudden sympathy for a madman mistreated on the streets of Valencia, it grew through the cooperation of many people. Interestingly, the priest created a brotherhood, which consisted not only of 100 priests but also of 600 laymen, of whom 300 were men and 300 were women. Popularly called the Hospital of Innocents, it received the approval of Pope Benedict XIII but functioned under the protection of the municipality of Valencia as a secular institution independent of the Royal Court through the king's approval. This mixture of national, religious, and private sponsorship created a pattern which extended not only from Spain to Mexico but could be found also in northern Europe and in Great Britain.[2]

The first hospital for the insane in England continues today as the Bethlem Royal Hospital in Beckenham, Kent. This institution was founded in 1247 when a former sheriff of London bequeathed his lands to the church of St. Mary of Bethlehem, not for a hospital but for a priory. By the following century financial pressures forced the city to establish a board of governors for supervision of what came to be known as a "hospital" or "hospice." Used by both wayfarers and the infirm, it came to be maintained increasingly for the latter. By 1402 it contained madmen, and continued to harbor them thereafter. When Henry VIII dissolved the religious orders, the hospital came completely under control of the city of London. In 1676 a new building doubled its capacity but also made it a popular pastime for visitors to observe the patients. During the late 17th and 18th centuries, therefore, the hospital received much publicity, as the notorious "Bedlam." In spite of this unsavory reputation, the movement for the establishment of hospitals as the preferred means of treatment for the acutely ill of all kinds moved inexorably onward.[3]

The 18th century produced many new hospitals in England—starting in 1716 in London, with many following in the city, and then spreading out to the provinces. However, a significant change was taking place in the character of the groups which were organizing these hospitals. The new movement had started with the destruction of the Catholic institutions by Henry VIII; by the 18th century it was largely but not exclusively secular. The founding members were usually upper-class and often wealthy. A broader governmental role was still to come. It was the century of popular charity and voluntary hospitals.[4]

The growth of English mental hospitals paralleled these developments. Proprietary hospitals conducted for profit began in the 17th century and grew to such numbers by the mid-19th century that their use and abuse came under public scrutiny, as William Parry-Jones has shown in his recent excellent book.[5] Private hospitals supported by public subscription were represented by such places as Bethel Hospital (Norwich, 1713), the wards for the insane at Guy's (1728), St. Luke's Hospital (London, 1751), and Manchester Lunatic Hospital (1766). County hospitals would not arrive until the next century, when they were given authorization under the County Asylums Act of 1808, which was a product of the governmental investigations of 1807 into the condition of criminal and pauper lunatics.

The religious sponsorship of new hospitals had essentially disappeared, with one notable exception. In 1791 a young Quaker girl had died under mysterious circumstances at the York Lunatic Asylum. Aroused by suspicions of mistreatment and abuse, the Quakers organized to found their own institution, the York Retreat. In many respects this establishment was paramedical. Managed by one of the founders, it placed its emphasis on optimism, kindness, and a firm ordering of the patient's life. Although a physician was available, little stress was placed on the use of medication. The York Retreat was to become an important model for the New World.[6]

As would be expected, the English colonies in North America developed their institutions along similar lines. The first general hospital in Philadelphia opened in 1752 on a voluntary, charitable basis and, right from the start, the Pennsylvania Hospital provided for the insane. Farther south in Williamsburg, Va., the colonial leaders established the first separate psychiatric hospital in the country, the Eastern Lunatic Asylum, in 1773.[7] Although the precedent had been established, it would be many years before any resurgence of the asylum movement occurred. The Friends' Asylum for the Insane in Philadelphia led the way in 1817, soon followed by three other voluntary hospitals: the McLean Asylum (1818), the Bloomingdale Asylum (1821), and the Hartford Retreat (1824). In the latter year the State of Kentucky opened its asylum and ushered in an era of state-hospital construction. Our focus, however, is on the McLean Asylum.

As Bostonians became aware that they lagged behind Philadelphia, New York, and Baltimore in the founding of hospitals, they started to plan as early as the late 1790s for a general hospital (which eventually opened in 1821 as the Massachusetts General Hospital) and a mental hospital. In 1811 a corporation was founded to solicit funds and to make proper plans for the two institutions. For a number of reasons it was decided to push ahead first with the asylum. Although led by certain eminent Bostonians and enlisting a wide range of citizens, it still was essentially an elite group. Undoubtedly the founders had difficulty in obtaining adequate guidelines for their planning. Benjamin Rush's *Diseases of the Mind* had been published in 1812 and was widely known; it had much useful information on clinical psychiatry but little to offer directly on the subject of hospitals. More useful would have been the edition of Samuel Tuke's *Description of the Retreat* (at York), reprinted in Philadelphia in 1813 as part of the campaign for founding the Friends' Asylum. Boston had its local expert in Dr. George Parkman, who had had some psychiatric training in Paris under the famed Dr. Philippe Pinel. Parkman had returned to Boston in 1813 and had opened his own small private institution for the treatment of the insane. Parkman offered his leadership for the proposed asylum, and in the process produced several minor publications; for complicated reasons his offer was never finally accepted by the Board of Trustees.[8]

The Massachusetts legislature granted a charter to the corporation on February 28, 1811. That governmental and popular forces, and not the medical profession, were primary in the organization, can be seen in the method by which the Board of Trustees was selected. Fifty-six distinguished citizens participated in the initial incorporation; they in turn selected eight of the 12 trustees. The remaining four were chosen by a special Board of Visitors consisting of the governor, lieutenant governor, president of the Senate, and speaker of the House, as well as the chaplains of both houses. The fact that the latter two were included reveals that although the role of the churches in the establishment of hospitals was diminishing they still were able to bring some influence to bear on the formation of new social institutions. Something of the flavor of the first meeting of the corporation may be seen in the fact that John Adams presided. The group quickly organized into committees and started an extensive fund-raising drive. A total of 1,047 subscribers was obtained from Boston and surrounding towns.[9] Obviously an interest in the project and the ability to contribute were the positive qualifications of these participators. With today's emphasis on increased community control of medical delivery systems, this early 19th century community involvement may seem a worthy predecessor. There were distinct differences, however; these were private funds, and I am certain that sociological analysis of the contributors would reveal the vast majority to have been of the upper class, members of an elitist group. Nonetheless, a considerable spectrum of individuals was involved in making these early Massachusetts institutions possible.

Having decided to go ahead with the insane asylum, the trustees had now to select a site and to arrange for construction of buildings. In December 1816, after a number of false starts, the trustees finally decided upon the so-called Barrell estate of some 18 acres situated on a beautiful promontory across the Charles River from Boston. Apart from financial considerations, two factors were predominant in the choice: 1) Its location across Craigie's Bridge (which Nina Fletcher Little describes well) placed it within easy access of the city. 2) The description of Bowditch as a "peaceful retreat" "beautifully situated" in "quiet precincts" gives us important clues to the therapeutic philosophy of those times. Most of these early hospitals were products of urban groups to whom a peaceful country setting was already appealing. More important, this was a period when romanticism was flourishing. The worship of nature was widespread; its adulation was led by the poets, but philosophers as well as men of simpler goals formed the chorus. Along with nature, natural man or the savage often seemed healthier than his brother hemmed in by the crowding bustle and stench of the cities. The tranquil site not only brought the promise of peace to the disturbed mind, but aided in breaking up old and unhealthful associations. Based on the developments of Lockean associationism in the 18th century, therapeutic programs were purposefully developed to aid in dismembering old and chaotic associations and replacing them with order and peace. All of the medical writers, who also believed in a Hallerian irritability of the body, sensitive to stimuli, stressed the need to take the patient away from his immediate environment and family, but it is endlessly fascinating to observe that none of them explored the detailed reasons why this should be necessary. The conceptual tools of communication, intrapsychic dynamics, and interpersonal relations had not yet been developed to the point of usefulness. At the same time there was a recognition, even though simplistic, that there was something harmful in the family and societal structure for many of their patients.

The Barrell property included a sumptuous house designed in the early 1790s by Charles Bulfinch, the eminent American architect, in the style of an English country manor. How then to use this as a hospital? The trustees engaged Bulfinch as a consultant and sent him off to visit the hospitals in New York, Philadelphia, and Baltimore for ideas. The trustees also formed their own building committee; one of their members, Ebenezer Francis, also made a trip to examine hospitals with particular attention to the Friends' Asylum, which had just opened outside Philadelphia at Frankford. From these various studies, it was decided to use the original building as the headquarters for the superintendent and his staff and to add two three-story wings, each to be connected to the main building by a covered arch. Mrs. Nina Fletcher Little in her book on the early years at McLean Hospital has shown her skills as historian of folk art by assembling an impressive collection of early plans and prints of the Massachusetts Lunatic Asylum (as it was sometimes called until renamed the McLean Asylum in 1826 as a result of the bequest of John McLean, a Boston merchant of some prominence). She has not, however, shown how this hospital fitted in with others of the time; fortunately, the material is available in a thorough recent study by Dr. Dieter Jetter.[10] Finally the additions were completed. A certain amount of the stonework was contributed by inmates of the prison, another institution just then becoming popular as a social facility.

In the meantime the trustees had turned down the only person with any psychiatric training, George Parkman, in favor of Dr. Rufus Wyman, a successful general practitioner who may have sought the position partly because ill health impelled him to seek a less arduous position. There is no evidence that he had any training in psychiatry or any inclination toward it. In spite of this inauspicious beginning, the trustees' choice turned out to be excellent. From his appointment in 1818 to his retirement, forced by ill health in 1835, Wyman served as a dedicated and superb superintendent and physician.[11]

Wyman and his counterpart at the Hartford Retreat, Dr. Eli Todd, by their excellent administration, humaneness, and therapeutic skills were to become inspirations for the psychiatrists who would follow them in the next 30 years.[12]

But their contributions must be seen as part of a team effort, even though they may have played the role of leaders. Wyman had a most active visiting committee. When the first applicant for admission was presented on October 6, 1818, the committee spent three hours interviewing him before they arranged for his admission. (He did well, was discharged as cured, and became a successful salesman.) The committee soon gave up its intake procedures as impractical but its members visited the asylum frequently and often spent entire afternoons in fulfilling their responsibilities. A set of detailed rules and regulations established before the asylum opened gave them their guidelines. The committee members made sure that these were followed properly. They not only evaluated the quality of the financial records and checked with the superintendent about administrative problems, but also reviewed the care which the individual patients were receiving. Dr. Wyman's administrative duties had been lightened in 1823 by the appointment of a steward and a matron. The steward ordered supplies, handled the finances, and hired the servants and attendants. By 1837 the servants included a chief cook, four assistants, two laundresses, and a wing girl. Whereas the asylum had started with one attendant each for the male and female wings, there were now nine men and seven women. Wyman had high expectations for the qualifications of his aides, but unfortunately was often disappointed in actual practice.

The final member of the therapeutic team was the closest assistant to Dr. Wyman: the apothecary. The person filling this position was required to have completed at least one year as a medical student. In return for his work he received specialized medical experience and was given his room and board. To this post George William Folsom (1803-1827) was appointed in 1825. He had gone to Phillips Exeter Academy before attending Harvard Medical College. As an eminent art historian engaged in tracing the brief career of Henry Folsom, the artist, Mrs. Little discovered a number of diaries of his brother George William Folsom, including those published here; these date from his period at the McLean Asylum. Folsom must have started at his post with some apprehension, for he later reported that he had found "crazy people much more pleasant than I expected" (page 29). From February 26 to December 31, 1825, he recorded the details of his new life. From his notes we learn a fair amount about his responsibilities at the asylum. He ordered the medicines, mixed them, and administered them but only in following Wyman's orders. Twice a day he visited the patients and spent much time conversing with them and participating in their activities. He also made entries in the four medical record books that were kept at the McLean Asylum on: 1) medical treatments used, 2) combinations of prescriptions, 3) individual case records, and 4) the pulse. He was not responsible for the two other records: the business accounts and the visitors' book.

Although his diary does allow glimpses of what life was like inside the McLean Asylum, it has sharp limitations for, as Walter Muir Whitehill says in his introduction, "the journal is no literary gem." This is a gross understatement: the writing is static and the sentences are incomplete and often approximate the character of a list, with no transition between topics. Despite the cryptic quality of Folsom's writing and its contents, Mrs. Little has done an excellent job of identifying various Boston figures and landmarks in it. The amount of illustrative material which she has been able to furnish is amazing, and she has done a superb bit of detective work in unraveling architectural details. Since Mrs. Little is not a medical historian, it may be unfair to carp on her failures in this area; but I wish she had used the medical material—the case and treatment books—to flush out the story of the patients, their problems, and their treatments. Folsom gives us only glimpses of these matters. Some of them are helpful (for example, the type of medical literature he studied) but the lack of an index makes it difficult to locate this information, for Folsom's manner of writing only motivates browsing, at most.

Folsom's diary ends late in 1825, but asylum records indicate his continued presence until August 1826. A year later his brief life was brought to an end by unknown medical causes. The apothecary position once occupied by Folsom was continued, but was renamed house physician in 1828, a term that seems much more familiar to us. By this time the asylum-building craze was nearing full force and the reform optimism of the 18th century enlightment seems to have reached fruition. The leaders of these new institutions vied with one another to produce better results, and what Albert Deutsch felicitously called "the cult of curability" was founded.[13] It is somewhat an apocryphal insiders' joke that Dr. William M. Awl of the Ohio Asylum was the first to report a staggering 100% of cures among recent patients, for which achievement he was knicknamed Dr. Cure-Awl. But in this happy occurrence there is a somber limitation. What happens to patients whose illness is not recent? The first of a number of dark clouds had appeared on the horizon.

W. L. Parry-Jones has made a thorough study of the private asylums in Great Britain which provides a backdrop for the various problems that were to arise also on the American scene. Abuses of patients' rights were one of the most common. Although probably not mistreated as frequently as in the setting of the general society, there were innumerable examples of less-than-adequate treatment, not to mention inadequate care, as well as neglect and, even worse, various degrees of brutalization. In these days of international concern about the misuse of mental hospitals as political instruments, it is useful to learn that wrongful detention is an old issue. A case occurred as early as 1706, but much more concern about this possibility was expressed as the 19th century progressed. The problem became a special concern of the reform movements, both in Great Britain and the United States after 1860. The victims were not political prisoners, but suffered as a result of power plays within families; undoubtedly there were also cases where careless evaluations led to unnecessary hospitalization. That this still exists as a definite risk can be seen in a recent provocative and disturbing study in which "sane people" were easily hospitalized after the mere verbal complaint of limited auditory hallucinations.[14] Although Parry-Jones pays primary attention to the private asylums he also notes the two other types of facilities provided: the public or county hospitals, which are equivalent to our state hospitals, and the registered hospitals, which resemble our voluntary hospitals. Paradoxically, the opening of all these institutions led to a second problem—inadequacy of the services offered. This always seems to be the result of offering a service which represents a great need in the community: the supply is quickly overrun by the demand. A third problem arose for the middle-class patient who was not eligible for the public hospital or affluent enough to afford private therapy. A fourth difficulty came from lack of clarity as to who should operate the private asylum. The very earliest private asylums at the dawn of the 17th century had been nonmedical. The first asylum run by a doctor opened about 1630 under Helkiah Crooke, a physician to both the Bethlehem Hospital and King James I, but this did not become the dominant fashion until well into the 19th century.[15] The private hospitals were run for reasons that ranged from pure profit-making to shining altruism; the leaders included clergymen, quacks, former keepers, and widows and daughters of former managers. By 1831 a survey indicated that nearly two thirds of the leaders were medically qualified. But even that figure must be used with caution, for numerous contemporary medical schools would issue doctoral degrees without any requirements for attendance at lectures or classes. Problems of proper qualification continue to plague us, as can be seen by the recent burst of publicity about certain psychologists in mental health clinics who had received their Ph.D. degrees from colleges that had only minimal requirements.[16]

Two other trends spelled trouble for the asylum system. All proponents recognized that early treatment led to better results, but campaigns to encourage early arrivals only aggravated the overcrowding. Added to this was the fact that in spite of all the expressed enthusiasm about the curability of insanity a fair number of patients never recovered enough to warrant discharge. A considerable number of so-called incurables were to live 50 years or more within the confines of the state hospitals. Such persons occupied beds steadily and increasingly, and provoked endless discussions as to how to deal with the problems they created for hospitals that planned for the restoration of health but were faced instead with a role of mere custodianship. Parry-Jones rightly points out that as the 19th century progressed, it became more and more obvious that the mental asylum was not adequately attaining the hopeful goals initially set.

The failure of the asylum is the object of a recent and thorough study by David Rothman,[17] whose focus is broad: the rise and decline of a large number of asylum-like institutions in the United States. These include not only the insane asylums, but asylums for the poor and the juvenile delinquent, workhouses for the rogue and vagabond, and prisons for the obvious criminal element. Rothman omits only schools for the idiots and the hospitals for the acutely ill; in a way it is regrettable that he did not use one of the latter as a model. Hospitals have a long institutional history; this makes them useful in understanding other asylums. Although Rothman is correct in stressing the boom in asylums which occurred during the Jacksonian era, he does relatively little to trace their origins, even though he devotes much space to other 18th century social systems for the care of dependents. Because of this approach he often conveys the feeling that the asylum was entirely the invention of the Jacksonians. At the same time he is correct in stating that most previous studies of such institutions—especially the medical institutions—have been written from a narrow internal viewpoint and therefore do not properly reflect the influences of broader social forces. Rothman planned his study from the social viewpoint and consequently has produced a useful book. In an initial chapter he traces the general thought of the 18th century, according to which the deviant and the dependent were considered a natural part of God's world; any remedies attempted were local and were implemented in the normal community setting. Those who were not obvious members of the community became no local burden but were "warned out." By the 19th century these same problems were seen to arise from "the faulty organization of the community." According to Rothman the new solution, the asylum, had a dual purpose: it attempted to rehabilitate the individual and to serve as an "example of right action for the larger society."

Rothman traces the history of various asylums into the latter part of the century. He constantly expresses amazement that the growing evidence of their failure led to little apparent change in the enthusiasm for such institutions. For the mental hospital, reform was on the way but it came slowly and discontinuously. One medical factor in the change was the growth of neurology after the 1860s and its application to patients suffering from a wide spectrum of emotional problems. With the discovery of the functioning patient even the hospitals started to open outpatient clinics, and much later the alienist and the neuropsychiatrist started to move out into society to practice their skills. The quality of life within the state hospital (as most of the former insane asylums came to be known) was subjected to frequent attack. We need only mention the short-lived National Association for the Protection of the Insane, the work of Clifford Beers (who started out to reform the hospital and ended by trying to prevent insanity through mental hygiene), and most recently the exposés of Albert Deutsch.[18] More than humanistic concern was needed to bring about a change.

Reform was made possible partly through the 20th century growth of sociology with its refined attention to institutions, roles, and social interaction. Two books are seminal, one published in 1954 and the other in 1961. The first, by the psychiatrist and sociologist team of Stanton and Schwartz, had a greater impact on the medical community through its careful study of what life was like within such an institution.[19] The second, by the sociologist Erwing Goffman, extended these studies by exploring the social roles that were imposed in various hospitals.[20] It seemed that the hospital was indeed a crazy place which helped manufacture madness. Roles had been revised; the world had been turned upside down. The trend continues. Madness is a sociological phenomenon; according to some it is even a higher form of life, an attempt by selected geniuses to live in a world that is crazy. The asylum has been turned inside out and has engulfed the world. Instead of being a microcosm defining what seemed in 1830 to be a proper paradigm of a family-like regimen for recovery, the asylum is now the community saying: "heal thyself." If only we possessed a time machine to transport us into the future to see where this trend is leading and what historians will be saying about it then!

The original asylum was planned as a peaceful retreat in the country, away from the stresses of urban life. As we have learned more of the biological, interpersonal, and societal factors in the various emotional and intellectual problems that plague man, the original goals may seem simplistic but not inappropriate. We must not condemn our predecessors for not having the information we have today (which the future in turn will undoubtedly find quite limited). Such criticism is not only scientifically contrahistorical; it is also unsportsmanlike at best. Changes occur on many levels. With the extensive urbanization creating a nonending megalopolis in many sections of the country, even the possibility of a rural retreat has been reduced steadily. This is well illustrated by the history of the psychiatric service of the second oldest hospital in the United States, the New York Hospital. At first the insane were housed in the semibasement, as at the Pennsylvania Hospital. As increasing numbers created additional demands, the construction of another wing was considered. Instead, a separate building was erected behind the main hospital. This building, which opened in 1808, helped in many ways but soon was rendered obsolete by pressures for a new institution. The new asylum was located several miles from the tip of Manhattan in a lovely setting called Bloomingdale, which commanded a beautiful view of the Hudson River. But this solution lasted only until the mid 1890s, when another move became mandatory because of exploding urbanization. Just about the time that the Bloomingdale Hospital was moving out to White Plains, the McLean Hospital was making a similar transfer from its original site to Waverly. But the trend to moving psychiatry back into both the general hospital and the community had developed to such an extent that when a new New York Hospital was erected through the generosity and foresight of Payne Whitney in 1932, a department of psychiatry was reestablished within the confines of the main hospital along with an active outpatient facility. The movement toward the community accelerated. Many forces were at work, but it was the American Psychiatric Association that took a lead in advocating community psychiatry in the 1950s. With the increasing attention to facilitation of the delivery of health services, broader questions came to the fore. Not only was the asylum under reevaluation, but the large teaching center as well.[21] There is no question that many medical problems are in flux; not the least is the role of the mental hospital. Although change is occurring for the McLean Hospital, as with all similar institutions, the facility is adapting creatively and still continues its long and proud tradition of service. The asylum is different: redefined but functioning well and hardly dead.

REFERENCES

1. Rumbaut, R.: Bernardino Alvarez: New world psychiatric pioneer. *Amer. J. Psychiat. 127*:1217-21, 1971.
2. Rumbaut, R.: The first psychiatric hospital of the Western world. *Amer. J. Psychiat. 128*:1305-09, 1972.
3. Allderidge, P. H.: Historical notes on the Bethlem Royal Hospital and the Maudsley Hospital. *Bull. N.Y. Acad. Med. 47*:1537-46, 1971.
4. Poynter, F. N. L., editor: *The Evolution of Hospitals in Britain.* London, Pitman, 1964.
5. Parry-Jones, W. L.: *The Trade in Lunacy: A Study of Private Madhouses in England in the Eighteenth and Nineteenth Centuries.* London, Routledge & Kegan Paul, 1972.
6. Tuke, S.: *Description of the Retreat, an Institution Near York* (York, 1813). London, Dawsons, 1964.
7. Dain, N.: *Disordered Minds: The First Century of the Eastern State Hospital in Williamsburg, Virginia, 1766-1866.* Charlottesville, Va., University Press of Virginia, 1971.
8. Carlson, E. T.: The unfortunate Dr. Parkman. *Amer. J. Psychiat. 123*:724-28, 1966.
9. Bowditch, N. I.: *A History of the Massachusetts General Hospital.* Boston, Wilson, 1851.
10. Jetter, D.: *Zur Typologie des Irrenhauses in Frankreich und Deutschland.* Wiesbaden, Steiner, 1971.
11. Carlson, E. T.: Dr. Rufus Wyman of the McLean Asylum. *Amer. J. Psychiat. 116*:1034-37, 1960.
12. Braceland, F. J.: *The Institute of Living: The Hartford Retreat, 1822-1972.* Hartford, Inst. of Living, 1972.
13. Deutsch, A.: *The Mentally Ill in America: A History of Their Care and Treatment from Colonial Times.* New York, Columbia University Press, 1949.
14. Rosenhan, D. L.: On being sane in insane places. *Science 179*:250-58, 1973.
15. Hunter, R. and Macalpine, I.: The Reverend John Ashbourne (c. 1611-61) and the origins of the private madhouse system. *Brit. Med. J. 2*:513-15, 1972.
16. Anonymous: Clinic shut; Ph.D. lack is at issue. *New York Times,* October 4, 1972.
17. Rothman, D. J.: *The Discovery of the Asylum: Social Order and Disorder in the New Republic.* Boston, Little, Brown, 1971.
18. Deutsch, A.: *The Shame of the States,* New York, Harcourt, Brace, 1948.
19. Stanton, A. H. and Schwartz, M. S.: *The Mental Hospital: A Study of Institutional Participation in Psychiatric Illness & Treatment.* New York, Basic Books, 1954.
20. Goffman, E.: *Asylums: Essays on the Social Situation of Mental Patients and Other Inmates.* Garden City, N.Y., Anchor, 1961.
21. New York Hospital Bicentennial Colloquium: *The Future Role of University-Based Metropolitan Medical Centers.* New York, Josiah Macy, Jr., Foundation, 1972.

THE SEARS ROEBUCK CATALOGUE OF 1897

In recent decades the writing of history has turned increasingly from the military and political sphere to the social sphere. More and more teachers and students have wondered how many French peasants in 1789 were really affected by the Revolution. How many Roman citizens, freedmen, or slaves were deviated from their daily routines by the fact that Rome declined and then fell?

With the expanded scope of historical writing there came a development of investigation into the affairs of the obscure citizen—his problems, his resources, his utensils, and his techniques. An interesting example was provided by Professor Charles C. Gillispie, who in 1959 reproduced 485 plates, mainly technological, from the famous encyclopedia of Denis Diderot. The pictures show us the tools, devices, and procedures that were used in 18th-century France. They also show us a little of the appearance and dress of French artisans although they depict these people as partly idealized figures, free from malnutrition, injury, and old age.

Recently some bright person was inspired to reprint the Sears Roebuck catalogue of 1897.[1] Evidently this is now a scarce item, most copies of the original having been used up in the houses, counting-houses, and outhouses of William McKinley's America.

The Sears Roebuck reprint contains about 800 ample pages of text[2] preceded by two engaging prefaces, one by the flippant and perceptive S. J. Perelman, the other by Richard Rovere, a writer whose essays have taught the layman some worthwhile facts of epidemiology.

Having read these attractive prefaces, the reader will plunge directly into the text proper of the catalogue. This starts with a variety of instructive fluff about the virtuous and efficient policies of the Sears Roebuck Company, about prices and methods of ordering, together with a disinterested bit labeled "How to Send Money." There is also a list of freight rates, which tells us that the charges for shipping 100 pounds of freight from Chicago were as follows: to New York City, 75 cents; to Los Angeles, $2.40; to Tampa, $2.77; to the "Indian Territory," $1.30 to $1.50; and to Flagstaff in the Arizona Territory, $3.90.

The introductory information concludes with testimonials from bankers. These statements reveal that Sears Roebuck had a fully paid-up capital of $150,000 and hence was worthy of confidence. His faith strengthened, the reader is now ready to confront the main text.

We need not pursue minutiae through the hundreds of pages which successively offer groceries, drugs, hardware, tools (including hog scrapers and sausage stuffers), stoves, agricultural implements (including windmills and equine treadmills), and on into clothing, household impedimenta, musical instruments, weapons, and vehicles.

It is a tradition in North American folklore that when the secluded sedentary thinker reached the chapter on harnesses it was time for him to send for a new catalogue. Investigation reveals that in 1897 the Department of Harness started on page 736, with only 7% of the text yet to come.

The section called Drug Department follows the Grocery Department. This sequence is reminiscent of the old alliance between the trade in drugs and that in spices. This union is preserved in the Italian word *speziale*, which means druggist and grocer.

The section on drugs extends for 20 pages and is followed by six pages on medical equipment. Under drugs we may notice a few items such as ague pills; arsenic complexion wafers; a cure to stop the drinking habit ("stops the craving for liquor instantly and stimulates the entire system to healthy action"); female pills composed of pennyroyal, tansy, and cottonroot bark; and a famous classic—Pink Pills for Pale People, "the great blood builder. Cures pale and sallow complexions. Suppression of the Periods. Rheumatism and all diseases arising from mental worry, overwork, early decay, etc."

Another engaging product is Dr. Pasteur's Microbe Killer, alleged to prevent "la Grippe, catarrh, consumption, malaria, blood poison, rheumatism, and all disorders of the blood. It acts as an antiseptic, killing the germs which are the cause of these diseases. This preparation of Dr. Pasteur's will eradicate any form of disease and purify the whole system." Half a gallon sold for 97 cents.

Under Special Family Remedies the catalogue presents not only essence of peppermint, sweet spirits of nitre, castor oil, and Seidlitz powders, but laudanum (10¢ an ounce) and paregoric (12¢ for two ounces). Another page lists a Cure for the Opium and Morphia Habit at 75 cents a bottle.

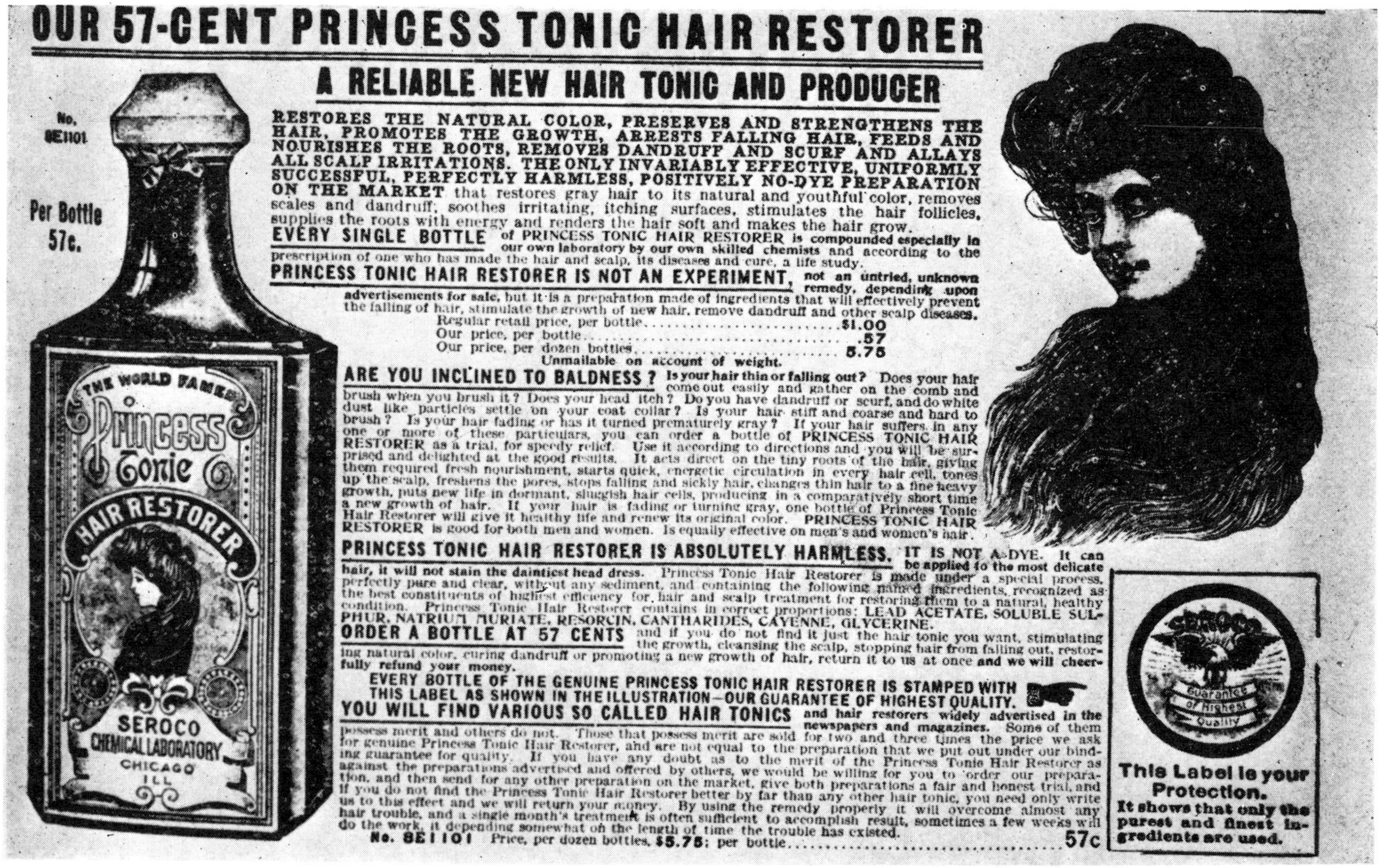
OUR 57-CENT PRINCESS TONIC HAIR RESTORER
A RELIABLE NEW HAIR TONIC AND PRODUCER
No. 8E1101
Per Bottle 57c.
THE WORLD FAMED
Princess Tonic
HAIR RESTORER
SEROCO
CHEMICAL LABORATORY
CHICAGO ILL
RESTORES THE NATURAL COLOR, PRESERVES AND STRENGTHENS THE HAIR, PROMOTES THE GROWTH, ARRESTS FALLING HAIR, FEEDS AND NOURISHES THE ROOTS, REMOVES DANDRUFF AND SCURF AND ALLAYS ALL SCALP IRRITATIONS. THE ONLY INVARIABLY EFFECTIVE, UNIFORMLY SUCCESSFUL, PERFECTLY HARMLESS, POSITIVELY NO-DYE PREPARATION ON THE MARKET that restores gray hair to its natural and youthful color, removes scales and dandruff; soothes irritating, itching surfaces, stimulates the hair follicles, supplies the roots with energy and renders the hair soft and makes the hair grow.
EVERY SINGLE BOTTLE of PRINCESS TONIC HAIR RESTORER is compounded especially in our own laboratory by our own skilled chemists and according to the prescription of one who has made the hair and scalp, its diseases and cure, a life study.
PRINCESS TONIC HAIR RESTORER IS NOT AN EXPERIMENT, not an untried, unknown remedy, depending upon advertisements for sale, but it is a preparation made of ingredients that will effectively prevent the falling of hair, stimulate the growth of new hair, remove dandruff and other scalp diseases.
Regular retail price, per bottle..........$1.00
Our price, per bottle..........57
Our price, per dozen bottles..........5.75
Unmailable on account of weight.
ARE YOU INCLINED TO BALDNESS? Is your hair thin or falling out? Does your hair come out easily and gather on the comb and brush when you brush it? Does your head itch? Do you have dandruff or scurf, and do white dust like particles settle on your coat collar? Is your hair stiff and coarse and hard to brush? Is your hair fading or has it turned prematurely gray? If your hair suffers in any one or more of these particulars, you can order a bottle of PRINCESS TONIC HAIR RESTORER as a trial, for speedy relief. Use it according to directions and you will be surprised and delighted at the good results. It acts direct on the tiny roots of the hair, giving them required fresh nourishment, starts quick, energetic circulation in every hair cell, tones up the scalp, freshens the pores, stops falling and sickly hair, changes thin hair to a fine heavy growth, puts new life in dormant, sluggish hair cells, producing in a comparatively short time a new growth of hair. If your hair is fading or turning gray, one bottle of Princess Tonic Hair Restorer will give it healthy life and renew its original color. PRINCESS TONIC HAIR RESTORER is good for both men and women. Is equally effective on men's and women's hair.
PRINCESS TONIC HAIR RESTORER IS ABSOLUTELY HARMLESS. IT IS NOT A DYE. It can be applied to the most delicate hair, it will not stain the daintiest head dress. Princess Tonic Hair Restorer is made under a special process, perfectly pure and clear, without any sediment, and containing the following named ingredients, recognized as the best constituents of highest efficiency for hair and scalp treatment for restoring them to a natural, healthy condition. Princess Tonic Hair Restorer contains in correct proportions: LEAD ACETATE, SOLUBLE SULPHUR, NATRIUM MURIATE, RESORCIN, CANTHARIDES, CAYENNE, GLYCERINE.
ORDER A BOTTLE AT 57 CENTS and if you do not find it just the hair tonic you want, stimulating the growth, cleansing the scalp, stopping hair from falling out, restoring natural color, curing dandruff or promoting a new growth of hair, return it to us at once and we will cheerfully refund your money.
EVERY BOTTLE OF THE GENUINE PRINCESS TONIC HAIR RESTORER IS STAMPED WITH THIS LABEL AS SHOWN IN THE ILLUSTRATION—OUR GUARANTEE OF HIGHEST QUALITY.
YOU WILL FIND VARIOUS SO CALLED HAIR TONICS and hair restorers widely advertised in the newspapers and magazines. Some of them possess merit and others do not. Those that possess merit are sold for two and three times the price we ask for genuine Princess Tonic Hair Restorer, and are not equal to the preparation that we put out under our binding guarantee for quality. If you have any doubt as to the merit of the Princess Tonic Hair Restorer as against the preparations advertised and offered by others, we would be willing for you to order our preparation, and then send for any other preparation on the market, give both preparations a fair and honest trial, and if you do not find the Princess Tonic Hair Restorer better by far than any other hair tonic, you need only write us to this effect and we will return your money. By using the remedy properly it will overcome almost any hair trouble, and a single month's treatment is often sufficient to accomplish result, sometimes a few weeks will do the work, it depending somewhat on the length of time the trouble has existed.
No. 8E1101 Price, per dozen bottles, $5.75; per bottle..........57c
SEROCO
Guarantee of Highest Quality
This Label is your Protection.
It shows that only the purest and finest ingredients are used.

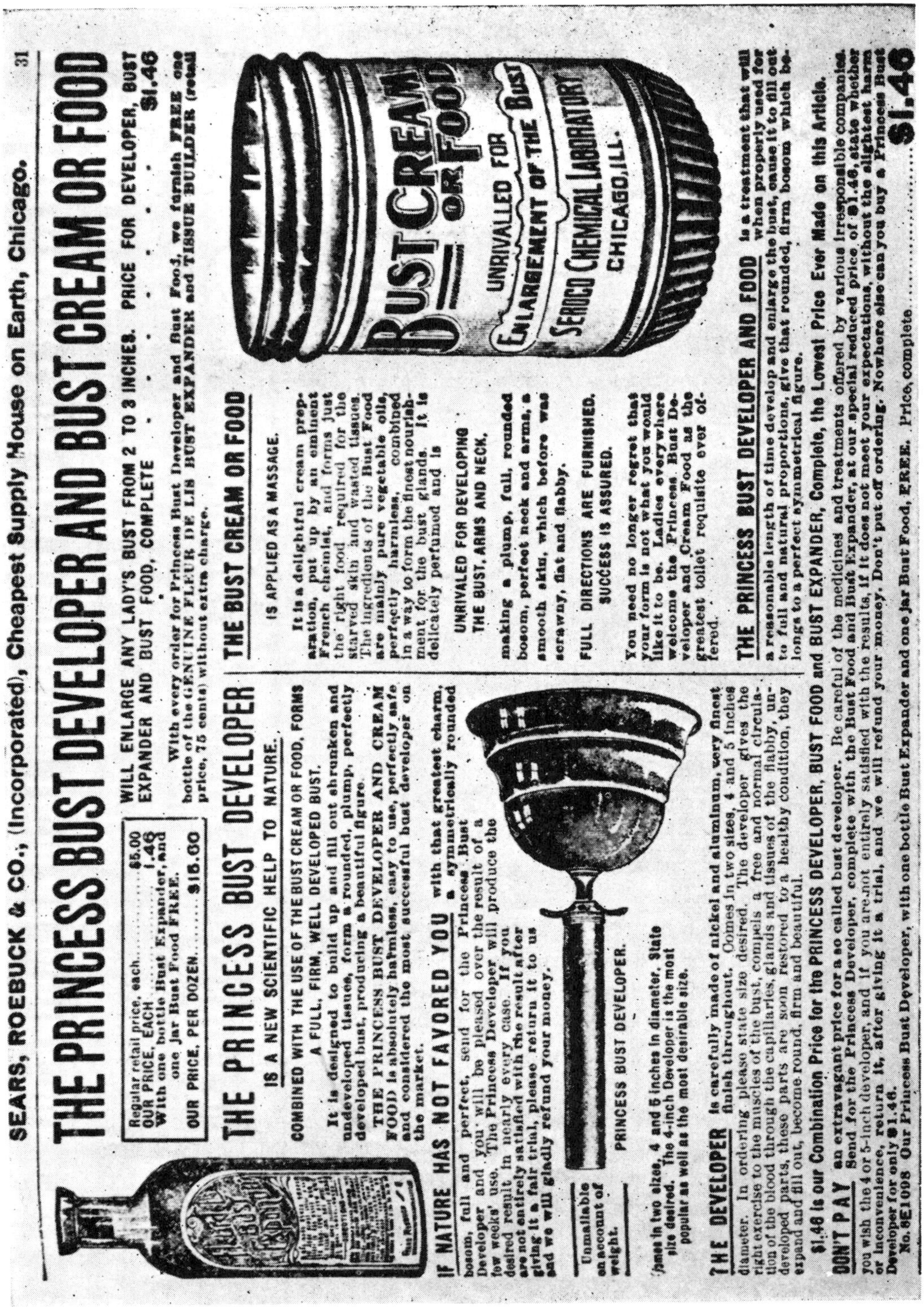
SEARS, ROEBUCK & CO., (Incorporated), Cheapest Supply House on Earth, Chicago. 31

THE PRINCESS BUST DEVELOPER AND BUST CREAM OR FOOD

Regular retail price, each..............$5.00
OUR PRICE, EACH....................1.46
With one bottle Bust Expander, and one jar Bust Food FREE.
OUR PRICE, PER DOZEN.........$15.60

WILL ENLARGE ANY LADY'S BUST FROM 2 TO 3 INCHES. PRICE FOR DEVELOPER, BUST EXPANDER AND BUST FOOD, COMPLETE $1.46

With every order for Princess Bust Developer and Bust Food, we furnish FREE one bottle of the GENUINE FLEUR DE LIS BUST EXPANDER and TISSUE BUILDER (retail price, 75 cents) without extra charge.

THE PRINCESS BUST DEVELOPER

IS A NEW SCIENTIFIC HELP TO NATURE.

COMBINED WITH THE USE OF THE BUST CREAM OR FOOD, FORMS A FULL, FIRM, WELL DEVELOPED BUST.

It is designed to build up and fill out shrunken and undeveloped tissues, form a rounded, plump, perfectly developed bust, producing a beautiful figure.

THE PRINCESS BUST DEVELOPER AND CREAM FOOD is absolutely harmless, easy to use, perfectly safe and considered the most successful bust developer on the market.

IF NATURE HAS NOT FAVORED YOU with that greatest charm, a symmetrically rounded bosom, full and perfect, send for the Princess Bust Developer and you will be pleased over the result of a few weeks' use. The Princess Developer will produce the desired result in nearly every case. If you are not entirely satisfied with the result after giving it a fair trial, please return it to us and we will gladly refund your money.

Unmailable on account of weight.

PRINCESS BUST DEVELOPER.

Comes in two sizes, 4 and 5 inches in diameter. State size desired. The 4-inch Developer is the most popular as well as the most desirable size.

THE DEVELOPER is carefully made of nickel and aluminum, very finest finish throughout. Comes in two sizes, 4 and 5 inches diameter. In ordering please state size desired. The developer gives the right exercise to the muscles of the bust, compels a free and normal circulation of the blood through the capillaries, glands and tissues of the flabby, undeveloped parts, these parts are soon restored to a healthy condition, they expand and fill out, become round, firm and beautiful.

THE BUST CREAM OR FOOD

IS APPLIED AS A MASSAGE.

It is a delightful cream preparation, put up by an eminent French chemist, and forms just the right food required for the starved skin and wasted tissues. The ingredients of the Bust Food are mainly pure vegetable oils, perfectly harmless, combined in a way to form the finest nourishment for the bust glands. It is delicately perfumed and is

UNRIVALED FOR DEVELOPING THE BUST, ARMS AND NECK,

making a plump, full, rounded bosom, perfect neck and arms, a smooth skin, which before was scrawny, flat and flabby.

FULL DIRECTIONS ARE FURNISHED. SUCCESS IS ASSURED.

You need no longer regret that your form is not what you would like it to be. Ladies everywhere welcome the Princess Bust Developer and Cream Food as the greatest toilet requisite ever offered.

BUST CREAM OR FOOD
UNRIVALLED FOR
ENLARGEMENT OF THE BUST
SEROCO CHEMICAL LABORATORY
CHICAGO, ILL.

THE PRINCESS BUST DEVELOPER AND FOOD is a treatment that will when properly used for a reasonable length of time develop and enlarge the bust, cause it to fill out to full and natural proportions, give that rounded, firm bosom which belongs to a perfect symmetrical figure.

$1.46 is our Combination Price for the PRINCESS DEVELOPER, BUST FOOD and BUST EXPANDER, Complete, the Lowest Price Ever Made on this Article.

DON'T PAY an extravagant price for a so called bust developer. Be careful of the medicines and treatments offered by various irresponsible companies. Send for the Princess Developer, complete with the Bust Food and Bust Expander, at our special reduced price of $1.46, state whether you wish the 4 or 5-inch developer, and if you are not entirely satisfied with the results, if it does not meet your expectations, without the slightest harm or inconvenience, return it, after giving it a trial, and we will refund your money. Don't put off ordering. Nowhere else can you buy a Princess Bust Developer for only $1.46.

No. 8E1098 Our Princess Bust Developer, with one bottle Bust Expander and one jar Bust Food, FREE. Price, complete..........................$1.46

Reprinted from *1897 Sears Roebuck Catalogue*. Copyright, 1968, by Chelsea House Publishers, New York, N. Y. Reprinted by permission. Reduced slightly.

For the most part the compound remedies are catalogued without mention of their ingredients, effective restrictive legislation being some distance in the future. The text includes a list of homeopathic products, arranged entirely according to symptoms, viz.:

D600 Cures rheumatism or rheumatic pains
D602 Cures fever and ague, intermittent fever, malaria
D604 Cures piles, blind or bleeding, external or internal.

Some of the notices in the catalogue contain statements about pathogenesis or semeiology. For example, under Curtis' Consumption Cure it is alleged that "tuberculous matter is nothing more or less than nourishment imperfectly organized. Now if with this remedy we can procure the organization of this food material . . . we can cure the disease."

In beating the drum for Dr. Echols' Australian Auriclo, a Newly Discovered Cure for Heart Trouble, the catalogue states that heart disease often causes sudden death. It then lists the following as some of the more common symptoms of heart disease:

Shortness of breath
Fluttering or palpitation
Pain or tenderness in the left breast, side or under the left shoulder blade between the shoulders
Irregular or intermittent pulse
Oppressed feeling in the chest
Choking sensation in the throat. . .
Dropsy. . .

This is a fair representation of doctrines prevalent before the work of James B. Herrick on coronary disease.

The medical section of the catalogue also advertises various items of equipment, such as The Princess Bust Developer ("If Nature Has Not Favored You"), which may be seen in the accompanying illustration.)

S. J.

REFERENCES

1. 1897 Sears Roebuck Catalogue, edited by Fred L. Israel. New York, Chelsea House Publishers, 1968, 786 pp. (plus unnumbered intercalated pages).
2. Some unnumbered pages have been included among the numbered pages.

VIENNESE SEROLOGICAL RESEARCH ABOUT THE YEAR 1900: ITS CONTRIBUTION TO THE DEVELOPMENT OF CLINICAL MEDICINE

Erna Lesky

Professor, Institute for the History of Medicine
University of Vienna
Vienna, Austria

It is true that immunological discoveries of the Vienna School, such as agglutination (1896), precipitation (1897), and blood groups (1900), as well as the final definition of the concept of allergy (1906), are mentioned in every medical textbook. However, they are registered there only as firsts and the dates are given. Thus far no one has tried to consider them as a unified complex or to draw attention to the fact that the creative impulses for all these discoveries came from the same background. What I want to attempt, therefore, is to treat these discoveries, which concern some of the most basic laws of immunology, in their genetic affiliation. Such an undertaking must necessarily involve something else. We must attempt to study the facilities offered for experimental research in clinical medicine at that time, using serology—then one of the most promising medical fields—as our case in point. As we have chosen one of the leading medical centers for our discussion we may expect exemplary results.

W. D. Foster[1] states that, in general, hospital laboratories did not come into existence before the end of the 19th century. At the center of clinical university medicine, the General Hospital of Vienna, laboratories were still rudimentary. The clinic of Professor Hermann Nothnagel, for example, had one scantily equipped laboratory room at its disposal, where routine analyses of urine and blood could be carried out. What went beyond that, in particular the reception and further development of new ideas in medical research, fell to the theoretical institutes in the School of Medicine. These, it is true, were equipped poorly enough. Everything depended on the inventiveness of the heads of the various theoretical institutes and on their ability to improvise and to secure the cooperation of the clinics.

Against this background the pioneer work of Max Gruber (1853-1927)[2] must be evaluated. Beginning in 1887, he carried on his research in the four poorly equipped rooms of the Vienna Institute of Hygiene. But the problems which he attacked there were so timely that he also attracted pupils from abroad. Among them was Herbert E. Durham (1866-1945)[3] of Guy's Hospital, London. Thus the Vienna Institute of Hygiene not only became seminal for Viennese serological research but, through the activities of Durham, also determined the work done in this field in London. Further, we owe the prototype of all serodiagnostic test methods, the agglutination test, to the joint efforts of Austrian and British scientists. This is not the place, however, to go into greater detail concerning the history of that discovery.[4] In our context it is of interest only insofar as it influenced clinical practice and as it helped to develop further serodiagnostic methods.

Concerning both, it is interesting to note, first, that as early as January or February 1896, Durham and Gruber discovered the double applicability of the agglutination test: that it can be used both to identify bacteria and to detect specific agglutinin in blood serum. In March 1896 Gruber sent another pupil to the clinic of Professor Nothnagel, to look for typhoid agglutinins in the serum of patients. The fact that this pupil of Gruber, whose name was Albert Sidney Grünbaum, also came from London is another evidence of the close connections that existed between Vienna and London.

Gruber also did something else. He attended the annual meeting of internists at Wiesbaden, and on April 9, 1896, he informed the assembled physicians about the possibility of early diagnosis of typhoid fever and cholera by means of the agglutination test.[5] In spite of these early contacts with the clinicians, Gruber and his English pupils nevertheless must share their priority rights in this respect with the Frenchman F. J. Widal (1862-1929). The two cases of typhoid fever at Nothnagel's clinic in the spring of 1896 offered too small a basis for publication. Paris furnished more typhoid cases and then, on April 15, the discoveries of Gruber and Durham were made public there in the *Semaine médicale*. Widal's publication on the clinical utilization of serodiagnosis in typhoid could therefore appear as early as June 26.

The agglutination test very soon entered the clinics as a routine test.[6] As early as August 1897 Widal was able to report at the 65th annual meeting of the British Medical Association in Montreal that there

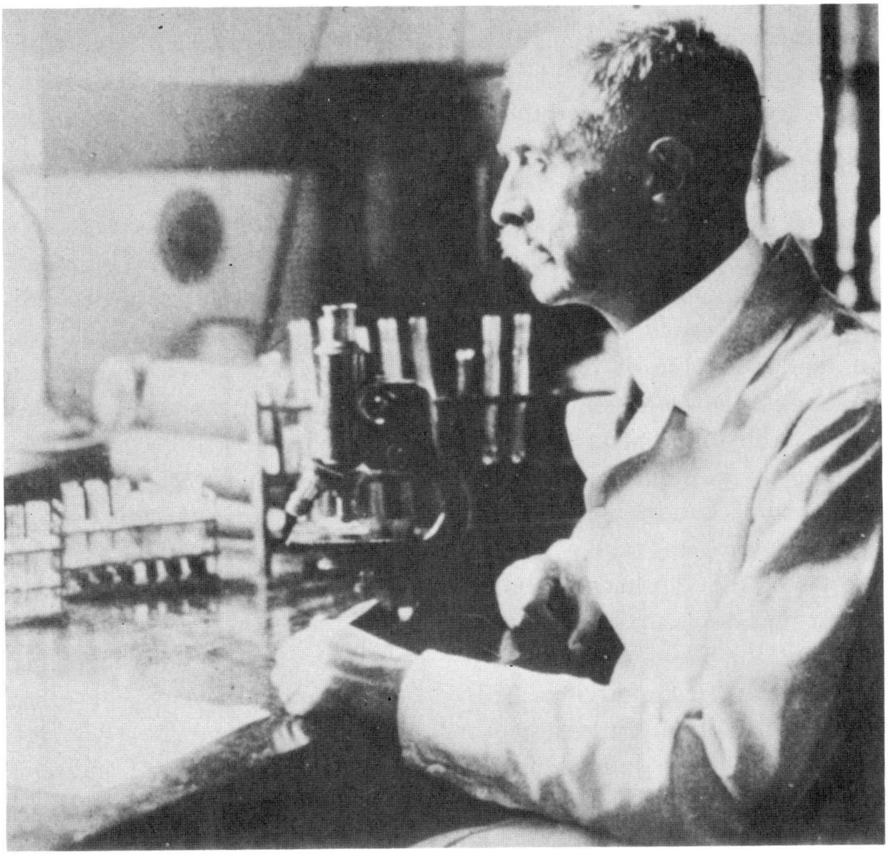

Fig. 1. Karl Landsteiner (1868-1943). All illustrations in this essay are based on original pictures in the archives of the Institute of the History of Medicine in Vienna.

were records of the test being done in several thousand cases.

While in 1896 the agglutination test, which later came to be called the Gruber-Widal test, began its triumphant advance through the clinics, its birthplace, the Institute of Hygiene in Vienna, witnessed preliminary experiments leading to another discovery of far-reaching importance. A young physician had entered the institute on January 1, 1896, as an assistant. He had previously concerned himself with chemical work alone, but in the new milieu he began to try his hand at serological experiments. This physician was Karl Landsteiner (1868-

1943),[7] (Figure 1) and we in no way undervalue his genius when we draw attention to the immediate connection between these discoveries. The discovery of the interagglutination of human sera, i.e., Landsteiner's theory of the human blood groups, was an outgrowth of Gruber's line of research and is based on the phenomenon of agglutination discovered by him and Durham. In 1900, when Landsteiner published his discovery of isoagglutination as a physiological phenomenon, he no longer was a member of the Institute of Hygiene. We are ignorant of the causes that made him give up a paid assistantship at the Institute of Hygiene to become an unsalaried volunteer at the Institute of Pathological Anatomy, which was headed by Anton Weichselbaum (1845-1920), the well-known discoverer of the *Diplococcus meningitidis*. We know, however, that the latter institute at the time of Landsteiner's transfer (1897) prided itself on a bacteriological laboratory that was well equipped according to the standards of the time. During the next 10 years (1897-1907), while Landsteiner worked there, this laboratory became a world-famous serological center. Landsteiner succeeded in interesting his colleagues at the Nothnagel clinic in his serological research. To what extent they took an active part in it is apparent from the famous publication on the blood groups (1901).[8] Two of Nothnagel's assistants mentioned there by Landsteiner, Alfred von Decastello-Rechtwehr (1872-1960) and Adriano Sturli, themselves defined the "no-type" AB blood group a year later. Julius Donath (1870-1919), with whom Landsteiner in 1904 clarified the pathophysiological mechanism of paroxysmal cold hemoglobinuria,[9] likewise came from the Northnagel clinic. Two years earlier, Landsteiner had cooperated with Josef Halban (1870-1937), who then was assistant at the First Gynaecological Clinic, in a study on immunity in the newborn.[10] In 1905-1906 Landsteiner, in cooperation with the venereologist Ernst Finger (1856-1939), succeeded in infecting monkeys with syphilis.[11] In 1907, together with Finger's assistant, Rudolf Müller (1877-1934), he explained the principle underlying the Wassermann reaction. These are some of the outstanding results which made Landsteiner's laboratory—in spite of its minimal size and utter simplicity of equipment, which seems almost incredible today—a center of immunological research connected with the Allgemeines Krankenhaus.

Before dealing with the third center of serological research in Vienna at the turn of the century, we must glance at the two other capitals of European medicine, Paris and Berlin, and inquire about the homes of

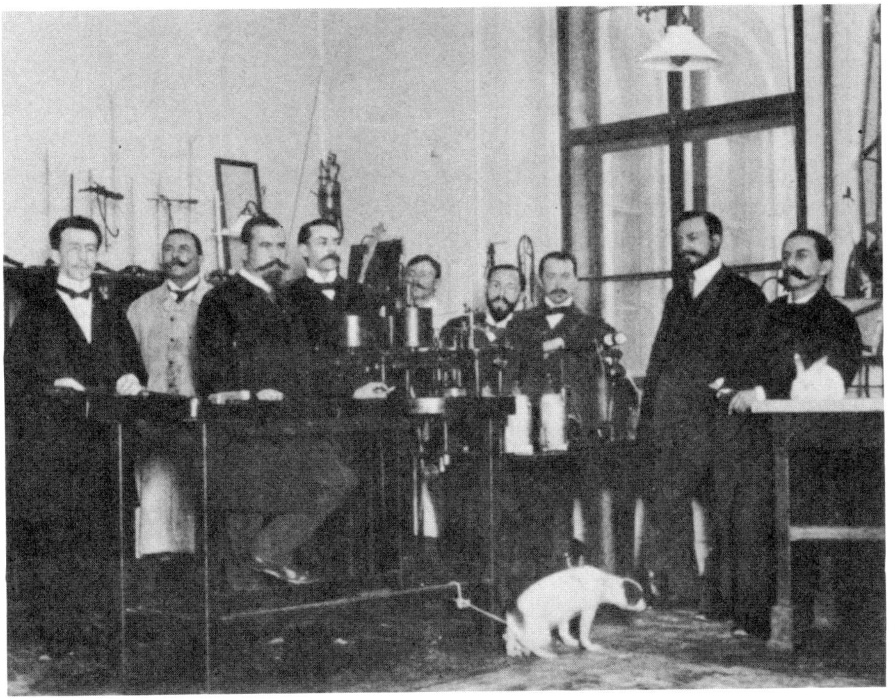

Fig. 2. Richard Paltauf (1858-1924) and his collaborators at the Institute of Experimental Pathology, Vienna. Photograph, 1905.

bacteriological and serological research there. We immediately think of the Institut Pasteur in Paris and the Institute for Infectious Diseases in Berlin, which was headed by Koch. In 1888 and 1891, respectively, the French nation and the German state had erected these institutes specifically for this new field, which proved equally important for therapy and prophylaxis; these institutes also had been equipped with the most modern facilities. We observe an essential difference. While this field of basic research received generous official support elsewhere, the Austrian pioneers Max Gruber and Karl Landsteiner were obliged to gain their results the hard way in laboratories in the Institute of Hygiene or the Institute of Pathological Anatomy that were improvised and possessed only modest means.

A change for the better finally came during the last years of the century. It is connected with the name of one man, Richard Paltauf (1858-1924)[12] (Figure 2). We cannot overestimate the fact that in 1894, when the therapeutic value of rabies antiserum and diphtheria serum could no longer be disregarded, a man appeared on the scene who founded a Rabies and Serotherapeutic Institute in Vienna. Paltauf's ultimate aim was the creation of a large research center with many departments, according to the Paris model. Paltauf was a pathological anatomist who, in 1893, became the head of the pathological anatomy department at the Rudolf Hospital. He proved to be a most successful large-scale organizer; from his skill not only this municipal hospital but also theoretical university medicine in general derived great benefit. Starting from the department of pathological anatomy in his home hospital, he built up in the course of a few years his "kingdom" of experimental medicine. This enterprise included the following institutions: the Rabies[13] and Serotherapeutic[14] Institute founded in 1894, the Serological Research Center of the department of pathological anatomy, the Histopathological Institute at the university and, since 1900, the Institute of General and Experimental Pathology.

In all these institutions Paltauf assembled a staff of gifted and even brilliant assistants. Among these we must mention first Rudolf Kraus (1868-1932)[15] and Robert Doerr (1871-1952);[16] the latter became professor of hygiene at Basel. These two men in turn attracted young clinicians not only from the Rudolf Hospital but also from the university clinics. Among those who worked at the serotherapeutic laboratory of the Rudolf Hospital were the pediatrician Clemens von Pirquet (1874-1929),[17] the surgeon Paul Clairmont, and the psychiatrists Wagner von Jauregg and Otto Pölzl—to mention only a few.

We see that a stage of serological research characterized by rapid development at the same time offered many powerful impulses to clinical therapy. In this connection I can give only a sketchy list of the most important of these influences. There is the discovery of the method of precipitation by Rudolf Kraus in 1897; this has become one of the indispensable routine tests in almost all fields of medicine.[18] There is the isolation of dysentery antitoxin, performed by Kraus in cooperation with Robert Doerr. This was followed by the production of antitoxic dysentery serum.[19] It was also in this group that, in the course of their search for useful sera, Ernst Lowenstein (1878-1949) and Michael Eisler-Terramare (1877-1970)[20] for the first time succeeded in preparing toxoids from tetanus toxin by means of formalin treatment. Eisler and Friedrich Silberstein put this tetanus toxoid to practical use in the production of tetanus serum, which became the model for Gaston Ramon (1886-1963) in the 1920s. Ramon produced diphtheria anatoxin in order to extract antitoxic immune sera and for the active immunization of humans.[21] As a last example I should like to mention gamma globulin. When this protein is used today hardly anyone remembers that we owe it to the biochemical pioneering work of Ernst Peter Pick (1872-1960).[22]

You will excuse this cursory enumeration, which serves merely to demonstrate the enormous scope of what was achieved under Paltauf. But I want to enlarge a little on a process which I can best characterize as a scientific chain reaction which seems especially apt to illustrate the interdependence of serological experiment and clinical diagnosis. I am thinking of Pirquet's conclusions about the nature of serum sickness (or the practice of vaccination) and the tuberculin test and their inclusion under the general concept of allergy.

Commentators[23] have rightly pointed to Pirquet's bold play of associations, which related far-off, long-known phenomena such as vaccination and newly found clinical phenomena (serum exanthema) to each other, and thus arrived at fundamental biological laws, such as the concept of allergy. Those who have been fascinated by the working of Pirquet's mind and have tried to follow his ideas have nevertheless neglected up to the present time to offer an adequate treatment of the laboratory foundations of his findings. Further, we must not fail to concentrate on the question of the part played by the serological laboratories of Paltauf and Rudolf Kraus in the immunological concepts of Pirquet (Figure 3).

In 1902 Rudolf Kraus, already famous as the discoverer of serological precipitation, published a study titled *Further Investigations Concerning Specific Precipitations*.[24] His collaborator was a young assistant in the pediatric clinic of the university, Clemens Pirquet. In this study Pirquet's own ideas are not yet apparent. He presents himself rather as an ardent pupil of Kraus, engaged in mastering Kraus' serological methods and concepts. The outward circumstances of this schooling were thus described by Pirquet's friend and colleague, Bela Schick (1877-

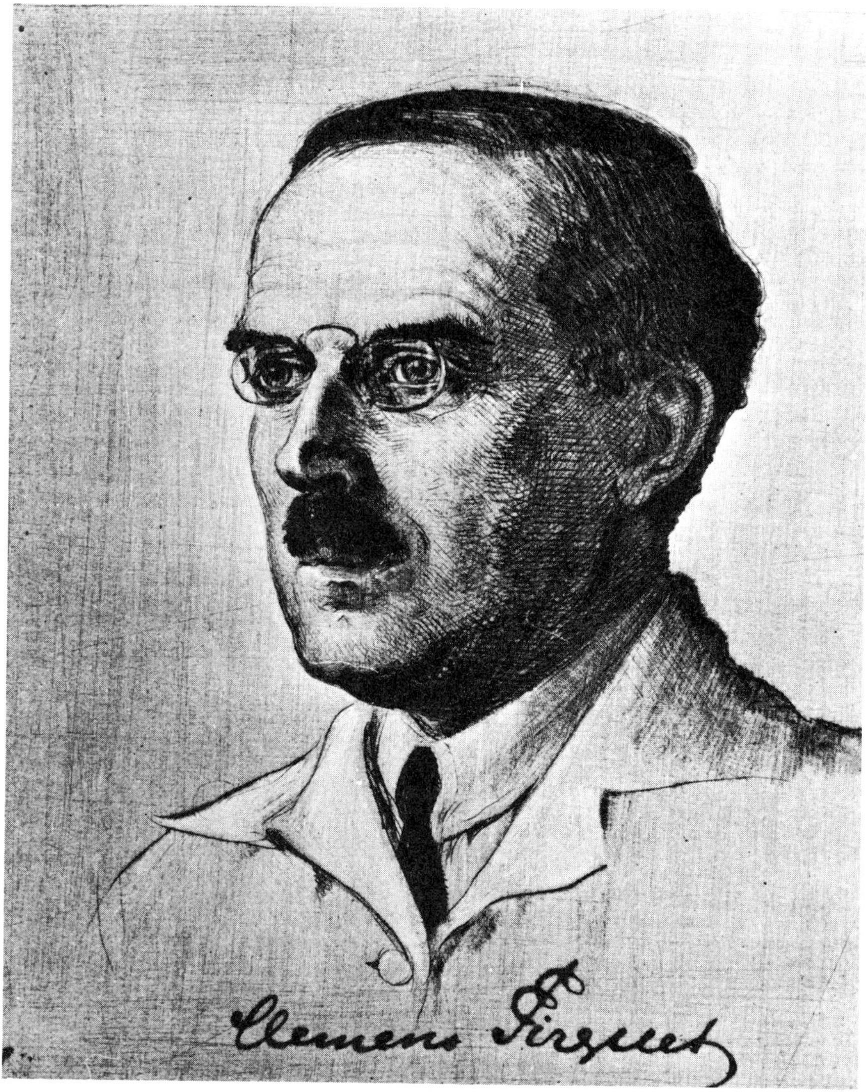

Fig. 3. Clemens von Pirquet (1874-1929). Unsigned etching.

1967):[25] "Immediately after lunch we all rushed by street car to the Serotherapeutisches Institut, where Paltauf and Rudolf Kraus worked. This institute was our laboratory. We had none in the clinic for several years."

In the same year, 1902, Paul Moser (1865-1924), first assistant at the pediatric clinic, came out with his scarlatinal antiserum.[26] Far from being an accidental coincidence, this achievement was evidence of the close cooperation that existed between the pediatric clinic and the Serotherapeutic Institute. The high dosages of Moser's serum that were used offered ample opportunities for Pirquet and Schick to study serum sickness, which they were the first to define as a separate syndrome.[27] Pirquet observed that when there was a second injection, the symptoms appeared at once or within a few hours, whereas after the first injection they took seven at 12 days to develop. This became the pivotal point for further considerations.[28]

With Pirquet putting the question about this reduction of the incubation period we have come to the mental processes which I have called a scientific chain reaction. Raising this question involves the raising of two further questions. These are Pirquet's very own: What is the nature of the incubation period, and what are the processes that induce the body to learn a different reaction: i.e., to acquire a new quality, for which Pirquet in 1906 devised the term allergy?[29] This is the crucial point in the statement of the problem. Here Pirquet the clinician most profitably became aware of everything Pirquet the serologist had learned from Kraus, the discoverer of serologic precipitation. The process of precipitation which he had so often observed in the test tube appeared to Pirquet to be a heuristic model. In the monograph on serum sickness,[30] which appeared in 1905, he explicitly refers to Kraus and his discovery. The reference occurs in the passage in which he expounds, at length and according to experiments, his hypothesis of the formation of precipitins to accord with his concept of serum sickness as an antigen-antibody reaction. When we read Pirquet's concluding remarks we find that the clinician has become one with the laboratory-centered serologist in an almost ideal way: "Just as the precipitate shows when we add one drop of horse serum to the serum containing antibody, the specific edema, the immediate reaction, occurs if an individual containing antibody is treated with horse serum."[31] The conclusion Pirquet draws from this analogy between the processes observed in the laboratory and in the clinic is contained in the following sentence in his book: "The reaction *in vivo* is as specific as that *in vitro*."[32]

This analogy was to be of the greatest consequence for clinical medicine. It suggested to Pirquet not only the explanation of the processes underlying revaccination, which had long been practiced, though its nature was not understood—Pirquet was able to explain it also as an antigen-antibody-reaction[33]—but also the tuberculin test that is known by his name.[34] If we for once consider this test in this way, the phenomena that appear in the skin become as plain as the phenomena that accompany serum sickness or revaccination. The characteristic reddening of the skin of persons infected with tuberculosis is caused by vaccination with tuberculin, just as the precipitate appears in the test tube filled with serum containing antibody when horse serum is added.

The tuberculin reaction was the crowning achievement of Pirquet's work. As this test dispenses with the test tube it represents the final transposition into the living body of the process observed in the test tube. A transformation of this kind could be achieved only by a scientist who, during his time in the laboratory, had also remained a true clinician.

Today the tuberculin test is performed all over the world. Apart from some modifications it has remained as conceived by Pirquet. Therefore we should not forget that, being an outgrowth of experiments conducted at the serological laboratory in Vienna, it offers one of the most impressive examples of the fertilizing influence of basic research on clinical medicine.

NOTES AND REFERENCES

1. Foster, W. D.: *A Short History of Clinical Pathology.* Edinburgh and London, Livingtone, 1961, p. 113.
2. Lesky, E.: *Die Wiener medizinische Schule im 19. Jahrhundert.* Graz-Köln, Böhlaus Nachf., 1965, p. 595 ff.
3. Foster, W. D., op. cit., p. 73 f.
4. On the history of agglutination see: Gruber, M.: Geschichte der Entdeckung der spezifischen Agglutination. In: *Handbuch der Immunitätsforschung und experimentellen Therapie,* Kraus, R. and Levaditi, C. editors. Jena, Lieferung, 1914, pp. 150-154. Reprinted under the title Agglutination in *Wien. Med. Wschr. 77*:742f, 1927. Paltauf, R.: Die Agglutination. In: *Handbuch d. pathog. Mikroorganismen,* Kolle, W. and Wassermann, A., editors. Jena, 1904, vol. 4, p. 645 ff. Bordet, J.: Geschichtlicher Überblick und allgemeine Anschauungen über Immunität. In: *Handbuch d. Immunitätsforschung und experimentellen Therapie,* Kraus, R. and Levaditi, editors. Jena, Lieferung, 1914, p. 43ff. Bulloch, W.: *The History of Bacteriology.* London, 1960, Oxford University Press, p. 266f.
5. Gruber, M.: Prioritätsanspruch. *Wien. Klin. Wschr. 9*:244, 1896.
6. Foster, W. D., op. cit., p. 76. By 1904 almost 1,000 scientific studies on agglutination had been published. Cf. Römer, P.: *Die Ehrlichsche Seitenket-*

tentheorie und ihre Bedeutung für die medizinische Wissenschaft. Wien, Hölder, 1904, p. 323.

7. Speiser, P.: *Karl Landsteiner.* Wien, 1961. Lesky, E., op. cit., p. 574. Simms, G. R.: *The scientific work of Karl Landsteiner.* Zürich, Med. Diss., 1965. Foster, W. D., op. cit., p. 107f. Schorr, M.: *Zur Geschichte der Bluttransfusion im 19. Jahrhundert.* Basel and Stuttgart, Basler Veröff. *Gesch. Med. Biol.,* Fasc. 7, 1956. Buess, H.: Der Ausbau der Blutttransfusion in neuester Zeit. *Bull. Schweiz. Akad. Med. Wiss. 9:*248-69, 1953.
8. Landsteiner, K.: Über Agglutinationserscheinungen normalen menschlichen Blutes. *Wien. Klin. Wschr. 14:*1132-34, 1901.
9. Donath, J. and Landsteiner, K..: Über paroxysmale Hämoglobinurie. *Münch. Med. Wschr. 51:*1590-93, 1904.
10. Halban, J. and Landsteiner, K.: Über Unterschiede des fötalen und mütterlichen Serums und über eine fällungshemmende Wirkung des Normalserums. *Münch. Med. Wschr. 49:*473-78, 1902.
11. Finger, E. and Landsteiner, K.: Untersuchungen über Syphilis an Affen. *Sitzb. Akad. Wiss. Wien.* 3, *114:*497-539, 1905; *115:*179-200, 1906; *Arch. Derm. Syph. 78:*335-68, 1906; *81:*147-66, 1906.
12. Lesky, E., op. cit., p. 577ff. Pick, E. P.: Richard Paltauf, seine Schule und ihre Forschungsergebnisse. *Wien. Klin. Wschr. 65,* 698-702, 1953.
13. Paltauf, R.: Die Errichtung der Anstalt zur Wuthschutzimpfung in der k.k. Krankenanstalt Rudolfsiftung. *Jahrb. Wien. Krank. 3:*912-29, 1894.
14. Paltauf, R.: Das staatliche Institut für Herstellung von Diphtherie Heilserum in Wien. Errichtung desselben und seine Tätigkeit im Jahre 1895. *Jahrb. Wien. Krank. 4:*1-52, 1895. Kraus, R.: Richard Paltauf und das Serotherapeutische Institut. *Wien. Med. Wschr. 77:*739-41, 1927. Teichmann, J.: *Bundesstaatliches Serotherapeutisches Institut Wien, 1894-1954.* Wien, Gruber, 1954.
15. Löwenstein, E. and Kraus, R. *Wien. Med. Wschr. 82:*1016f, 1932. Eisler, M.: *Wien. Klin. Wschr. 45:*1072f, 1932. Teichmann, J.: Zum 100. Geburtstag Rudolf Krans'. *Wien. Med Wschr. 118:* 869-72, 1968.
16. Reuter, F.: In memoriam R. Doerr. *Wien. Klin. Wschr. 64:*129f, 1952.
17. In this connection another two-man team should be mentioned. At the same time, in 1903, Pirquet had been connected with Max Gruber, who was already in Munich.
18. Kraus, R.: 30 Jahre Präzipitinlehre. *Wien. Med. Wschr. 77:*743f, 1927. Teichmann, J.: 70 Jahre Präzipitation. *Wien. Klin. Wschr. 79:*281-84, 1967.
19. Kraus, R. and Doerr, R.: Das Dysenterieserum. *Wien. Klin. Wschr. 19:*929f, 1906.
20. Teichmann, J.: Prof. Dr. M. Eisler-Terramare zum 80. Geburtstag. *Wien. Klin. Wschr. 69:*52f, 1957. Idem: Prof. Eisler-Terramare und sein Wirken am Serotherapeutischen Institut. *Mitt. Öst. Sanitäts-Verwaltung 58:*147-50, 1957.
21. Dagoquet, F.: L'immunité, histoire et méthode. *Conférence donnée au Palais de la Découverte.* D. 94. Paris o.J., 1964, p. 17 ff. Parish, H. J.: *A History of Immunization.* Edinburgh and London, Livingstone, 1965. p. 141f.
22. Pick, E. P.; *Wien, Klin. Wschr. 65:* 699, 1953; Brücke, F. T.: Ernst Peter Pick. Nachruf. *Alman. Öst. Akad. Wiss. 110:*446-59, 1960.
23. Wagner, R. *Clemens von Pirquet: His Life and Work.* Baltimore, Johns Hopkins Press, 1968, p. 16. Idem: Clemens von Pirquet, discoverer of the concept of allergy. *Bull. N.Y. Acad. Med. 40:*229-35, 1964.
24. *Centralblatt f. Bakteriologie, Parasitenkunde und Infectionskrankheiten 32:*60-74, 1902.
25. Schick, B.: Pediatrics in Vienna at the beginning of the century. *J. Ped. 50:* 119, 1957.
26. Schick, B. (op. cit., p. 119) speaks about the amazing results obtained with this serum. It becomes clear therefore that R. Kraus advocated calling the antitoxic scarlet fever antiserum according to Moser-Dick (Berechtigung, das antitoxische Scharlachserum Moser-Dick zu benennen. *Wien. Med. Wschr. 77:*745f,

1927) after the good results obtained with the Dick-Dochez serum in America became known. Cf. also Parish, H. J., op. cit., p. 198ff. Wagner, R., op. cit., p. 29.

27. This was in the monograph *Die Serumkrankheit,* Vienna, 1905, which he published with Bela Schick.

28. After Schick, B. (op. cit., p. 120) the first observation was made by Pirquet on December 2, 1902. Cf. von Pirquet, C. and Schick, B.: *Die Serumkrankheit.* Vienna, 1905, p. 77.

29. Pirquet, C. v.: Allergie. *Münch. Med. Wschr. 53*:1457-58, 1906. Idem: Zur Geschichte der Allergie. *Wien. Med. Wschr. 27*:745-48, 1927. Doerr, B.: Ueber Anaphylaxie. *Wien. Klin. Wschr. 27*:415-22, 1908. Idem: "Die Anaphylaxie." In: *Die Immunitätsforschung,* vol. 6. Wien, Springer, 1950. Idem: Die Allergie. Ibid., vol. 8. Wien, 1951. Blittersdorf, F.: Zur Geschichte der Serumkrankheit. *Sudhoffs Arch. Gesch. Med. 36*:149-58, 1943. Pache, H. D.: 50 Jahre Allergie in der Kinderheilkunde. *Münch. Med. Wschr. 98*:1233-36, 1956. Schadewaldt, H.: Die geschichtliche Bedeutung der Pädiatrie für die Entwicklung der Allergie. *Die Med.:* 14-15, 1959. Wagner, R., op. cit.[23] Parish, H. J., op. cit., p. 133.

30. Pirquet states that his coassistants, Hamburger and Moro, were the first to observe precipitation in the human body after an injection of horse serum. Pirquet, however, was not able to prove congruity between the concentration of precipitin and serum sickness either in humans or in rabbits. Pirquet therefore distinguished the antibodies causing serum sickness as "antibodies of vital reactions," different from the precipitins.

31. *Die Serumkrankheit,* p. 113f.

32. Pirquet, C.v.: *Klinische Studien über Vakzination und vakzinale Allergie.* Leipzig and Wien, 1907.

33. Following up these new lines of research, Pirquet even tried to explain the smallpox exanthem on the basis of agglutinins. How far he had now departed from the teachings of his original mentor becomes clear from the polemics into which Kraus entered against Pirquet in the Society of Physicans. Cf. Wagner, R., op. cit., p. 48.

34. First published under the title: Tuberkulindiagnose durch cutane Impfung. *Berl. Klin. Wschr. 44*:644f., 1907. Cf. *Wien. Med. Wschr. 57*:1369-1374, 1907; *Wien. Klin. Wschr. 20*:1123-28, 1907. Wagner, R., op. cit., p. 66.

SIX HUNDRED YEARS OF MEDICINE IN VIENNA*

A HISTORY OF THE VIENNA SCHOOL OF MEDICINE

ALFRED VOGL

Professor of Clinical Medicine, New York University
President of the Pirquet Society of Clinical Medicine
New York, N. Y.

THE University of Vienna, Austria, which is celebrating the 600th anniversary of its founding, has been the alma mater of many of the members of this audience. In pausing on this occasion to look back over the centuries from the vantage point of 1965, it may be wise not just to reminisce nostalgically about the good old times, but rather to examine critically the kaleidoscopic events of these centuries.

In so doing, we may not only recall the influences to which we were exposed during our formative years, and thus expose the roots of our intellectual development, of our motivations, beliefs, and prejudices, but we may also become aware of some of those related and causal factors in the political, economic, and cultural world of Austria and Europe that shaped the history of the Vienna Medical School.

From such a review we may derive insight, understanding, and a keener appreciation of those factors and forces that over the years have tended either to inhibit or to further the growth of learning in institutions such as the Vienna Medical School. The lessons learned should help us in the search for direction for future goals for ourselves and our younger friends here and abroad.

On March 12, 1365, Duke Rudolf IV of Austria (Figure 1), bynamed the Founder (*der Stifter*), obtained permission from Pope Clement VI to establish a university in Vienna. In the words of the papal charter, this act converted the ancient School of St. Stephen's "into a university according to the ordinances and customs observed first at Athens, then at Rome, and after that at Paris."

*Presented at a special meeting of the Pirquet Society of Clinical Medicine, New York, N. Y., on the occasion of 600th anniversary of the founding of the University of Vienna, held at The New York Academy of Medicine, October 13, 1965.

From its inception this new university had a bona fide medical faculty. However, as the historian Josef von Aschbach stated 100 years ago, ". . . it was not much of a medical school during the first 400 years of its existence." In the beginning, the reason was the sorry state of medicine in general in the later middle ages and the paralyzing effect of scholasticism on all learning. Later on, in the 16th and 17th centuries, it was the lack of interest in any scientific endeavors in the war-torn and plague-ridden Vienna of that epoch.

In those early days of the medical school, teaching consisted merely in the reading to the students of some ancient treatises prescribed by the authorities of the university. There were three masters to whom the texts were assigned by drawing lots. The books used were the "*ars parva*" by the Greco-Roman physican Galen, written in the second century A.D., and the "*Canon*" of Avicenna and the "*liber medicinalis*" by Rhazes, both 10th-century Persian-Arabian physician-philosophers. These writings were based essentially on the works of Hippocrates. Criticism or deviations from these doctrines were inadmissible.

The entire study of medicine consisted in memorizing the teachings of Galen and of his commentators (Figure 2). After 2 years of study the successful student would receive his B.A. without ever having seen a patient or the dissection of a body.

The contact of the student with patients began in the third year when he had to accompany a practicing physician on his rounds, watching his master's way of observing the patient, inspecting the ever-present urinal, giving long-winded discourses on the nature of disease and, finally, composing the traditionally very complicated prescriptions. After 2 to 3 years of apprenticeship the bachelor of arts was entitled to obtain a doctor's degree by giving a dissertation on one of the aphorisms of Hippocrates.

The faculty consisted of all the doctors licensed to practice in Vienna and its suburbs. From the early records it becomes apparent that its members were mainly concerned with establishing a professional guild capable of eliminating competition by quacks and foreign graduates and enforcing their more or less important claims, such as that for a privileged spot in the Corpus Christi procession (*Fronleichnams-Prozession*) or exemption from city taxes. They would resolve not to treat any pharmacist who had supplied drugs to a quack, or a patient

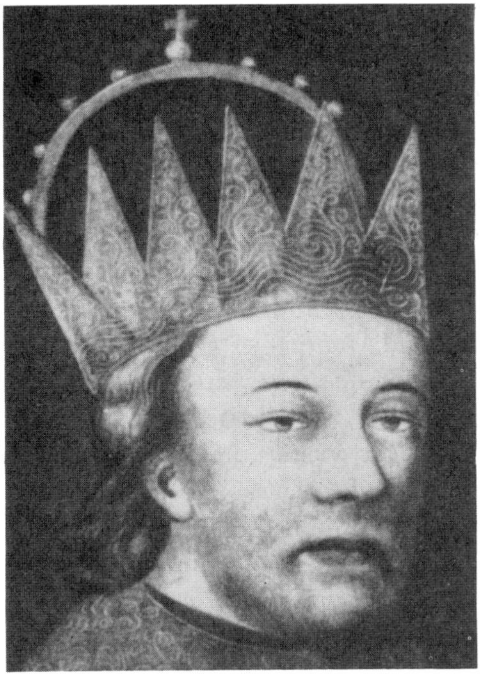

Fig. 1. Duke Rudolf IV, *der Stifter,* 1339-1365.

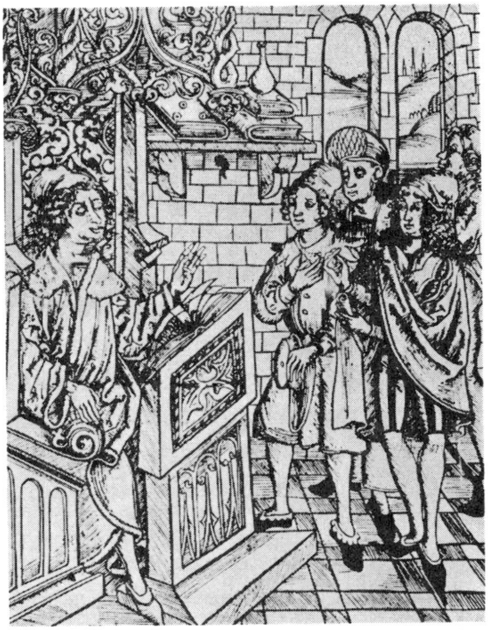

Fig. 2. Teaching of medicine in the 15th century.

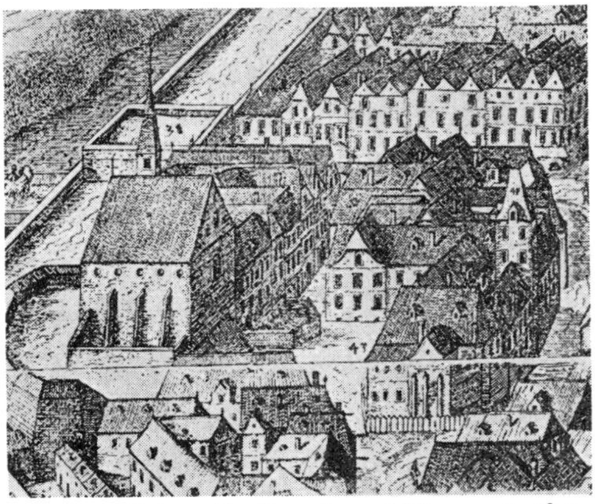

Fig. 3. University Quarter of Vienna in the 14th century.

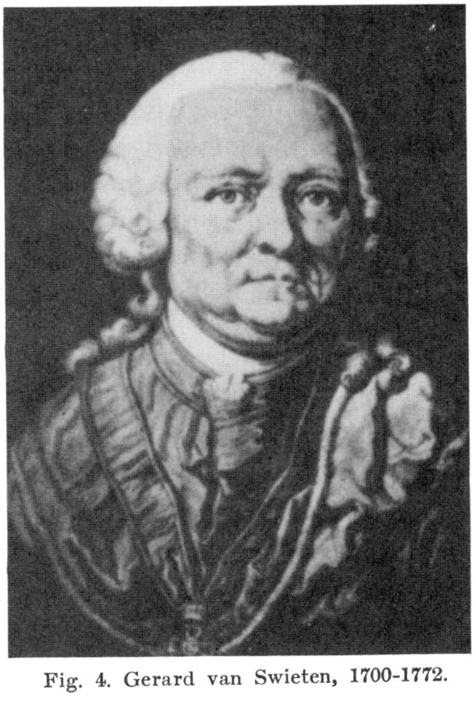

Fig. 4. Gerard van Swieten, 1700-1772.

who had previously been under the care of a nonlicensed healer. Since all other faculties had patron saints, the medical faculty chose two saints, St. Cosmas and St. Damian, as their own protectors and established for them an annual solemn mass at St. Stephen's.

The members of the faculty considered surgical procedures as being below the dignity of a learned doctor and they left cataract, hernia, and stone operations to the migrant healing artists. This attitude prevailed in Vienna at a time when surgery was already developing into a highly respected profession and an important branch of teaching at the faculties of Padua in Italy and Montpellier in France.

The university buildings and the student quarters were located in a cramped area of the city (Figure 3). Later this district had to be walled off in order to prevent the frequent vicious fights between the unruly students and the hostile burghers of Vienna.

Even at the time when the Renaissance and humanism changed the course of Western civilization (around 1500) and produced revolutionary figures on the medical scene, such as Vesalius in Padua, Guy de Chauliac in Montpellier, Lanfranc in Paris, Paracelsus in Basel and Harvey in London, no fresh breeze penetrated the stagnant atmosphere of the medical faculty at Vienna. Here economic and political conditions were at a desperately low level as the result of the religious wars marked by wanton destruction of life, property, and cultural goods.

In 1629, in line with the pious spirit of that time, the university was put under the authority of the College of Jesuits by Emperor Ferdinand II. Under this oppressive regimen the medical faculty remained in its state of lethargy and standstill. Foreign students did not come to Vienna and wealthy Austrians sent their sons abroad to study at the flourishing universities of Italy and France. In 1703 an imperial order suspended the conferral of medical degrees in Vienna because of the poor quality of teaching. The Medical School had reached its lowest status.

During the 17th century only a few members of the faculty are noteworthy for their activities. Among them were Managetta and de Sorbait.

Johann Wilhelm von Managetta, personal physician to three emperors, a man of wide educational background, took vigorous measures to improve the deplorable state of sanitation in Lower Austria and conceived, in an age dominated by the most absurd superstitions, sensible regulations to combat the disastrous epidemics ravaging the country. In Vienna he made himself immortal by inventing the *Wiener Trankel*, a laxative that is still popular there.

Paul de Sorbait, who succeeded Managetta and remained chief of the medical faculty for 25 years, finally managed, against the stubborn resistance of the College of Jesuits, to introduce the teaching of anatomy, which was already well advanced in other medical schools.

The delay in upgrading the medical school in the late 17th and early 18th centuries is difficult to understand. This was an epoch of political and military glory for Austria following the defeat of the Turkish invaders and the victory in the Spanish Wars of Succession. Those were the days of feverish construction of magnificent baroque palaces and churches and of resplendent festivities at the courts of the emperor and the high aristocracy. However, the esteem for university teachers was very low in the same influential circles, and the salaries offered were so inadequate that no man of distinction sought these positions.

It was Empress Maria Theresa who changed this situation radically after her ascendance to the throne in 1740. She must have been painfully aware of the deplorable level of medicine in Vienna and felt the need for vigorous measures to change the conditions. It will be remembered that Maria Theresa's Austria dominated not only a great part of the ancient Holy Roman Empire but also Italy and the Netherlands, two countries in which medical schools were flourishing at that time. They were the regions from which a regeneration of Austrian medicine had to come.

In Italy, around the year 1600, at the University of Padua, Montanus had revived the Hippocratic method of teaching medicine at the bedside. Italian physicians introduced this system to the Netherlands where similar ideas, propagated by the great British clinician Thomas Sydenham, had fallen on fertile ground. In Holland, at the University of Leyden, Hermann Boerhaave was professor of medicine. He was an enthusiastic follower of Montanus' and Sydenham's precepts and had succeeded in making the medical school of Leyden the leading institution of his time by teaching according to the three basic rules of Hippocrates: use common sense instead of unfounded speculations; observe the patient carefully; and rely upon the healing power of nature. The empress turned for advice to Boerhaave who recommended his outstanding disciple, Gerard van Swieten, for the dual position of personal physician to the empress and of protomedicus in charge of medical education in Austria (Figure 4).

Van Swieten's appointment, almost 400 years after the founding of the university, marks the actual beginning of the Vienna Medical School as one of the leading institutions of its kind.

Van Swieten started by removing the obstructive influence of the College of Jesuits, an action that finally made possible systematic instruction in anatomy with regular dissections. The decisive impact of this innovation upon the level of medical education can hardly be realized today. Van Swieten also created the first teaching hospital, even though a modest one, with beds for six males and six females, in the old Burgerspital. He also added to the curriculum the teaching of obstetrics and eye diseases, and appointed another pupil of Boerhaave's, Anton de Haen, as professor of medicine and chief of the new clinic.

De Haen, a devoted teacher, created a clinical school in which new practices were taught, such as attention to all the qualities of the pulse, the taking of a thorough history, and the use of the thermometer. He also laid the very foundation for meaningful clinical investigation by introducing the keeping of detailed case records. De Haen tried to ban the ridiculous polypharmacy customary in the 17th and 18th centuries, and to replace it with diets and hygienic regimes. His teachings had a lasting influence upon the therapeutic orientation of the Vienna medical school, which henceforth required establishment of an exact diagnosis prior to the institution of therapy, and favored a sober and critical approach to any kind of treatment.

It is regrettable that de Haen, although outstanding as a teacher, was too conservative and opinionated to recognize new discoveries; he failed to see the merits of smallpox vaccination or of the most important diagnostic advance of his period: the work of Leopold Auenbrugger (Figure 5). Auenbrugger had invented the method of diagnosing chest disorders by percussion and had described it in a little book *Inventum Novum* in 1761. However, when the influential de Haen belittled this strange new technique of knocking with fingers at the patient's chest and refused to introduce it in his clinic, the whole faculty followed suit and the art of percussion was officially buried. For many years it was practiced only by Auenbrugger and his friends, among them de Haen's successor, Maximilian Stoll. In order to be accepted, percussion had to wait 47 years until Corvisart, Napoleon's

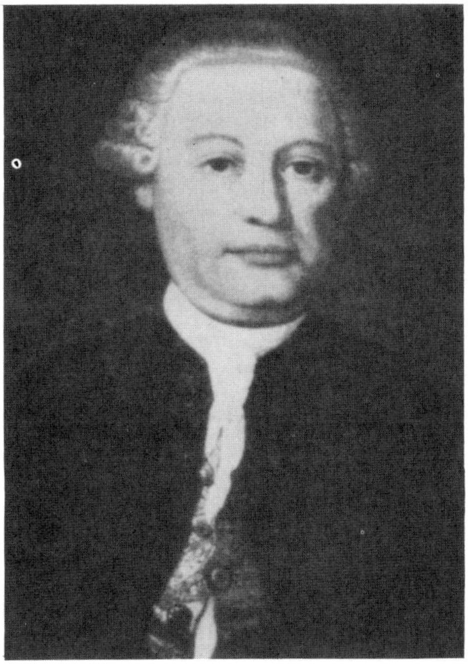

Fig. 5. Joseph Leopold von Auenbrugger, 1722-1809.

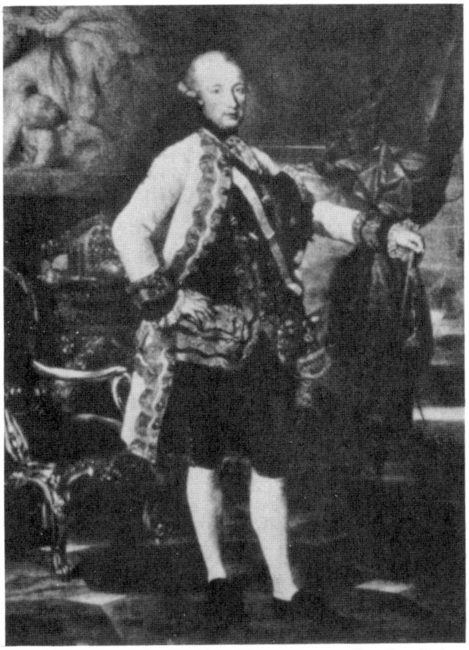

Fig. 6. Joseph II, Emperor of Austria, 1780-1790.

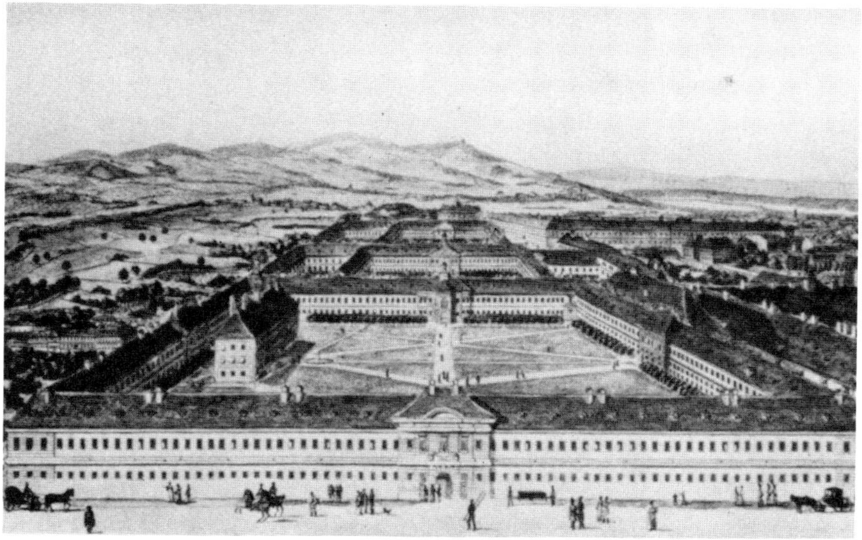

Fig. 7. Allgemeines Krankenhaus in Vienna, about 1800.

personal physician, published a French translation of Auenbrugger's book with favorable comments. Only then was percussion acclaimed as the first real advance in physical diagnosis since the times of Hippocrates. Auenbrugger, incidentally, never received an appointment to the teaching staff of the faculty.

The rise of the Vienna Medical School received a decisive impulse from Emperor Joseph II (Figure 6). He took probably more personal interest in questions of public health and of medical education than any ruler of a large country has ever done before or after him. The creation of the Vienna General Hospital (*das Allgemeine Krankenhaus* shown in Figure 7) was Emperor Joseph's favorite personal project. It was destined to become one of the most famous medical institutions of the civilized world and the home for the Vienna Medical School during its best period. A decision that also had great impact on teaching and studying of medicine in Vienna was Emperor Joseph II's Act of Tolerance, which granted for the first time the admission of Jewish students to the University. This decree not only opened the medical career to a new group of eager and talented students from many parts of Europe, it also changed the composition of the faculty during the following 150 years. During this long period Jewish physicians and investigators made major contributions to medicine and thus enhanced the name of the Vienna Medical School.

The leading physician during Emperor Joseph's regime was Johann Peter Frank. He expounded the then novel idea of the responsibility of the state for maintaining the health of its population. His book, titled *Medizinische Polizey*, was the first comprehensive text on preventive medicine and public hygiene. During his many active years in Vienna he brought about an intimate and fertile relationship with the then eminent Italian medical schools. In the *Allgemeine Krankenhaus*, of which he was director, he founded a pathologic-anatomical museum, and he introduced as an important innovation the isolation of patients with infectious diseases.

The 60-year period between 1745, when van Swieten started his reforms, and 1805, when Johann Peter Frank was forced to resign his position, was an exciting era of progress, which historians later designated the First Vienna Medical School.

This memorable epoch was followed by an abrupt decline, not due to any lack of men of ability but solely because of the oppressive political atmosphere that had settled upon Vienna and Austria. This was the time of all-out reaction against the liberal spirit that had been promoted by Emperor Joseph, it was a period of thought control and mutual distrust, the era of Prince Metternich and of the Biedermeier style with its surface calm and its hated secret police: in short, the era of the Vormärz. The position of head of medical education of Austria fell into the hands of a Baron Stifft, an arch-reactionary who during the 40 years of his dictatorship succeeded in removing virtually all eminent or promising men from their positions and replacing them with servile and politically trustworthy nonentities.

The very few men who survived this purge were able to uphold a certain standard in the faculty despite the discouraging atmosphere permeating it. Among them were two skillful and imaginative surgeons, Vinzenz von Kern and Joseph Wattmann, and the obstetrician Lukas Boer who introduced the teaching of obstetrics as an independent branch of medicine and had the courage to expose the dangers of the then fashionable meddlesome practices of his colleagues.

Shortly after 1840 a miracle happened: out of this political and scientific wilderness, almost suddenly, the Second Vienna Medical School rose like a phoenix from the ashes and brought with it the

Golden Age of medicine in Vienna. This time it was not the doing of a great administrator or reformer, nor had the stifling political atmosphere yet begun to clear. It was solely the result of the fortuitous appearance of the constellation of a few men of genius, endowed also with energy, perseverance, and unlimited devotion to their work. They had converged on the capital of the large Austro-Hungarian Empire from various parts of the multilingual monarchy. Their names were Rokitansky, Skoda, and Hebra.

Carl Rokitansky (Figure 8), born in Koeniggraetz in Bohemia, is one of the great pioneers in medicine and, with Giovanni Battista Morgagni (in Italy) and Rudolf Virchow (in Germany), he became the cofounder of pathologic anatomy as the basis for scientific medicine by correlating autopsy findings with the clinical manifestations of the disease. Rokitansky drew his brilliant descriptions and definitions of morbid entities, many of them previously unknown or misunderstood, from about 100,000 autopsies performed during his career. He recorded his vast knowledge in his *Handbuch der Pathologischen Anatomie,* whose first edition appeared in 1842. This widely read text and his personal teaching for over 40 years had direct influence upon the thinking and practice of medicine of two generations, and the impact of his concepts is still felt in pathology today.

At the same time another Bohemian, Joseph Skoda (Figure 9), born in Pilsen, raised the field of clinical diagnosis to astounding heights by making ingenious use of the newly introduced method of percussion (Auenbrugger) and auscultation (Laennec). He checked his physical findings with the aid of his friend and mentor Rokitansky at the autopsy table and was in this way able to develop a new clinical system of the pathology of the heart and lungs. Skoda's description and interpretation of physical findings in chest diseases were so exact that they are as valid and useful today as they were 150 years ago. This pathfinding work found recognition by his contemporaries only slowly and against the stubborn resistance of the medical authorities in power. They disliked Skoda's fancy and time-consuming methods of physical examination as well as what they called his "therapeutic nihilism," particularly when it became known to have lower mortality than their "active methods of treatment" consisting of blood-letting, purges, and emetics. His opponents succeeded in preventing Skoda from obtaining the chair in medicine until 1846, when he was finally

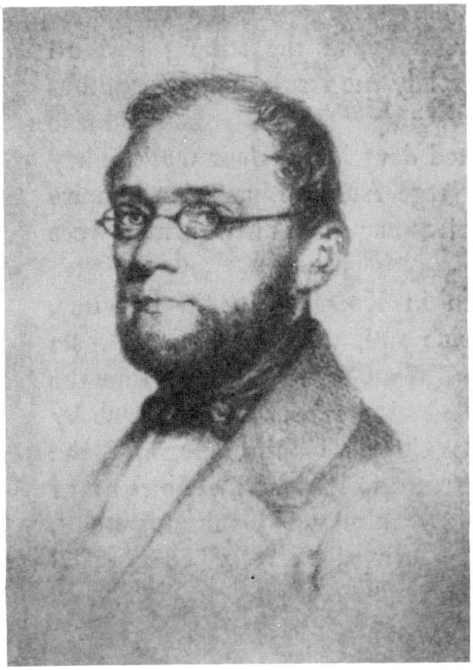

Fig. 8. Carl von Rokitansky, 1804-1878.

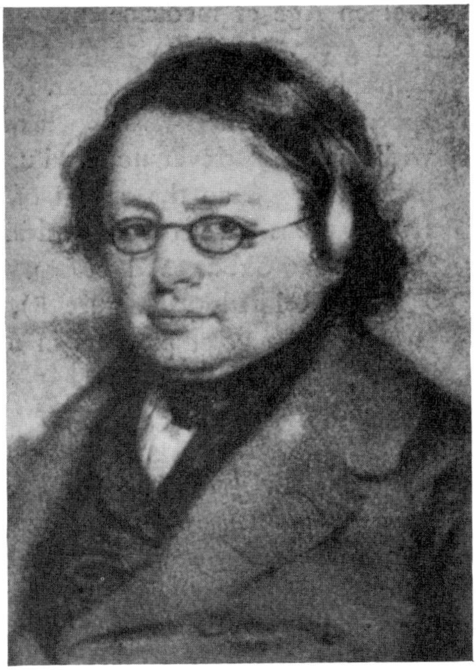

Fig. 9. Joseph L. Skoda, 1805-1881.

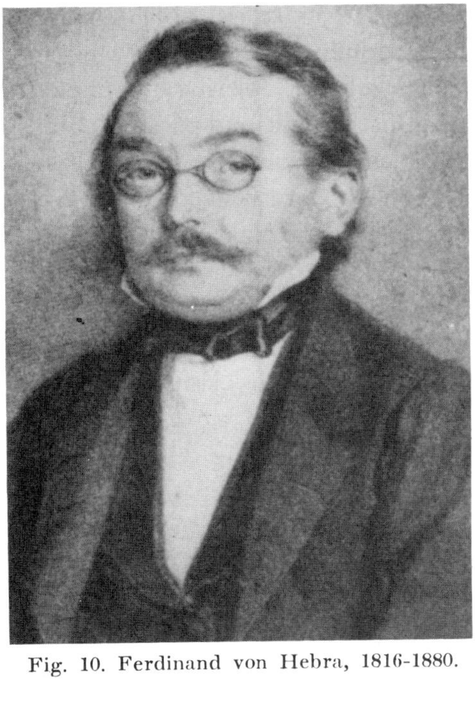

Fig. 10. Ferdinand von Hebra, 1816-1880.

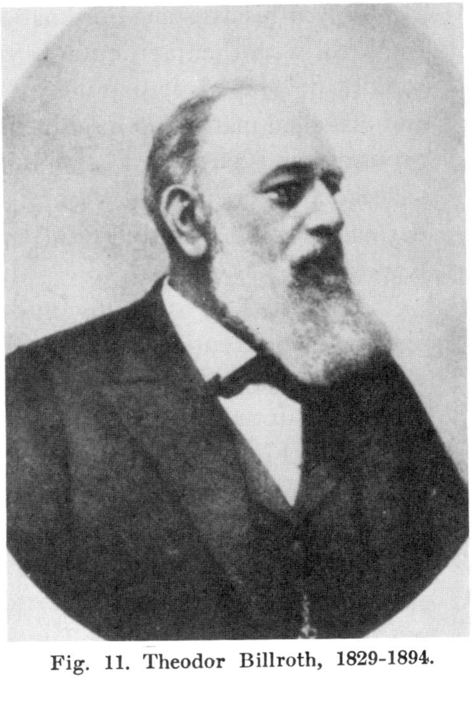

Fig. 11. Theodor Billroth, 1829-1894.

appointed through the energetic intervention of Rokitansky with the help of Archduke Ludwig.

Another great Bohemian of this era was Johannes von Oppolzer who, at Skoda's recommendation, became the chief of the newly created Second Medical Clinic. In contrast to the essentially anatomical concepts of his colleagues Rokitansky and Skoda, Oppolzer emphasized the disturbance of physiologic function in the pathogenesis of disease. This orientation promoted logically a more positive attitude towards active and individualizing therapy, while at Skoda's clinic the guiding principle was still "*primum non nocere*": refrain from any action that might interfere with the natural healing power of the human organism.

Also the development of surgery was decisively influenced by the teachings of Skoda and Rokitansky. Franz Schuh, who was professor of surgery, raised the standard of his specialty when he insisted on pathologic evaluation of operative findings. He evoked the admiration of his colleagues when he performed aspiration of pleural and pericardial exudates, the presence of which had been recognized through physical examination.

A new branch of medicine was born when Skoda entrusted his wards of patients with skin diseases (generally referred to as *Krätzekranke*) to his assistant Ferdinand von Hebra (Figure 10), a Moravian by birth, with the instruction to study the pathology of the skin. Hebra rapidly developed dermatology to a high level. He described, defined, and classified many skin diseases on clinical, pathologic, and parasitologic grounds, and published a monumental atlas of skin diseases. Hebra succeeded in creating in Vienna an internationally renowned school of dermatology. It remained at the same level under his pupil Moritz Kaposi.

The chairs of anatomy and physiology were also occupied by teachers and scientists of outstanding quality: Hyrtl and Brücke. They were colorful characters who were known often to clash violently in their differing estimation of each other's fields and capacities.

Joseph Hyrtl, a Burgenlander, won admiration as one of the great teachers of anatomy, especially of surgical (topographic) anatomy. His text book passed through 22 editions and remained the Bible of anatomy all over the world for two generations.

Under Ernst von Brücke, who had come from Heidelberg, the teaching of physiology developed from virtual nonexistence to an essential part of medical education. During the 40 years of his professorship he trained innumerable students in the fast-expanding field of physiology and in methods of physiologic research. In this way he created the necessary balance against the then prevalent anatomical orientation of the Vienna Medical School.

The attitude of the government towards the leaders in medicine had changed completely during this period. Many professors were honored by the emperor with titles and decorations, and were raised to nobility and appointed members of the Upper House of Parliament.

However, even during this splendid period of progress the voices of reaction were not silenced, and the power of entrenched office holders was still strong. A sad, almost incredible illustration of this fact is the story of Ignaz Philipp Semmelweis. As a young doctor Semmelweis, through keen bedside and autopsy observation, recognized the infectious nature and manner of transmission of childbed fever, the killer of thousands of young women at that time. He reported his findings and recommendations to the Society of Physicians in Vienna in 1847 and again, in a monograph, 14 years later. However, he found himself involved in an unequal battle against a solid front of the obstetricians of the faculty. They were outraged by the effrontery of the young Hungarian who tried to discredit their theories and thus undermine their positions. Despite the active support of Rokitansky and Skoda he was forced out of his position in Vienna, suffered a mental breakdown, and died at the age of 47 in an insane asylum. More thousands of women were to die from childbed fever before Semmelweis' concept gained universal acceptance years after his death.

This cruel interlude is evidence that even during the heroic phase of the School, prejudice, inertia and selfishness were still powerful forces that might easily have led to another decline of the medical faculty at the time when the group of ingenious men who had been in the forefront of progress were getting old. Fortunately, these very same men used the weight of their prestige to have the best possible candidates for any opening at the faculty called to Vienna, no matter what their origin or background. Thus it happened that, through Rokitansky's insistence and against violent opposition, Theodor Billroth (Figure 11), a North German of Swedish ancestry, became professor of surgery in Vienna. With him the school of surgery reached its very

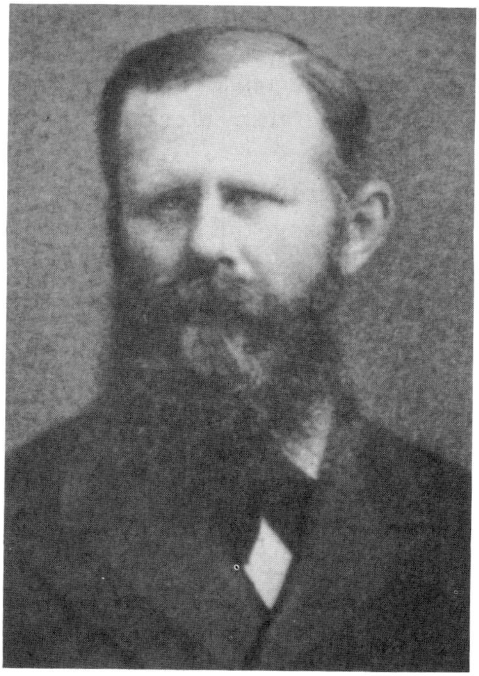

Fig. 12. Hermann Nothnagel, 1841-1905.

culmination. Research and practice advanced brilliantly under his leadership. Elaborate animal experiments were carried out and led to revolutionary progress in operations on the larynx, the esophagus, the stomach, and the bowels. The reputation of Billroth's clinic soon made it an international center for training in surgery, and his assistants were much in demand for leading positions at many universities in Europe.

Billroth, as a teacher, pioneer in surgery, and powerful personality, stood out like a giant within the medical faculty. Fortunately, the other branches of medicine were also represented by eminent men during his time.

To mention only a few:

Hermann Nothnagel (Figure 12), born in Berlin, was one of the last men to master the entire knowledge in internal medicine and neurology of his time. He made significant contributions, especially in the field of gastroenterology and pharmacology, and he had the reputation of being one of the greatest teachers of this period. From Nothnagel's staff came many excellent internists and neurologists who enhanced the reputation of Vienna as a medical mecca around the turn of the century. But outside his scientific achievements, Nothnagel will always be remembered as a fighter for the highest professional standards and as the fearless defender of human rights against the hydra of political anti-Semitism that began to raise its ugly head during his time.

Salomon Stricker, the first professor of experimental pathology, became a legendary figure because of his unorthodox teaching methods and his fascinating lectures during which he demonstrated animal experiments.

Adam Politzer, founder of a prominent school of otologists, developed his field from simple beginnings and wrote a textbook of otology that became a classic.

Hans Horst Meyer, born in East Prussia, was one of the founders of experimental pharmacology and thereby one of the pioneers of rational therapy. His work contributed enormously to the clarification of the action and the value of numerous drugs that had previously been used empirically. Meyer's textbook, *Experimental Pharmacology*, remained the standard text for several decades.

Theodor Meynert, professor of neurology and psychiatry, initiated the study of microscopic changes of the central nervous system, and his successor, Richard von Krafft-Ebing, was the first psychiatrist who ventured to delve into the problems of the psychology of sexual life and its deviations.

The life and work of these men whose activities extended toward or beyond the turn of the century, led into what, for many of us, has been contemporary medicine, the age of increasing specialization. Until World War I, Vienna remained one of the foremost centers of medicine, recognized as a school with a remarkable tradition, staffed with eminent experts, who were highly respected as teachers, investigators, and practitioners. Some of the men whose teachings made a lasting impression upon the older generations of living Vienna graduates were the anatomists Emil Zuckerkandl and Julius Tandler, the pathologists Richard Paltauf and Jakob Erdheim, the surgeons Anton von Eiselsberg and Julius von Hochenegg, the ophthalmologist Ernst Fuchs, the orthopedist Adolf Lorenz, the radiologist Guido Holzknecht, the psychiatrist Julius Wagner-Jauregg, the neuropathologist Constantin von Economo, the gynecologist Ernst Wertheim, and the pediatrician Clemens von Pirquet, the father of the science of allergy.

These men, of a caliber high above average, were able to maintain the reputation of the Vienna Medical School in its increasingly difficult competition with rival schools abroad. All this glory, alas, came to an abrupt end with the outbreak of World War I and the postwar dissolution of the once powerful and wealthy Austro-Hungarian empire.

The small new Austria and its overgrown capital Vienna were too poor to provide the ever-increasing expenses for facilities and salaries of a first-class medical school, and Vienna could no longer attract outstanding scientists from abroad. It was therefore the difficult task of the surviving members of the prewar faculty to maintain its reputation. Perhaps the only prominent newcomer from abroad was the Dutchman Karel Frederick Wenckebach, who promoted the development of cardiology in Vienna. Most of the vacant chairs were filled with pupils of their former occupants, some of them recognized leaders in their field, such as Ernst Peter Pick in pharmacology, Otto Poetzl in neuropsychiatry, and Heinrich von Neumann in otology. Many other appointments made during that period, however, were based more on political expediency than on scientific qualifications. Thus many first-rate candidates for leading positions were not appointed, as for instance the gynecologist and pioneer in endocrinology Josef von Halban, or the innovator of fracture treatment Lorenz Boehler. Many others went abroad and found recognition, among them Carl Landsteiner, the discoverer of the blood groups and Nobel prize laureate, Béla Schick, whose diphtheria skin test had a profound impact on the theory and practice of immunization, Paul Klemperer, the pathologist who originated the concept of connective tissue disease, and Robert Barany, who received the Nobel prize for his work on the physiology and pathology of the organs of equilibrium.

In this period between the two World Wars, in which minor lumina dominated the medical faculty, there lived and worked in Vienna one man whose ideas and teachings had developed outside the official circle of the faculty but were finding a resounding response throughout the civilized world: Sigmund Freud, the revolutionary thinker and creator of psychoanalysis. While the faculty pointedly ignored him and some of its members publicly derided his concepts, Freud stayed on in Vienna and thereby made it the focus of the steadily increasing international attention to the new science. He no doubt attracted personally more disciples, students, and patients to Vienna than any other single clinician in official position at that time.

The continuing deterioration of the level of the medical school in the pre-Nazi era and its disintegration during the Nazi regime and World War II are matters of common knowledge.

After the war little was left but shambles of an old tradition. Out of these and against tremendous odds, a few courageous and devoted men, such as the highly respected internist Ernst von Lauda, tried to rebuild the Vienna Medical School. With total disruption of the continuity of teaching staff and students this was, indeed, a Herculean task. During this relatively short period of reconstruction, no personalities of exceptional rank as teachers or scientists have as yet emerged and no scientific work of outstanding significance has been published. It may take another constellation of the Rokitansky-Skoda-Hebra type to guide the Medical School to new heights.

No one should try to predict the future. The age of "great medical schools" may be over altogether. The leveling influence of easy and rapid communication throughout the scientific world and the free intercourse and exchange of teaching and research staffs of universities will make it increasingly unlikely that any one medical school as such can be greatly superior to others. However, whatever differences there will always be between various schools will depend on the quality of the physical facilities as well as the ability of the teaching staff. The quality of the facilities will necessarily depend on the existing economic conditions, the interest, and the generosity of the community. The quality of the teachers, on the other hand, will depend less on available funds than upon the principles that determine their selection.

With these facts in mind, can we draw any lesson from the history of the Vienna Medical School as to its quality in the future? The rise of the School has in all its phases been associated with times of economic prosperity, with a liberal and progressive atmosphere and with a far-seeing, unprejudiced, and independent policy in the selection of the teaching staff.

Conversely, the School has gone down whenever the country was poor, the atmosphere oppressive, and the choice of men for leading positions dictated by political, nationalistic, or religious motives. The pool of talents from which a small country can draw its leaders naturally is limited. The future can therefore look bright only if every opportunity is given to the most gifted men and if, at the same time, the horizon is searched constantly for new stars. Apathy, jealousy, bias, and the unwillingness to part with the comfortable past have done tremendous harm to the Vienna Medical School again and again, and they would do the same in the future.

In the best tradition of the Vienna Medical School there has been devotion to research by its members and great pride in their discoveries but, at the same time, there has been the firm resolution to remain first and foremost a school in which students are to be educated to become good doctors. These principles must remain the hallmark of the School if it is to regain its position among the best institutions of medical learning of the world.

We salute the Vienna University tonight and wish its Medical School a future true to the ideals of its glorious past.

Acknowledgments

Figures 1, 3 to 6, and 8 to 12, from Schönberg, L., *Das Medizinische Wien,* 2d. ed. Vienna, Urban & Schwarzenberg, 1947. Reproduced by permission.

Figure 2 is from Castiglioni, A., *A History of Medicine,* 2nd ed. New York, Knopf, 1947. Reproduced by permission.

Figure 7 is reproduced from a colored print by Artaria & Co., Vienna (n.d.). Reproduced by permission.

BIBLIOGRAPHY

Clinical Symposia, vol. 9. Summit, N. J., Ciba, 1957.

Schrauf, Karl. *Studien zur Geschichte der Wiener Universität im Mittelalter.* Vienna, Selbstverlag, 1904.

Von Aschbach, Josef. *Geschichte der Wiener Universität im ersten Jahrhunderte ihres Bestehens.* Vienna, K. K. Universitätsverlag, 1865.

Wunderlich, Carl R. A. *Ein Beitrag zur Geschichte und Beurtheilung der gegenwärtigen Heilkunde in Deutschland und Frankreich.* Stuttgart, Ebner, Senkert, 1841.

DOCTORS' RIOT, NEW YORK, 1788

WHITFIELD J. BELL, JR. Ph.D.

President
American Association for the History of Medicine

Librarian
American Philosophical Society
Philadelphia, Pa.

THE Doctors' Riot in New York City on April 13-15, 1788, was one of the many episodes which marked the history of medical instruction in the United States and Britain before the passage of the anatomy acts in the 19th century. Though its story has been told often,* the following contemporary, nearly first-hand account contains interesting details. Colonel William Heth, author of the letter, had been an officer of the Virginia troops in the Revolution. Edmund Randolph was governor of Virginia. The letter was found in Executive Papers, Box 53, Folio April 11-20, 1788, in the Virginia State Library, by Herbert A. Johnson, coeditor of *The Papers of John Marshall*, of the Institute of Early American History, Williamsburg, Va.

Only that part of the letter which relates to the riot is printed. Double punctuation has been eliminated, and each sentence made to begin with a capital letter.

WILLIAM HETH TO EDMUND RANDOLPH

New York 16th April 1788

Sir

. . . . We have been in a state of great tumult for a day or two past—The causes of which, as well as I can digest them from various accounts, are as follows. The Young students of Physic, have for some time past, been loudly complained of, for their very frequent and wanton trespasses in the burial grounds of this City. The Corpse of a Young gentleman from the West Indias, was lately taken up—the grave left open, & the funeral clothing scatterd about. A very hand-

*Pomerantz, S. I.: *New York: An American City, 1783-1803,* New York, 1938; Packard, F. R.: *History of Medicine in the United States.* New York, 1931, I, pp. 236-37; Headley, J. T.: *The Great Riots of New York, 1712-1873.* New York, 1873, pp. 56-65.

some & much esteemd young lady, of good connections was also, recently carryd off. These—with various other acts of a similar kind—inflamed the minds of people exceedingly, and the young members of the faculty, as well as the Mansions of the dead, have been closely watchd. On Sunday last, as some people were strolling by the hospital, they discovered *a something* hanging up at one of the windows, which excited their curiosity, and making use of a stick to satisfy that curiosity, part of a mans arm or leg tumbled out upon them. The cry of barbarity &c was soon spread—the young sons of Galen fled in every direction—one took refuge up a chimney—the mob raisd—and the Hospital appartments were ransacked. In the Anatomy room, were found three fresh bodies—one, boiling in a kettle, and two others cuting up—with certain parts of the two sex's hanging up in a most brutal position. These circumstances, together with the wanton & apparent inhuman complexion of the room, exasperated the Mob beyond all bounds—to the total destruction of every anatomy in the hospital, one of which, was of so much value & utility, that it is justly esteemd a great public loss having been prepared in a way, which costs much time & attention, and requires great Skill to accomplish.

On Monday morning, the mob assembled again, and encreased thro' the day, to an alarming size. Vengeance was denouncd [?] against the faculty in general, but more particularly against certain individuals. Not a man of the Profession thought himself safe. An innocent Person got beat & abused, for being *only dressed in black*. Two, of the young tribe were unfortunate enough to fall into their hands. But the Mayor obtaind them, upon a promise of sending to gaol—a measure, to which in their rage, they submitted—not reflecting, that *sending them to gaol,* would secure them from their violence & resentment. And therefore, so soon as they found themselves defeated in their furious intentions, respecting their captives they repaird to the goal, & commenc'd their attack (with all that intemperence & folly, which ever marks the conduct of People assembled in that way)—vainly endeavouring to break in—when they could do nothing more than break windows &c which they will be tax'd to repair. The militia were orderd out—small parties were sent to disperse them, but they instantly disarmd these detachments, & broke their guns to pieces, & made them scamper to save their lives. The evening advanced a pace—& the affair became very serious. The Governor, after trudging about all day—first *with* the Mob in the Morning, endeavouring to pacify and accommodate; and in the afternoon, to assemble a body respectable enough to preserve the Gaol, & to restore peace & good order—advanced about dark, with a number of the Citizens, but without any kind of order, or without any other than a few *side arms* & canes—while the Adjutant Genl of the Militia about 300 yards in his rear, led up in very good order, about 150 Men—(tho' not more than half with fire arms) among whom, were many gentlemen of the City & strangers volunteers. This body were not long before the goal, before the bricks & stones from the Mob, provoked several to fire—& perhaps, their [sic] might on the whole have been 60 guns discharged—but this is mere guess. This body, made their way into the goal, where a party remained all night—but a sally of 60 or 70 were defeated. Three of the mob were killd on the spot & one has since died of his wounds, & several were wounded. One of them was bayoneted on attempting to force into a window of the Prison, which he saw filld with armd Men—a proof, of the astonishing lengths to which popular rage will sometimes carry Men. Numbers on the Governors side, besides himself, are severely bruised. Baron Steuben recd a wound first above the corner of his left eye & nose—from which he lost a great deal of blood. Mr. Jay got his scull almost crackd—and are both now laid up. Genl. Armstrong has got a bruis'd leg—but is able to go out.

Yesterday, the Militia turn'd out again, made a respectable appearance, & paraded about exceedingly—both *Horse & foot*—but it must be observd, *that the enemy were not to be heard of*. In truth, numbers who were *in the Mob on Monday evening*—turn'd out *yesterday to support government*. . . .

A HISTORY OF THE LEGAL REGULATION OF MEDICAL PRACTICE IN NEW YORK STATE

JOHN BARRY BARDO

Yale University, New Haven, Conn.*

REGULATION of the practice of medicine in New York was recognized as necessary early in the history of the colony and state. A colonial law in 1684 prohibited the practice of medicine "without the advice and consent of such as are skillful in the said Arts." In 1760 another colonial law provided for the regulation of medicine in New York City through the examination and licensure of candidates by specified magistrates. After the Revolution, examination by a magistrate was made contingent on the possession of certain educational qualifications. Legislation enacted in 1797 provided a measure of regulation of medicine; it permitted magistrates to license individuals by indorsing certificates of study issued by reputable physicians and surgeons.

The law of 1760 had not been retroactive, and the irregular practitioners already in the city were therefore unaffected by it, but the laws of 1797 required that:

> ...no person practicing physic or surgery at the time of the passage of the Act should continue to so practice without satisfactory proof to the Chancellor, a judge of the Supreme Court, a master in chancery, or a Judge of the Court of Common Pleas, that he had practiced for two years . . . or had studied that time with a reputable physician or surgeon, and had filed a certificate to that effect with the County Clerk.

The act further required that no other person should practice physic or surgery without a certificate from one or more physicians or surgeons that he had studied medicine for four years under the preceptors signing it, and that he was qualified to practice.[1] Applicants were not required to pass examinations. Legislation passed in 1806 made the pro-

*Presently at the Tufts University School of Medicine, Boston, Mass.

fession itself responsible for the regulation of "physic and surgery."[2] The law permitted incorporation of medical societies in each county and authorized the officers of the county and state societies to examine and license candidates. Candidates for licensure could appeal the decisions of local bodies. This law, the object of which was to obtain incorporation for a medical society for "the suppression of empiricism and the encouragement of regular practitioners,"[3] was intended to secure independence for the State Medical Society and the county medical societies, while the newly incorporated State Medical Society was recognized as the more important body insofar as it could pass on the refusal of a county society to grant a medical license to a properly qualified student, and could grant this privilege in countermand to the action of the county societies.[4] In subsequent years laws were enacted requiring the registration of practitioners with the county clerk, and penalties were imposed for the illegal practice of medicine.

An important step in the regulation of medical practice occurred when the University of the State of New York, through its Board of Regents, was authorized in 1809 to incorporate colleges, and empowered such colleges to grant the degree of doctor of medicine without examination by the censor. This degree constituted a license to practice. Incorporated colleges with the approval of the regents could also endorse degrees conferred by colleges outside the state.

The period from 1806 to 1872 appears to have been a difficult one for the regulation of medical practice; three forces then contended for control of the power of licensure. These were the organized medical profession, the medical colleges, and the University of the State of New York, acting through its regents. Under the law of 1806, the only penalty for practicing without a license was the inability to collect fees by action at law. A further revision of this law in 1813 omitted all penalties for practicing without authority. The Revised Statutes of the State, passed in 1827, were designed to

> forbid the practice of physic and surgery to any one not a member of a county society, and not only to regulate the licensing of practitioners, but to provide for the good behavior of licentiates by prescribing a legal method of expelling members of county societies for forfeiting their right to practice medicine for gross ignorance or misconduct in his profession or immoral conduct or habits.[5]

Under this law no one could practice unless he had a license or a diploma from an incorporated medical society of the state or had the degree of M.D. from a university. If he was authorized to practice in another state or country and had a license or diploma from a medical society in such a state or country he was required to file a copy of his license or diploma with the county clerk, and to give the medical society of the county satisfactory proof of his having followed the plan of study prescribed for students in New York State.[6]

Further confusion arose when the penal clause of the 1827 statutes, which make an unlicensed practitioner guilty of a misdemeanor, was repealed.

The laws became even more inefficient and confused. An act passed in 1844 made it a misdemeanor to practice without a license in cases of gross ignorance, malpractice, or immoral conduct.[7]

In 1872 the regents were first empowered to appoint "one or more boards to consist of not less than seven members who shall have been licensed to practice physic and surgery in this State."[8] Under the law three separate boards of examiners were appointed to examine and license candidates in the schools of medicine then in existence. Although this law first established the principle that licenses should be granted by a state department and not by those engaged in teaching and practicing medicine, the principle was limited in application, and the other sources of licensure—the medical societies and the colleges—continued to hold their powers. By an 1880 statute, however, the societies were divested of their legal right to issue licenses, and that power now was divided between the regents and the colleges. Further streamlining of regulations came in 1890, when the medical degree no longer sufficed as a license to practice and the power to grant licenses was granted solely to the regents. Candidates for licensure were required to have specified preprofessional education and to have attended only medical schools registered by the University. Another significant provision of this law created a Board of Medical Examiners that represented the regular medical profession, the homeopathic, and the eclectic schools; these boards were charged with the responsibility for examining and licensing candidates.[9]

In 1893 the laws relative to medical practice were consolidated into the Public Health Law. The next major statutory change occurred in 1907 when the three separate boards of examiners were replaced by one board that was made responsible for medical licensure and of the enforcement law. To assist the board, the regents were empowered to appoint a secretary.[10] The same statute for the first time recognized osteopathy as one of the schools of medicine.

After 1907 there were still provisions in the law that permitted various kinds of medical sects. Still prevalent, according to J. J. Walsh, were sellers of false cures and remedies: "We still permit the compounder of medicine, even more impudent in his ignorance and almost without pretense of knowledge of his avocation, just as he did in the eighteenth century."[11]

Between 1893 and 1926 charges of illegal practice were commonly prosecuted by counsels for the various medical societies and, pursuant to the Public Health Law,[12] fines imposed for convictions were paid to the county medical societies, which in turn used these fines to pay their lawyers. Defense lawyers protested that the prosecuting attorneys were motivated to conduct successful prosecutions more by prospective fines than by an intention to maintain high standards of medical practice. An outcry arose demanding prosecution of such cases by public attorneys and, in practice, the New York County Medical Society, which had made it a policy to refuse fines from convictions for illegal practice, began to use the services of the district attorney of New York County in such prosecutions. This practice was based on the fact that violation of statutes of the Public Health Law regarding medicine constituted a misdemeanor and that, as such, it should be prosecuted by the law officers of each county, namely the district attorneys. This practice became so widespread that a demand arose for intervention by the attorney general.[13]

Between 1907 and 1927, the statutory responsibility for professional licensure and law enforcement was vested in the New York State Board of Medical Examiners. This Board hired medical investigators, who supervised the licensing examinations prepared and rated by the Board; these investigators were charged with the responsibility for enforcement of medical professional laws. They gathered evidence based on complaints submitted to the secretary of the Board who, if the evidence seemed sufficient, referred it to attorneys who instituted criminal prosecution of the alleged violators.[14]

However, as indicated by the prosecution of cases of illegal practice by lawyers from county medical societies, the burden of professional law enforcement became too great for the limited agency of the Board of Medical Examiners.

Inadequate enforcement of the Public Health Law and of the Education Law[15] that related to medicine resulted in a convocation of doctors and lawyers representative of the several county medical societies of New York State. The purpose of this meeting, held at The New York Academy of Medicine in 1926 and 1927, was to obtain repeal of the medical regulatory statutes of the Public Health Law and to draft the so-called Medical Practice Act, Article 131 of the Education Law.

The Medical Practice Act prohibits the practice of medicine or the use of the title of doctor by an unlicensed individual.[16] Illegal practice constitutes a misdemeanor. The attorney general and, in some instances, the district attorney, are required to prosecute such cases in courts of specified jurisdiction. Under the Medical Practice Act no license is required of an intern or member of the resident staff of a legally incorporated hospital or of any resident physician serving in a state institution or in an institution of political subdivisions of the state, provided the physician has completed specified courses in a registered medical school in the United States or Canada, or in a foreign medical school that has maintained standards not lower than those prescribed for medical schools in New York State.[17]

The 11 articles of the Education Law that establish minimum requirements for entrance into the professions also postulate certain standards for professional conduct on the part of licensed practitioners. Violation of these statutory prohibitions may result in the revocation or suspension of a license or in a censure or reprimand. The final authority for the imposition of these sanctions, as established in the Education Law, is the Board of Regents. Section 211 of the New York State Education Law establishes the Board of Regents as the executor of all determinations regarding the discipline of violators. As prescribed by the Medical Practice Act, grounds for initiation of disciplinary proceedings are: fraud or deceit in admission to practice; conviction of a crime; failure to register where failure is not satisfactorily explained; fraud or deceit in practice; unprofessional conduct; immoral conduct; failure to become a citizen within a specified period; advertising for patronage by means of handbills, posters, circulars, letters, stereopticon slides, motion pictures, radio, or magazines; the use of secret methods, cure, or treatment in practice; criminal abortion or complicity in it; fee-splitting; alcoholism; drug addiction; and insanity.[18]

The Medical Practice Act authorized the action of the attorney general in enforcement.[19] The act specifically imposed upon the attorney general the duty of prosecuting all illegal practitioners of medicine. At the time the Education Bureau of the Department of Law (the attorney general) estimated on the basis of investigation that "of every four individuals practicing medicine within New York State, at least one was an unqualified charlatan."[20] The Department stated:

> An integral part of the proper administrative machinery for clearing the state of illegal quacks and charlatans is the assignment of a deputy attorney general to devote his entire time to the important work of prosecuting these cases on behalf of the citizens of the state.[21]

And while providing for prosecution of unlicensed individuals under the Education Law, the Medical Practice Act also created a Medical Grievance Committee separate from the Board of Medical Examiners. This Committee was charged with the duty of conducting hearings involving disciplinary charges against licensed practitioners. It was formed:

> To eliminate this licensed unethical group. This committee . . . modeled upon the grievance committee of the Bar, for the discipline of licensed physicians . . . has authority to investigate all charges of unprofessional conduct on the part of practicing physicians and to recommend to the Board of Regents the revocation of a physician's license, and the annulment of his registration or any other form of discipline.[22]

The Medical Practice Act provided: a means for uniform criminal prosecution of illegal practitioners, standards for entrance into the profession for professional conduct, and a mechanism by which those statutory standards might be enforced. Also it designated the Board of Regents of the University of the State of New York as executors of decisions in cases involving charges made against a doctor in regard to the legality of his licence.

While this most important statutory change promised increased effectiveness in professional law enforcement, such a condition was not immediately forthcoming. Although the attorney general of the State of New York had been made responsible for prosecutions of illegal practice of medicine, as already mentioned, the investigative body for professional law enforcement was still the State Board of Medical Examiners, whose funds for operation, in fact, came from the yearly registration fees paid by licensed doctors in the state. And the institution of the separate Medical Grievance Committee charged with the duty of hearing disciplinary cases did little to ease the burden carried by the investigators of the Board of Medical Examiners.[23]

In 1938 an investigation focused upon abortion rings and on the effectiveness of the State Education Department in dealing with them. Disciplinary action was instituted in Kings County under the direction of John Amen, an assistant attorney general. Preliminary findings of this investigation disclosed a discouraging picture of disciplining abortionists who were physicians. Statistics showed that during the entire existence of the Medical Grievance Committee, 52 of 77 formal charges involving abortion or attempted abortion were dismissed. In the 25 cases in which guilt was found, 7 licenses were revoked and 14 suspended; 4 physicians were censured.[24]

Until the fall of 1938 responsibility for the investigations of violations of the professional statutes rested on both the Division of Professional Education and the secretaries of the professional Boards of Examiners in medicine, dentistry, and pharmacy, who were under the direct supervision of the associate commissioner for Higher and Professional Education. These secretaries reported the results of their investigations to the assistant attorney general assigned to the department, who then instituted and conducted formal hearings before these bodies, including the Medical Grievance Committee.

At that time the regents created a new position bearing the title of executive secretary of the Division of Professional Conduct. The duties of this functionary included responsibility for investigation of all complaints, of all unprofessional conduct or illegal practice in any of the licensed professions and, as well, of supervision of the New York office responsible for the administration of laws that dealt with the professions. The intent to provide the public and the professions with more efficient and systematic enforcement of the acts that dealt with professional practice was further implemented in 1940, when the regents established the Division of Law Enforcement. The regents attached all professional investigators and inspectors to this division and installed the executive secretary of the Division of Professional Conduct as director. This newly established division was mandated to secure evidence stemming from complaints and to prepare cases based upon such complaints.[25]

The secretaries of the medical and dental boards were administratively divested of all responsibility in relation to investigations and the gathering of evidence, despite their objections. The statutes that fixed responsibility for investigations on these secretaries remained unchanged.

The associate commissioner for Higher and Professional Education reported: "one of the outcomes of this new procedure has been the striking increase in the number of cases prepared and presented to the Medical Grievance Committee."[26]

The second major administrative change that took place during this period occurred in 1941 when, the statute notwithstanding, the function of registering physicians, osteopaths, and physiotherapists was transferred from the secretary of the State Board of Medical Examiners to a central registration unit.

Although there was subsequent modification of the machinery for enforcing the laws relating to the professions, including medicine, the objectives of the Division of Law Enforcement (now called the Division of Professional Conduct) have remained the same; these are to suppress the practice of professions by unlicensed and unregistered individuals and to prevent the violation of professional laws by licensed practitioners. The policy of the division, since its inception in 1940, has been to obtain voluntary compliance with the Education Law and to educate both licensed and unlicensed persons as to the provisions of regulatory statutes.[27] And while disciplinary action against professional practitioners is the most severe form of action and is taken, in most cases, as a last resort, it is significant to the history of the regulation of medical practice in New York State to understand the aims of the machinery of the New York State Education Department and of allied officials and organizations.

In order to curtail and suppress the unlawful practice of medicine by unlicensed and unregistered persons and to prevent and detect the violation of the statutes by licensed and registered practitioners, the Division of Professional Conduct performs the following functions: 1) it investigates complaints alleging violations of the professional laws; 2) it dismisses complaints lacking merit; 3) it appears at hearings of the professional boards and grievance committees; and 4) it supplies stenographic assistance to the assistant attorney general and to the hearing boards and grievance committees.[28]

The objective of the assistant attorney general in the Bureau of Education is to assist in the enforcement of the laws that deal with the professions and to suppress illegal practice and unprofessional conduct. The assistant attorney general evaluates investigations made by the Division of Professional Conduct and prosecutes disciplinary and criminal cases. When satisfied as to the adequacy of evidence gathered by the Division of Professional Conduct, the assistant attorney general prepares formal charges and initiates the administrative hearings. He acts as legal adviser to the Division of Professional Conduct and is, in turn, dependent upon the effectiveness of the Education Department in obtaining evidence with which he can proceed with successful prosecutions and thus discharge the responsibility given him by the statute.

The disciplinary mechanism is set in motion by complaints from patients or physicians or from other sources. Complaints of illegal or unprofessional conduct are commonly made in writing to the offices of the New York State Education Department, the office of the attorney general, or to the offices of the state or county medical societies. After referral to the Division of Professional Conduct, all complaints are reviewed, investigated, and either dismissed or acted upon in the following ways:

In disciplinary cases, the assistant attorney general in the Education Bureau prepares formal charges against the practitioner after he is satisfied with the evidence against the alleged violator. The charges specify the provisions of the Medical Practice Act allegedly violated, and itemize the violations in detail. Arrangements for hearing of the case before a subcommittee of the Medical Grievance Committee are made in conjunction with the director of the Division of Professional Conduct. At hearings of the subcommittee, the assistant attorney general presents the evidence to sustain the charges. During the course of the hearings, the assistant attorney general does not participate in deliberations of the hearing body, but is consulted in connection with the findings of the hearing body, and he prepares the findings and recommendations of the grievance committee pursuant to its instructions. In medicine he appears informally before the full Grievance Committee only to read and explain the findings and recommendations of the subcommittee. Where the full grievance committee rejects a finding of guilty, the case comes to an end. The assistant attorney general has no power to appeal to the regents. Where the finding of guilt is affirmed by the full Grievance Committee, the assistant attorney general and the respondent appear before the Regents' Committee on Discipline.

The objective of the hearing body in medical disciplinary proceedings is to protect the public by eliminating unprofessional and unethical conduct. To achieve this objective it hears charges and makes recommendations to the Board of Regents with regard to revocation of licenses or other disciplinary action.

In formal hearings held before the Medical Grievance subcommittee or the full Committee, the accused practitioner has the right to appear in person or by counsel, to cross-examine witnesses, and to question the evidence. The evidence for the case is first presented by the assistant attorney general, then by counsel for the respondent. Then witnesses are examined and cross-examined. During the hearing the assistant attorney general may be called upon to advise members of the Grievance Committee or subcommittee as to the admissibility of evidence and motions, and to give legal advice to members of the hearing body if necessary. The findings of the subcommittee are then submitted to the secretary of the full Medical Grievance Committee, which meets quarterly. In medicine, a finding of guilt may result only from a unanimous vote of the 16 members of the committee. The respondent is not present, and no testimony is taken at the meetings of the full Medical Grievance Committee. The full Committee has available a transcript of the record of the hearing held before the subcommittee. In addition to the record, it is customary procedure for the full Committee to question the subcommittee and the assistant attorney general. The full Committee usually follows the recommendation of the subcommittee. The minutes of the subcommittee hearing, as transcribed by the hearing reporter provided by the Division of Professional Conduct, are sent by the assistant attorney general to the assistant commissioner for Professional Education in Albany, who then sends the complete record and a memorandum for each case, including a brief biographical sketch of the alleged violator, to the three members of the Regents' Committee on Discipline. The Committee is sent the case record and the memorandum including a brief biographical sketch of the accused doctor and verbatim excerpts from the charges, findings, and recommendations of the Medical Grievance Committee. At hearings of the Regents' Committee on Discipline, the respondent and his counsel, the assistant attorney general, the director of the Division of Professional Conduct, the assistant commissioner for professional education and the secretary of the Medical Grievance Committee are present. Following deliberations by the Regents' Committee on Discipline, in which only the members participate, the commitee instructs the assistant commissioner for Professional Education to prepare its report and recommendations for the full Board of Regents. The members of the Committee then sign this report and submit it, through the assistant commissioner for Professional Education, to the secretary of the Board of Regents.

The full Board of Regents hears each case on the basis of a copy of the report of the Regents' Committee on Discipline and a copy of the assistant commissioner's memorandum on the accused practitioner citing the charges, findings, and recommendations. The record of the hearing by the subcommittee is submitted to the regents who, by formal vote, approve, modify, reject, or remand the report of the Committee on Discipline and empower and direct the Commissioner for Professional Education to execute an order carrying out their decisions. The order is prepared by the departmental counsel and served by the Division of Professional Conduct. An order becomes effective only when served personally on the accused; this is by departmental policy, not by law.

A physician may appeal from any disciplinary penalty imposed by the regents through the medium of a judicial review under the provisions of article 78 of the Civil Practice Law and Rules. In recent years the possible scope of judicial review has been expanded to include the severity of the penalty imposed, and a review of judicial determinations has indicated that in a few instances the courts have felt that the quantum of punishment assessed by the regents has been too severe. Appeals taken from final action of the regents must be brought in the Appellate Division of the Supreme Court, Third Judicial Department, in Albany. Since the attorney general conducts the hearings upon which disciplinary penalties are predicated, the Appeals Bureau of the Department of Law argues all the appeals under Section 78 of the *Civil Practice Law and Rules*.[29]

We may summarize the life history of a complaint by listing sequentially the steps involved:

1) Formal complaint received at offices of Division of Professional Conduct.

2) Investigation ordered by director of the Division of Professional Conduct, who makes recommendation as to necessity for further action, dismissal of complaint, or formal disciplinary proceedings.

3) Subcommittee of Medical Grievance Committee designates cases in which formal charges are to be presented, based upon facts revealed in investigation and after recommendation from the director of the Division of Professional Conduct.

4) Assistant attorney general prepares charges.

5) Subcommittee of Medical Grievance Committee holds hearings, makes recommendations to the

6) Medical Grievance Committee, which makes its decision based on subcommittee recommendation.

7) Assistant attorney general sends case record to assistant commissioner for Professional Education, who then sends case record and memorandum to the

8) Regents' Committee on Discipline, which makes its recommendations, sending them through the

9) Assistant commissioner for Professional Education to the

10) Board of Regents, who approve, modify, reject or remand the report of the Committee on Discipline. The decision of the Board of Regents is carried out by the

11) Commissioner of Professional Education, who acts through the Division of Professional Conduct.

12) Possible judicial review in the Appellate Division, Third Department, argued by the Appeals Bureau, Department of Law.

It is of interest to note, after delineating the process of formal medical disciplinary proceedings, that hearings on charges are held before members of the medical profession, so composed on the assumption that only members of the profession are qualified to understand and judge the technical facts presented. However, *most* questions presented before the Medical Grievance Committee are issues of simple fact and are not really complicated technical questions. Even questions involving abortions and drug addiction ultimately rest on an issue of fact: whether something that is contrary to the provisions of the law has or has not been done.[30]

Although external to the mechanism of the New York State Education Department, the various county medical societies in the state play an important adjunctive role in investigation of complaints against doctors. The county medical societies attempt to resolve complaints lodged by patients or other physicians against member physicians.

Grievance committees of the societies function primarily to adjust complaints of negligence or excessively high fees. Such complaints, commonly based on inadequate physician-to-patient communication, are mediated by the grievance committees of county medical societies.

The county medical societies' boards of censors act upon complaints of violation of medical ethics.

These committees of county medical societies act to maintain the code of ethics of the society and to maintain good physician-patient relations. Furthermore, the vigilance of these bodies may serve to deter doctors from possible legal action when charges that question the validity of the medical license, not solely the privileges of medical society membership, would be involved.

While the actions of committees of county medical societies are limited to members of a particular society, and while their authority is limited to censure and to suspension or revocation of society membership, such committees assist in the legal regulation of medicine, as such, by providing records and testimony helpful in obtaining prosecution through the Division of Professional Conduct of the New York State Education Department for professional misconduct.[31]

A criticism of the system within the State Education Department was that of the time-lag in prosecuting cases. In 22 medical cases studied from 1945 to 1947 the average lapse of time between preferment of charges and their eventual resolution was 411 days; the median time lapse was 352 days.[32] This delay may have reflected the point raised earlier, that disciplinary proceedings are held before a body of busy physicians. The determination of many cases may not require the medical knowledge of the Medical Grievance Committee, although it is for those cases in which a professional judgment is required that the body exists. No complete solution to the problem of delay has yet been proposed by doctors, lawyers, or members of the State Education Department.

However, despite an increasing professional population, the State Education Department facilities for enforcement have kept pace with the growing number of professionals and with the concomitant increase

TABLE I.*

	Disciplinary complaints received by Division of Professional Conduct		*Cases closed*			
			By Division		*By Board of Regents*	
	Total	*Medical*	*Total*	*Medical*	*Total*	*Medical*
1965-1966	3836	193	4353	553	83	29
1962-1963	1289	909	521	112	66	38
1959-1960	701	144	817	91	50	24
1956-1957	1168	247	1096	278	47	23
1953-1954	696	118	644	148	59	27
1950-1951	448	96	268	62	34	20
1947-1948	190	63	198	91	49	34
1944-1945	469	96	529	148	58	32

*From records of the Division of Professional Conduct, New York State Education Department, Albany, N. Y.

in the bases of disciplinary and criminal action relating to the professional statutes. An increasing case load achievement of the Division of Professional Conduct has been attained through: 1) improvement in administrative procedures, including a 1961 increase from 10 to 20 investigators; 2) centralization of investigation; 3) pooling of investigators for service in all professions; and 4) increased field work. For a brief statistical sketch of the total and medical case loads of the Division of Professional Conduct and the Board of Regents since 1944 see Table I.[33] Medical disciplinary cases recorded from July 1, 1965, to June 30, 1966, appear in Table II.

While no determination of the average or median time lapse has been made in recent years, the lapse has been greatly reduced from that earlier mentioned. The increased case load achievement and decreased time lapse have been achieved in the face of a professional population that has grown from approximately 140,000 licensed persons in 1940, including roughly 35,000 medical practitioners, to 340,000 total professional licensees, including 42,000 licensed practitioners, in 1966.[33]

Regulation of medical practice has retained the character of supervision by legislation. The 19th century conflict regarding the seat of authority for licensure resulted in the establishment in 1890 of the principle that medical licenses be granted by the Board of Regents of the University of the State of New York. The Medical Grievance

TABLE II.*

Received by Division		Closed by Board of Regents	
Disciplinary	167	*Disciplinary:*	
Probation	24	Censure and reprimand	10
Restoration	2	Revocation	3
	193	Suspension	6
Investigation	209	Resignation accepted	1
	402	Revocation stayed—probation	9
			29
		Investigation	
Closed by Division		Restoration denied	2
Disciplinary	553	License restored	3
Investigation	236	Revocation stayed—probation	1
	789		6

*From records of the Division of Professional Licensing Services, New York State Education Department, Albany, N. Y., as of August 1, 1966.

Committee invoked the use of a panel of physicians in disciplining other physicians. Criminal prosecution of the unlicensed practitioners, previously the domain of district and other attorneys, became the responsibility of an assistant attorney general attached to the State Education Department. The investigative function now lies solely with the Division of Professional Conduct which, together with the assistant attorney general, is responsible for enforcement of the professional statutes.

Presently the provisions of the Education Law provide standards of qualification for practice, methods of examination, certification, registration of candidates, grounds for illegal practice, penalties, and disciplinary hearing proceedings. The procedures described above are the means by which the provisions of the law are enforced.

NOTES AND REFERENCES

1. Provisions of act quoted from Walsh, J. J., *History of Medicine in New York,* 5 vols. New York, Nat. Americana Soc., 1919, vol. 1, p. 82.
2. *Laws of the State of New York,* 29th session. An act to incorporate Medical Societies for the purpose of regulating the practice of physic and surgery in this state. Albany, Barber, 1806, chap. 138.
3. Shaftel, N. History of the Medical Society of the State of New York, 1807-1957, *New York J. Med. 57*:446-47, 1957.
4. *Ibid.,* p. 447.
5. Purrington, W. A., quoted in Walsh, J. J., *op. cit.,* vol. 1, p. 85.
6. *Ibid.,* p. 86.
7. *Ibid.*
8. *Laws of the State of New York,* 95th session. An act relating to the examina-

tion of candidates for the degree of doctor of medicine. Albany, Brown, 1872, Chap. 746.

9. *Laws of the State of New York,* 113th session. An act to establish boards of medical examiners of the State of New York for the examination and licensing of practitioners of medicine and surgery; to further regulate the practice of medicine and surgery. Albany, Bank Bros., 1890.
10. *Laws of the State of New York,* 130th session. An act to regulate the practice of medicine, and to repeal Article 8 of Chapter 661 of the laws of 1893 and acts amendatory thereof. Albany, Lyon, 1907.
11. Walsh, J. J., *op. cit.,* vol. 1, p. 92.
12. Public Health Law of 1893. In: *Laws of the State of New York,* 116th session. Albany, Lyon, 1893, vol. 1, chap. 661, sec. 153.
13. *Ibid.;* and from conversations with Reed Dawson, legal counsel for the New York County Medical Society, held November 30, 1965, and August 21, 1966.
14. This and further discussion of the function of the State Board of Medical Examiners was supplemented by conversation with J. McCullough, senior investigator of the Division of Professional Conduct of the New York State Department and one of five medical investigators for the New York State Board of Medical Examiners, February 1933 to January 1937. Conversation held November 23, 1965.
15. The Education Law of 1910, sec. 1263, contained provisions that paralleled those relating to medicine in the Public Health Law of 1893, sec. 153.
16. Methods of obtaining a medical license in New York State as established by the Medical Practice Act of 1927 (art. 131, Education law): 1) passed by a state licensing examination prepared by the Board of Medical Examiners; 2) by the endorsement of a license issued by another jurisdiction; 3) by passing an examination given by the National Board of Medical Examiners; and 4) by acceptance by the Board of Regents of the applicant's "conceded eminence and authority" in his profession.
17. Prior to 1958 the standards of foreign medical schools were deemed unacceptable by an examining committee that made visits to foreign medical schools. This committee was composed chiefly not of doctors but of nonmedical educators, who returned to New York and printed lists of "approved" foreign medical schools. Since 1958, however, 40 of the 55 state and territorial jurisdictions in the United States have required that physicians trained in foreign countries other than Canada pass an examination given by the Educational Council for Foreign Medical Graduates as a prerequisite to admission to their licensing examinations.
18. *Report of the Temporary State Commission on Coordination of State Activities.* Albany, Williams, 1948, appendix D, pp. 414-15; and the *New York State Education Law,* sec. 153, in: *The Consolidated Laws of New York,* annotated, Eldridge, H. N. and Bronaugh, M., eds. Northport, N. Y., Thompson, 1928.
19. *New York State Education Law,* sec. 6513, subdiv. 5.
20. *Annual Report of the New York State Education Department,* 1927, p. 79. Albany, Univ. State of N. Y., 1928, p. 79.
21. *Ibid.,* p. 82.
22. *Ibid.*
23. *Laws of the State of New York,* 150th session, Albany, Lyon, 1927, chap. 85; an act to amend the education law to conform to the state department's law, in relation to the practice of medicine, dentistry, veterinary medicine and surgery, pharmacy, nursing and trained attendance, chiropody, optometry, engineering and surveying, architecture, public accounting and shorthand reporting, and repealing articles 8, 9, 10, 11, 12, 13 and 15 of the public health law and articles 4A, 7A, 8 and 8A of the general business law relating thereto; Article 8: Practice of Medicine, secs. 140 to 153; and from a conversation with J. McCullough.
24. Amen, J. H. *Report of the Kings County Investigation, 1938-1942,* p. 82.

25. *Thirty-sixth Annual Report of the State Education Department, 1940.* Albany, Univ. State of N.Y., 1941, vol. 1, p. 173; and *Thirty-seventh Annual Report of the State Education Department, 1941,* Albany, Univ. State of N.Y., 1942, vol. 1, pp. 186, 226-27.
26. *Thirty-seventh Annual Report of the State Education Department, 1941,* Albany, Univ. State of N.Y. 1942, vol. 1, p. 186.
27. The professions regulated by the Division of Professional Conduct now include: architecture, landscape architecture, certified shorthand reporting, chiropractic, dentistry, dental hygiene, osteopathy, physiotherapy, nursing (registered and practical), ophthalmic dispensing, optometry, podiatry, psychology, veterinary medicine, and social work.
28. *Report of the Temporary State Commission on coordination of State Activities, Second Interim Report.* Albany, Williams, 1948, p. 109.
29. *New York State Education Law,* sec. 6515, subdiv. 5.
30. From conversations with Reed Dawson.
31. From conversations with Reed Dawson.
32. *Report of the Temporary State Commission on Coordination of State Activities,* Table 24, p. 151.
33. From records of the Division of Professional Licensing Services, New York State Education Department, Albany, N.Y., as of August 1, 1966.

ONE HUNDRED YEARS OF HEALTH: NEW YORK CITY, 1866-1966*

Leona Baumgartner

Visiting Professor of Social Medicine
Harvard Medical School
Boston, Mass.

The health of a people is influenced by many factors in the immediate environment and in society at large. The history and influence of any one institution becomes more meaningful if attention is paid to the usually larger forces that have contributed to its success or failure. To evaluate the contributions made by the Board of Health and the Department of Health of the City of New York to the physical well-being of all New Yorkers in the past century, one must be constantly aware of the influences of a host of other factors, including:

1) Better standards of living with concomitant improvements in diets, living conditions, and education.

2) A great increase in scientific knowledge.

3) An enormous growth of the medical establishment, i.e., hospitals, doctors, nurses, other technical personnel, voluntary health and professional agencies, laboratories, the pharmaceutical industry, etc.

4) A relative public apathy or concern and varying degrees of social responsibility for the state of health of the people.

5) The leadership, concern, and effectiveness of local, state, and federal governmental and political leaders.

6) The social climate of the times and the money made available for health activities.

Despite the importance of these factors I believe that without those remarkably viable and creative institutions, the Board of Health and the Department of Health,† the physical well-being of the people they serve would have suffered. Despite the ups and downs of these two

*Presented at a meeting celebrating the centennial of the Board of Health and of the Department of Health of the City of New York, New York, N. Y., held at The New York Academy of Medicine, November 10, 1966.

†Other governmental agencies have made their contributions too but cannot be included here. Notable in recent years has been the Department of Hospitals, the Office of the Medical Examiner, and the Mental Health Board. The presence of so many professional schools and voluntary, civic, and professional groups interested in health has been of great influence, as has, on many occasions, the assistance of the mass media.

agencies—and there have been many—their eternal vigilance and their willingness to change has meant that millions of persons have continued to live more safely in the potentially hazardous environment of this unique city.*

Early Years (1657-1866)

Concern for the health of all New Yorkers did not begin 100 years ago; it began almost as soon as the Dutch settled here. In 1657 Peter Stuyvesant enacted an ordinance that forbade anyone to throw garbage and refuse into the street. Thus began the fight, still not successful, to clear the city of pollution and to maintain a sanitary environment. Soon thereafter attempts were made to control the spread of infectious disease through quarantine measures. These twin concerns, the state of sanitation, particularly of living quarters, and the control of epidemic disease were to dominate the scene for more than 200 years.

Epidemics of cholera and yellow fever struck suddenly, affected the whole population, and threatened the economic life of the city. These facts probably made control of specific diseases easier than creating and maintaining a clean environment.

The struggle to cope with both of these problems was related to what George Rosen has called the epidemiological conundrum, i.e., miasma versus contagion as the explanation of the origin and spread of infectious disease. Reformers held to the first theory to justify their endeavors at sanitary improvements. Some health workers, influenced by William Budd and John Snow in England, held to their strict contagionist point of view. Others, such as John Simon and Max von Pettenkoffer, held to a third position: they admitted that infectious diseases were due to contagia, but held that these factors acted in conjunction with other elements, such as pollution of the atmosphere or soil, or even social factors. The battle raged and New Yorkers benefited, for gains were made on both points.

Some developments in these early years set patterns for the future. In 1796, for example, physicians were required to report infectious diseases; this initiated an early partnership of public and private effort which is still characteristic of the attacks on health problems made by the Department of Health. In the same year the state legislature em-

*This account gives inadequate attention to the improvement of milk and water supplies, in which the city, state, and federal governments have collaborated, and to which the Board of Health and the Department of Health have made important contributions.

powered the Common Council, then the chief institution of municipal government, to make its own sanitary ordinances; in 1805 it authorized the creation of a local board of health. Thus major control of local health affairs began to shift from the state to the city.

For the next 60 years the public management of health affairs was essentially unchanged. Various officials were added; the composition of the board was changed; work was divided and redivided among several offices; "health wardens" were appointed to inspect houses, lots, and noxious trades. The city inspector developed schemes for collecting and compiling vital statistics. The commissioners of health prevented the importation of disease as well as they could, and they were often called on to provide care for the sick poor. During epidemics, with the help of various eminent practicing physicians the board became very active; it mobilized medical talent, established hospitals, and enacted new regulations. But essentially, between epidemics there was no organization to carry on a vigorous health program. The social climate of the time did not demand or support it.

Members of the Board of Health for much of this period were also members of the Common Council, a body elected for purposes other than to protect the health of the citizenry. They gave major attention to other affairs and were often beholden to powerful interests, many of whose activities were sometimes detrimental to the public health. Year after year attention was called to unsanitary conditions, bad housing, noxious trades, contaminated milk, etc., to little avail. The city inspectors and health wardens were sometimes able to report limited successes. The worst nuisances were cleaned up, at least for a time. One bright spot was the continuing and ever better record of vital statistics and the analyses made from them. Out of comparisons made for different areas of the city grew a concept of preventable disease, not just control of epidemic disease.

But conditions were still deplorable; they called for reform, and the time for reform was ripe. The 1840's had brought a social and sanitary awakening in England. Cholera and typhus epidemics and slum conditions that followed industrialization had led to John Howard's studies of hospitals and prisons, Thomas Percival's investigation of fever, and studies of the operation of the Poor Laws. Most important of all was the publication of Sir Edwin Chadwick's *Sanitary Conditions of the Labouring Population of Great Britain* in 1842, which became a bible for sanitation reformers. Just as New York doctors-to-be in those years went to study in Europe, designers copied the latest fashions in clothes and in furniture; in this way new ideas were imported.

As pressures for reform mounted in New York City, the new health laws of England were studied. A private organization, the New York Asssociation for Improving the Condition of the Poor, later merged with the Charity Organization Society, today called the Community Service Society. Soon a number of influential persons in the city became alarmed. Peter Cooper, the merchant-prince-philanthropist, William Cullen Bryant, poet and editor of the *New York Evening Post*, Stephen Smith, and Norman B. Eaton, a lawyer, took over the task of collecting the facts on sanitary conditions in the tenement house district. Reform was demanded. The New York Academy of Medicine put pressure on the legislature. Smith's appeals to the legislature were in vivid, lurid, and human terms. One legislator cried, "Why, I believe I have got smallpox, for I begin to itch all over," as he heard a description of how wholesale dealers sold clothing manufactured in homes where the clothes had covered the beds of children with smallpox and remembered that he had just bought a suit from one of these dealers.

The reformers were helped by the threat of a new epidemic of cholera. Finally, they overcame the long-standing opposition of a corrupt alliance of Tammany Democrats and upstate Republicans, whose legislation had failed to handle effectively the growing threats to the health of the people in the city. A new administrative structure was set up by the state legislature in 1866 as part of an effort to achieve reform in all phases of municipal government.

A New Organization Gets Under Way

Thus the Metropolitan Sanitary District and the Board of Health came into being. They covered about the same areas as the city does today. The city had a million inhabitants. The new Board of Health received authority over all matters related to the health of the people, and authority so far essentially unchallenged by legislative or judicial act. For a few years members of the board were appointed by the state to circumvent the then corrupt Tammany organization, but were later appointed by the mayor. There was a Sanitary Bureau, headed by a physician, and a Bureau of Vital Statistics. Most of the sanitation inspectors were doctors. There was an engineer and a legal staff.

The new organization handled the next cholera epidemic (1866) with unprecedented success. This made possible a vigorous sanitary campaign in which many long-sought improvements were made. A chemical laboratory directed by Charles F. Chandler, professor of chemistry at Columbia University, examined water, milk, and food supplies. The results of these scientific analyses became the basis for administrative action. The reporting of diseases by physicians was extended to include cholera, typhus, typhoid, smallpox, scarlet fever, diphtheria, and measles. Each case was investigated and, when necessary, hospitalized. Disinfection was emphasized as a means of control.

The Board of Health initiated inquiries into a variety of health hazards: ventilation, heating, and overcrowding in public schools, conditions in foundling asylums and nurseries, venereal disease and prostitution, the condition of meat and cosmetics, explosions of kerosene lamps, safety measures along the waterfront, etc. Administrative and legislative actions were taken. Elisha Harris, the new registrar, advocated widespread health education, but the time was not yet ripe for acceptance of this revolutionary idea of teaching people about their own health.

It is significant that progress came in those years not through new laws but through the attempts "being made to execute existing law," as the attorney for the new board emphasized. In four years the board showed what could be done by able and determined men freed from the domination of corrupt politicians. In 1870 the Department of Health was put back under the control of the city and of "Boss" William M. Tweed, but the administrative pattern was set. Professionally competent physicians and other specially qualified persons had established an organization that self-seeking politicians feared to eradicate. The day-to-day work was carried on by those whose real values were their professional pride and the service they could render to the people. Since 1870 the tradition of noninterference by political leaders in health affairs has seldom been ignored.

Twenty Years of Slow Growth: Hospitals and Health in One Department

After the first spurt of activity following the establishment of the new board and department, the next 20 years were filled with a variety of activities, including the development of the first sanitary code; greater accuracy in reporting births and causes of deaths; regulation of the practice of medicine and surgery (1874); an attack on the excessive deaths of infants through a "summer corps" of doctors who visited tenements to care for the sick and to teach prevention; the establishment of a laboratory to make smallpox vaccine and to sell the surplus; the distribution of pamphlets, particularly on control of contagious disease and on the care of infants; the surveillance of rabid dogs; and inspection and provision of some medical care for children in schools and in children's institutions. Great emphasis was put on conditions in tenement housing, general sanitation in the streets, and regulation of noxious trades. The use of the worst cellars for living quarters was eliminated, and plumbing in new buildings had to meet new specifications of the Department of Health.

Control of city-operated hospitals was transferred to the new department. There is little evidence of effort to integrate the work of the rest of the health department with that of the hospitals, except in infectious diseases. But this problem of relating the care of the sick, the inpatient, to ambulatory care or the prevention of disease and disability is still to be solved.

Progress was slow. A sufficient staff was never provided; a clear scientific basis for action was often missing; the poor, who suffered the most, had no machinery through which they could make their needs known; and improvements necessary to clean up the mess in housing too often cut profits.

The Bacteriological Era

The next great forward thrust in health affairs in New York City came in the 1890's with the leadership of Herman M. Biggs and the widespread application of the new discoveries in bacteriology and immunology. Dr. Biggs, a man of unusual intellect and great charm, was a practicing physician who first became a consulting pathologist to the Department of Health in 1888. He was well acquainted with the scientific work of Koch, Pasteur, and others in European laboratories, work which had opened up new ways of treating and controlling infectious disease. The American scene had been dominated by those who thought dirt per se caused disease and so emphasized sanitation. Now a specific way to prevent disease was opened.

A first step was taken in 1892 after an outbreak of cholera in Hamburg, Germany. These were the years of immigration; the first infected ship arrived on August 31 of that year. Physicians began to report cases. The department had long sought funds for a bacteriological laboratory. Under pressure of the threatened epidemic, funds were finally provided, within 10 days of a renewed request, and Biggs became its first chief. It was not the first municipal laboratory in the world, but it was the first to be used for the routine diagnosis of disease, a service available to all physicians. As such, it set a precedent for other governments to follow.

In May 1893, Biggs brought William Hallock Park to the laboratory. Dr. Park's studies on diphtheria were well known, but the results had to be more widely applied if the disease were to be controlled. Within eight months doctors for the first time were able to make accurate diagnoses. The next summer Biggs went on one of his almost annual trips to Europe for a vacation and to observe medical developments there. This time it was to find out how effective was the newly announced diphtheria antitoxin. It was good enough for him to cable Dr. Park to begin the inoculation of horses that were already waiting. And with the help of funds raised by a local newspaper antitoxin was soon supplied to Willard Parker Hospital, the contagious disease hospital, and to private physicians. Here another step important to the rest of the country was established: the idea of making therapeutic sera available at a reasonable cost or providing them free to the poor. Years later E. J. Lederle, a retired commissioner of health, was to start the commercial manufacture of biological products in his own company. This paved the way for departments of health to withdraw from producing these items and also led to a vast new development in the pharmaceutical industry.

Bacteriological and chemical examinations and sanitary investigations in the field were soon combined. The famous Croton water supply was shown to be polluted. The reformers now had a firm scientific base for obtaining legislation to abate nuisance in watersheds. By 1911 chlorination of water supplies was initiated after a fight between the water and health departments; this anticipated the fluoridation battle of later years. Pasteurization of milk came in 1912. The laboratory proved essential in both cases.

The laboratory was important not only as a manufacturing and diagnostic center but as a research center; for years it was one of the few truly medical research centers in the country. This was before medical research was a part of medical-school and hospital activities, and before the Rockefeller Institute or any similar research institute had any impact.

In later years the public health laboratory added the control of private laboratories and, as new tests became available, it helped in diagnosing disease. Manufacture of all but very rare diagnostic sera was given up by 1955, for commercial laboratories could now carry the load.

Tuberculosis is Attacked: Continuing Care of Patients Begun

"The most common and fatal disease which prevails in New York is both communicable and preventable," said Biggs to the Board of Health in 1893. Biggs was talking about tuberculosis, which caused more than 6,000 deaths a year and did not disappear from the list of the 10 leading causes of death until 1959. Collection and destruction of sputum, disinfection of eating utensils and clothing, the avoidance of excessive contact with cases, and rigid governmental inspection of meat and milk were instituted. Within 10 years Biggs had added much more to the department's antituberculosis activities: medical inspectors who visited homes of patients to instruct families and to consult with physicians; free bacteriological diagnosis; hospitalization of patients and registry of cases; and, finally, over the opposition of the profession, compulsory reporting of cases by private physicians. A decade later ambulatory clinics for diagnosis and treatment were established in all boroughs and tuberculin testing was established. In later years, as evidence indicated their value, treatment by new drugs, BGC vaccination, and rehabilitation measures were added. Bit by bit, complete care for patients with long-term illnesses was provided. The city still spends about 40 million dollars on the control of tuberculosis, which has been a major activity of the department for decades.

Two More "Firsts" in Public Health: Nursing in the Home and Health Services for Mothers and Children

Two important developments took place shortly after the turn of the century: increased attention to children and the employment of the world's first public-health nurse, Lina Rogers. Another wave of reform had begun. This was the time of Theodore Roosevelt and of trust busting, women's suffrage, pure food and drug laws, workmen's compensation, and the establishment of settlement houses and child-labor laws. "Somehow," as William Allen White put it, "there came a realization that society must give the underdog a better kennel." But rich and poor babies died alike. Year after year in New York each summer the iron-tired funeral carts clattered through the streets bearing their small white caskets. Flies lit everywhere on uncovered foods, and the quality of milk was as poor in Gramercy Park as in Essex Street. One summer an experiment showed that 30 public-health nurses could teach immigrant mothers of newborn babies that there were new hygienic ways of caring for them: breast or boiled milk, clean hands, isolation from sick babies, etc. In one tenement area, where the nurses visited, 1,200 babies who should have been dead, if the usual statistics held, were still alive at the end of the summer.

Faced with these facts, the city fathers in 1908 created the first municipal unit in the world devoted to the health protection of mothers and children. Headed by another dynamic and articulate practicing physician, Josephine Baker, it absorbed the previous medical, nursing, and educational activities in this field and expanded rapidly. Infant and maternal death rates decreased; dental services for children began; medical care, including tonsillectomies, were provided; school health procedures were revised; midwifery improved; institutions that provided day care and other services for children were inspected; and girls and boys of school age were taught child care to help their immigrant mothers learn to cope with problems in the city. Children in these years bounced their balls to the tune of a well-known ditty:

Marguerite, go wash your feet
The Board of Health's across the street.

Other cities and states formed similar bureaus of maternal and child health. Four years later, the federal Children's Bureau was established by an act of Congress.

The Value of Health Education and of Regionalization Recognized

Another milestone in these years was the creation in 1916 of the Bureau of Health Education as the first such unit in the world that was affiliated with a public-health department. Under the guidance of Charles Bolduan, its many activities were widely copied. In the same year, Haven Emerson instituted the requirement of full-time service for all department officials. His reactivated Sanitary Bureau also removed from the streets 14,956 dead horses, 2,105 steers, and sundry mules, deer, monkeys, and camels—not to mention 50,000 dogs and cats! Plans for regionalization of health services in the city were begun. All maternity care was surveyed. But Emerson's bold ideas, worked out so imaginatively with Dr. Goldwater, died aborning.

World War I and a Slump

World War I brought a lull in municipal health affairs. Partisan politics had reentered the department with a new mayor. The whole era was one of social reaction, conformity, repression, and a low ebb of interest in social and human welfare. Plans for decentralizing health services and for bringing them closer to the people were dropped. Branch offices with tuberculosis clinics were closed. Publicity for the control of venereal disease ceased. And a clinic designed to test the values of periodic health examinations was short-lived. There was little innovation. But with federal funds 12 prenatal clinics were established, apparently the only lasting contribution of these years.

Renewed Activities and New Leaders: Formation of a Department of Hospitals

With another change in administration and the appointment in 1926 of Louis A. Harris, a new commissioner, things began to hum again. Corruption in the inspection services of milk and food was liquidated. This was to be the last time any important charge of corruption in the Department of Health service was substantiated. A new staff was recruited. Modern x-ray equipment was put into refurbished tuberculosis clinics. Cooperation with private physicians and other groups was sought once again. Shirley Wynn, another commissioner, initiated a large city-wide campaign for immunization against diphtheria led by Thomas W. Lamont, the prominent financier. An independent and strong Bureau of Nursing was established in 1928.

In the same year the Department of Hospitals was formed; this brought together those hospitals operated by the Department of Health, the Bellevue complex, and the city "charity" groups. The new agency was without an advisory or regulatory board until 1950. The importance of closer collaboration with other health-care agencies, of preventing the further fragmentation of medical care, was not seen until much later. Prevention and cure of disease were more or less independent activities. Only a few professional public-health experts were interested in medical care. City officials listened to the pleas of separate vested interests;

boards and departments to handle these interests began to proliferate.

City contributions to voluntary hospitals continued outside the jurisdiction of the new department; such contributions have yet to be subjected routinely to critical professional appraisal.

With the stock-market crash of 1929 and the revelation of corruption in the regime of Mayor James J. Walker, the department suffered; it revived again with the election of Fiorello H. LaGuardia in 1932. Mayor LaGuardia's genuine interest in people and their welfare and his close connections with George Baehr, his personal physician, and with that remarkable scientist and physician, Thomas Rivers of the Rockefeller Institute, both members of the Board of Health, made a rare combination. The spirit of the times encouraged change. Franklin D. Roosevelt's New Deal responded to the desperate needs of the people: needs that resulted from the country's economic collapse. The Social Security Act of 1935 and revisions of the Public Health Act made funds available for specific types of local health work. Surgeon General Thomas Parran, Jr., led new nationwide crusades, notably for the control of venereal diseases, and established the National Institutes of Health, which strengthened the nation's efforts in health research. He noted that "people in general are beginning to take it for granted that an equal opportunity for health is a basic American right." This utterance marked another step—granted, a long one—in wiping out the double standard for medical care—one for the rich and one for the poor—but the direction was clear.

Neighborhood Health Centers and Problems of Decentralization

The idea of bringing health services closer to the people through neighborhood centers received much attention again. An experimental health district had been set up in the lower East Side as early as 1914. Strong, centralized, and specialized control had been replaced by a system of local administration under one district chief but, by 1918, the plan had been dropped. The idea, however, was kept alive in part by privately financed agencies, particularly the Milbank Memorial Fund and the Red Cross, at the Judson, East Harlem, Mulberry, and Bellevue Yorkville health centers. In 1929 the Department of Health appointed the Committee on Neighborhood Health Development, composed of citizens and professionals, to formulate plans for providing the entire city with neighborhood health centers. A master plan was adopted in

1930. Seven permanent buildings were completed in seven years; by 1960, when the over-all plan was modified, 22 more health centers and six smaller ones had been completed and staffed.

The city's plan for neighborhood or district health centers was based on census tracts, natural cultural boundaries, local needs, and transportation facilities; each area had a population of about 200,000. For 30 years these units were centers of departmental interest and concern. Here were housed voluntary health agencies, health educators, public-health nurses, case-finding in chronic-disease control, and certain health services for the rich and the poor. The success of these centers is hard to measure. The caliber of the health officer and the length of his tenure in the same area made a difference. The lines between preventive and curative medicine, between public and private effort, between hospital and out-of-hospital care, between welfare and other medical care were still sharply drawn in those years, so that continuing and comprehensive care for families was not achieved. Lack of money curtailed services. Moreover, the continuing contentious, all-or-none arguments about centralization versus decentralization took too much energy. Criteria of what should or could be decentralized and what should or could not were lacking. Not until the mid-1950's was an apparently reasonable truce established. But despite many criticisms the district health centers served millions of New Yorkers and set the stage for today's more vigorous efforts to help the poor. It is seldom recognized that these centers have maintained over the years the world's largest outpatient department. Through them and through the efforts of private physicians, the city's remarkably successful control of tuberculosis, venereal disease, poliomyelitis, diphtheria, smallpox, and now pertussis and measles, has been achieved. Here one third of the infants born each year have received pediatric care and have been helped with problems of behavior and development. Some centers developed extensive aftercare for patients discharged from mental hospitals. Others set up services for the cerebral-palsied child, combined well- and sick-baby care, and have been sources of many other creative health demonstrations.

More Activity under LaGuardia

But let us go back to the first years of the LaGuardia regime. The findings of an exhaustive appraisal of the department made by the

American Public Health Association and John L. Rice, of New Haven, the new commissioner of health, started another era in the department. Federal funds became available via the state to expand certain health activities. Full-time professionally qualified leaders were put in charge of bureaus and districts; incompetents were retired or put where they could do no harm. Emphasis was on quality and efficiency. In-service training was built up through courses and demonstration-teaching centers; old-time employees were sent to universities; about 1,800 employees were reached in two and one half years in the course of the largest educational effort ever made by the department.

The tuberculosis services were modernized; a more vigorous campaign against venereal disease was begun. The maternal mortality study of the early 1930's, done jointly with The New York Academy of Medicine, showed that two thirds of maternal deaths were preventable. A professional advisory committee, the first of many, was formed to advise the commissioners of health and hospitals exactly what to do. By the mid-1940's the death rate had been reduced by the two thirds that the 1930's study had suggested was possible.

Thomas Duffield, a dynamic registrar of records, followed in the footsteps of his predecessors, the city investigators, and developed a supplementary medical report that was attached to birth and death certificates. The report was treated as confidential, and its tables of statistics have given scientists new and valuable tools which have added greatly to the knowledge of the true prevalence of certain diseases, the complications of pregnancy, and the causes of infant death. The term "fetal death," now adopted by the World Health Organization, was first used by the Department of Health in 1939. Trained statisticians began to watch routine departmental activities.

But the greatest contribution of the 1930's and early 1940's was probably the recruitment of a relatively large number of extremely well-qualified physicians on whom the department was to depend for many years. During the depression, public service appealed to more socially-minded professionals who found work in the department challenging and attractive. There was so much to do.

The first qualified pediatricians were put in charge of the services for mothers, infants, and school children. Scientific studies were made of how best to operate these services. The Astoria School Health Study, for example, set up a new system for the protection of school children, and it was widely copied throughout the country. The annual routine examination was replaced by a more careful one given every four years. When possible, the examination made by the child's own physician was used in school. Efforts were made to get parents to take the child to his own physician or to find some other medical care for him. But the most important advance was made by helping teachers to observe the child's condition on a day-to-day basis. This information was used as a guide to select those children who should see a doctor or a nurse. The new plan solved some of the problems of the time. Emphasis was put on the more urgent health problems of the children. Better use was made of staff, but the basic problem of what to do with the school health services was not solved. Mental health, so-called child guidance, was already a separate service. Medical care was fragmented. Health education stood apart. And so the situation still is—and not only in New York City, where services still are probably better than in many cities. But how to handle effectively the health problems of all school-age children is a major problem yet to be solved.

Change came too in the supervision of well babies in those latter days of 1930. Pediatricians were hired to supervise the services. A so-called research and training center was inaugurated at the department's Kip's Bay Health Center. Here doctors and nurses studied the problem of what could be done to improve services. Leading pediatricians, child psychiatrists, and nutritionists conferred on new developments in pediatrics, on what psychiatry had to bring to the care of the newborn child and his family, on treatment of minor illnesses, on nutritious low-cost diets, and on the behavior problems so troublesome to parents. A baby book was written and distributed with birth certificates. Pamphlets on feeding and on common behavior problems were developed with the help of mothers and were widely copied. Here Benjamin Spock taught and gathered material for his now famous "Baby Book": *Baby and Child Care.* Since World War II, the center's expanded work in mental health, known as the Attitude Study Project, has been recognized nationally and internationally. The World Health Organization uses its material.

Complete Medical Care for Some

The care of premature babies was an early chapter in the development of the comprehensive medical care to be so widely advocated in the mid-1960's. In the late 1930's prematurity had become the leading cause of infant mortality. A professional advisory committee made up of leading pediatricians, nurses, and departmental leaders surveyed all existing services. It recommended what needed to be done. Its advice was followed. "Premature centers" were developed. These were staffed with specially trained nurses and were equipped with incubators, oxygen, and blood, and were able to give all the care that a baby might need. Such centers taught the mothers how to care for their babies before the mothers were sent home; nurses made house visits before and after babies went home to see that mothers and homes were ready for the babies and that all went well. Also created was a special follow-up service in the hospital so that the baby would be seen by those who knew his condition, if he was not cared for by his own doctor. Part of the scheme was an ambulance service, with specially trained nurses that could transport the baby prematurely born at home or in a hospital without proper facilities to a "premature center." All the specialized services needed were established, not overnight, but a step at a time; these have helped to save the lives of thousands of babies, rich and poor alike, for there has been no discrimination. The services have been financed by parents, by the city, and by state and federal funds through the Crippled Children's program. Parents paid what they could, but all were cared for in the same way. More centers were established as needed, but not in every hospital.

This pattern of government as a leader, a catalyzer, a planner (though the word was not widely accepted in health circles at that time) and not an operator, worked well. The Department of Health with the help of experts surveyed the field, identified centers of strength as well as gaps, and exercised the leadership necessary to mobilize resources. Since it did not tell doctors or hospitals what to do, it aroused no cry of government interference. It decided the kind of services it would purchase with tax dollars and helped expand them. "Run your own affairs," the department said, "but this is the only kind of service we will buy." The policy resembled the setting up of specifications for the municipal purchase of soap or automobiles. This practice of setting standards for medical care for which tax funds would be paid has been extended to cover other areas. It could stand wider consideration in these days of expanding government activity in medical affairs.

The revision of the care of crippled children is another chapter in developing such integrated services of medical care. Families had received financial help to pay for hospital care, braces, etc., from the courts. Parents had to appear in court to petition for such help. Delays were interminable. Outpatient and inpatient care were not coordinated. A child might lie in a hospital bed for months before a brace arrived. He might never see the specialist who was in the hospital. In 1945 the service was transferred to the Department of Health. Again, with the help of federal and state money, a whole new system was inaugurated. Centers that met standards were set up by leaders in various fields, such as cerebral palsy, hearing, orthopedic disability, and were approved for support. All hospitals were encouraged to provide comprehensive service, to give the child what he needed for maximum rehabilitation, but payment from public funds was made only to those centers which met standards. Two new elements came into the planning for these services: the strong voluntary agencies concerned with some of the diseases that led to the crippling, and the parents of those who were afflicted. So the voice of the consumer was beginning to be heard, though more faintly than in the mid-1960's. These services did little to increase the skills of the neighborhood physician or of the poorer hospital from whom many patients sought care.

Special Problems during World War II

Another important forerunner of today's medical-care programs was that conducted during World War II under the National Emergency Maternal and Infant Care Program (EMIC) through which the infants and pregnant wives of men serving in the first four classes of the armed services were taken care of during pregnancy and for the first year of the baby's life. The enterprise reached out beyond the specialized hospital or doctor to all facilities in a community. Nearly 53,000 infants and mothers were taken care of in about four years. The average payment for the mother was about $120 and the average for the baby was $80. However, there was no maximum on what might be spent. One case cost $2,000. The important fact was that the patient received whatever was needed medically. Obstetric and pediatric consultants were encouraged. Standards for qualified consultants in all medical specialties were established with the assistance of the advisory committee and the county medical societies. Ten per cent of patients were seen by qualified medical consultants—a much higher percentage than prevailed generally. Standards were also set up for hospitals that would be approved for the care of EMIC patients. Ninety of the 110 hospitals with maternity services finally received sufficient approval for most pregnant women in the city to benefit from the improved services. Institutes were held for the professional staffs of hospitals in order to help them attain higher standards.

Other problems loomed large during World War II. Only two can be mentioned: venereal disease and day care for children. John Mahoney of the United States Public Health Service, later commissioner of health, discovered that penicillin could cure syphilis in 1943; thus began a new era of control. The city's vigorous "V.D." campaign was essential to the health, not only of New Yorkers, but to the millions who passed through the city in those war years. Retrospect indicates that continued public education about syphilis, a more extensive campaign among homosexuals, and improved cooperation from the private physician with respect to follow-ups might have prevented the subsequent resurgence of the disease; however, newly organized attacks are bringing the disease under better control once again in the mid-1960's.

A whole new era of protection for preschool children was created by the "door-key" children, whose mothers went off to work. A new Day Care Unit in the Department of Health inventoried nurseries and day-care centers and helped them expand and improve the care they gave. New Sanitary Code regulations and standards were soon copied elsewhere. The unit had teams of educators, nurses, pediatricians, social workers, nutritionists, and sanitarians, who worked not only in the centers where children were cared for but with the institutions which trained groups formed by the state, churches, schools, and private organizations.

In 1947 the city reached an all-time peak of 171,174 births; meanwhile it established a new low rate for infant mortality. The rate for maternal mortality dropped too. Midwives began to disappear; their licenses dropped from 193 in 1941 to 19 in 1947. New midwives were not trained; doctors had taken over. Nurse midwives later replaced the older type. New York City today is the only city in the country that licenses and supervises this new kind of midwife. Only two states do the same. With the growing interest in and use of nurse midwives in maternity care, the city is fortunate in that no legal barriers stand in the way of their employment.

Immediate Postwar Years

After LaGuardia, mayors for some years showed little interest in health affairs. Four commissioners of health came and went in seven years. Certain activities were strengthened; the department staff was strong and could carry on, but the pinch of low salaries and shortages in personnel began to be felt. One successful experiment was a forerunner of the wider use of the allied or paramedical professionals so widely heralded in the 1960's. So-called "public health assistants" (a new title), persons with no more than a high-school diploma but with special training, took over much of the work that more extensively trained persons had done previously.

Better diagnostic services, including x ray for patients who were cared for by private physicians but were unable to afford modern diagnostic services were set up in some "diagnostic centers" in the health centers. Physicians would not refer such patients to the larger hospitals because they seldom saw them again. Many of these doctors were not on hospital staffs. As a department report said at that time, "the services will thus occupy a position midway between governmental assumption of responsibility for medical care, on the one hand, and on the other a laissez-faire attitude in the care of the needy." There was an extension as well of the diagnostic testing for chronic disease in the Bureau of Laboratories. The new services were poorly financed, opposed by medical societies, and finally abandoned. But they were needed and they were to return in another guise later.

A bureau of nutrition under the scientific direction of an expert was established in 1949. As early as 1932 a nutritionist had acted as a consultant to doctors and nurses, preparing low-cost diets and providing other services. An extensive radio and TV program was later developed. Much of this work, as with other services, was maintained initially by private funds.

New Interests and Leadership

In 1954 Robert Wagner, the new mayor, brought a special knowledge of health affairs to City Hall. In the next 12 years many new experiments were initiated under the guidance of Leona Baumgartner, George James, Ross Kandle, and Paul Densen, experienced public-health leaders who were commissioners or deputies in those years. The staff included gifted and well-trained persons. Much reorganization took place; salaries were increased; persons with new skills were brought in; in-service training began again. The pressure of problems brought an air of excitement. A time for change had come.

Infectious diseases were largely under control. The limited goals of current public health needed stretching. Chronic diseases had come to the fore; continuing care was accordingly essential. Research knowledge was waiting to be more widely applied. With more scientific knowledge and specialization medical care had become more and more fragmented. The specialist was replacing the general practitioner; even nursing and social work had their specialties. The poor often received miserable care or none. Bureaucratic minutiae accumulated in a welfare department ill-equipped to handle the complicated problems of providing modern medical care; antiquated methods dominated the procedures by which the poor could get care. Health insurance and group practice were proving their value. Machines were taking over personal tasks. Medical costs were mounting. Health care was becoming a big business. The need for change was clear but change would not come quickly. Step by step, however, foundations for major changes were laid, and often were built on sound practices of the past.

The Interdepartmental Council Explores New Patterns ..

The Interdepartmental Health Council, composed of commissioners of hospitals, health, and welfare (later of mental health also), had been established in 1952.This council might have become a major force for effective coordination of public and private efforts but it failed to do so. The turnover in hospital commissioners was great in those years; departments were swamped with their own day-to-day problems; hospital and welfare departments lacked the professional personnel to plan or deal with major changes.

The council had little power to make radical alterations. The personalities and differing interests of the several commissioners who came and went affected its operation. The council finally secured an executive secretary. Representatives of other city agencies and voluntary agencies often met with it and with its various subcommittees. They worked on problems of the aged, on rehabilitation, maternal care, hospital-based comprehensive-care clinics in a few neighborhoods, prepaid group practice for selected groups of welfare patients, standards for nursing homes, care of amputees, and other problems. Standard setting was followed by the development of "approved" services from which the city would purchase care for the indigent. In the early 1960's care for well and for sick infants was successfully combined in some poverty-stricken areas and experiments like the one at the Gouverneur Health Center were under way; these were precursors for the well-publicized neighborhood centers of the programs that were to deal with poverty of the later 1960's.

The staff of the four departments worked jointly on projects. The council worked quietly; it seemed best that way. The stage was obviously being set for change, for more integration of services. One important lever was lacking—money to pay for care. Funds became available with the federal legislation of 1966.

The need for a total reorganization of the so-called system of delivery of personal health services was perceived and discussed in and out of the department, but vested interests, entrenched bureaucracy in and out of government, and lack of funds and of economic incentive to change made major moves unrealistic. Committees and commissions came and went. Each added its bit to the mounting piles of evidence that the unstructured, unplanned, inefficient, overlapping, obsolete facilities, the tradition-bound roles and stances of the health professionals, the confused welter of legal restrictions, the multiple sources of governmental funds and powers of different layers of government made the effective delivery of modern medical care to New York's millions more and more unattainable. The machinery was not built to carry the load. But some things could be done—patchwork perhaps, but each improvement brought some new knowledge of obstacles to be overcome. Sometimes there were major breakthroughs when the old machinery worked—as when a vigorous use of the new vaccine and control of oxygen given to premature babies were to cause the disappearance in record time of poliomyelitis and of retrolental fibroplasia, a major cause of blindness.

Two possibilities of change were repeatedly discussed. One was a merger of the public agencies concerned with health, including their several boards. The other was the formation of a quasi-public-private authority or corporation of some kind with freedom from restrictive civil service and budgetary regulations, with the ability to transfer public funds under strict accountability to voluntary nonprofit health organizations, or even to effect under the new organization one system of medical care that included both tax-supported and voluntary institutions. The Department of Hospitals did move toward "affiliation agreements," which paid medical schools and other strong teaching hospitals for carrying the responsibility for certain services in city hospitals. But this scheme carried certain problems with it and was comprehensive enough only to strengthen the leadership in certain major services in certain city hospitals.

More Activity in Control of Chronic Diseases

After the mid-1950's the Department of Health increased its work in the field of chronic disease and medical care. Early case-finding would cut down disability and even prevent death. Why not begin here? Better use of existing resources could provide the means. Why not intensify efforts in this direction?

The first center for the detection and prevention of cancer had been opened in 1947 as a cooperative venture of Cornell Medical College, Memorial Hospital, the New York City Cancer Commission, and the Department of Health. Cancer of the cervix, which caused 400 deaths a year, came first. Epidemiologists knew that this form of cancer was more prevalent among certain groups of women than among others. Devising simple techniques that could be used in mass surveys took much time. The self-operated vaginal-smear technique and more automatic screening of slides were tried, but the technology involved was not sufficiently advanced. Nevertheless mass screening was expanded. Screening for diabetes and glaucoma in special groups with high incidence was also initiated.

There was still too much tuberculosis. Instead of waiting to have the disease reported or relying on checking contacts mobile x-ray units were sent into the areas where tuberculosis rates were high. BCG vaccine was more widely used. Earlier rehabilitation for arthritic and stroke patients was sought in a variety of small experiments and demonstrations.

The relation of diet to coronary artery disease, a major cause of death and disability, was tackled through scientific studies which were to be widely copied later. The possibility of devising a low-cholesterol diet, palatable and easy to procure, was shown. Blood-cholesterol levels came down for those who remained on the diet. The many factors involved in the development of coronary disease are still not clear enough to be certain that control of diet per se suffices for prevention. An interesting by-product of these activities was collaboration with different segments of the food industry to produce margarines, ice creams, and other foods with a decreased content of highly saturated fats.

However it was obvious that, as a 1960 report said, "Were comprehensive and continuing medical care of a high-quality being received by most New Yorkers, many of these conditions would not be found." Better logistics for the delivery and management of medical care were sought in demonstrations for selected groups; for the most part existing facilities and personnel were used. One such project was carried out in a low-income housing project, another for older people in a housing project in Queens County, still another for all persons in the Gouverneur area in the Lower East Side. These projects brought services closer to the people and clearly led to earlier case finding and continued care. Each program had built into it some kind of evaluation, for it was as important to learn as to do.

Other ventures aimed at improved care for larger groups. The commissioners of welfare and health established a joint position in both departments whereby the expertise of both could be used in an attempt to obtain better medical care for the indigent. A joint venture with the Health Insurance Plan of Greater New York showed that hospitalization could be cut down through continuing care from an organized group. Another experiment, financed by research funds (see below), compared care given by a large teaching hospital, The New York Hospital, with that furnished through the usual fragmented service previously provided through welfare channels.

The problem of providing care for the indigent in proprietary hospitals and nursing homes was surveyed. With the help of physicians, nutritionists, and sanitarians the department developed regulations for these institutions that were later adopted by the Board of Hospitals. Thus, step-by-step, one problem at a time, better management of the health-care system was being effected; the time for major changes had not yet arrived.

Mental Health

The Department of Health had pursued mental-health activities after the 1930's. The care of the mentally ill was a state function. Pediatricians in the department in the late 1930's saw the importance of handling the so-called behavior problems in infants and young children and established training and consultation programs for well-child clinics (see above). The Board of Education operated a Bureau of Child Guidance for school-age children. In 1949 the department established three adult psychiatric services in health centers. Follow-up of those who were released from state hospitals was tried. In the mid-1950's the state legislature established local mental-health boards which carried with them state-matching funds, just as public health in the city had long been supported by state reimbursement. The pressure to create an independent organization to handle mental-health affairs was great, and so, at the price of further fragmentation of medical care a new agency, the Community Health Board, was formed under a plan formulated by the state legislature. It has extended services largely through contracts with public and private agencies. Again, the time for integration with other health services was not ripe.

New Environmental Hazards

Through those years, hazards from the environment were not forgotten. Eternal vigilance was maintained by sanitarians who were watching food, milk, and water supplies, and fighting filth and smoke: their units were always understaffed and were always fighting vested interests of one sort or another. Success was often hard to see. But for years there has been no outbreak of food poisoning or of intestinal disease traced to food or water, other than minor episodes due to the preparation of food at home or by social groups. Clearing major pollution in the waters around the city moved slowly; studies pinpointing important sources proved helpful. Effective handling of this problem requires a major concern about pollution on a tri-state basis and large financial support.

Other man-made hazards were being recognized. Certain deadly hazards were eliminated. Carbon-monoxide poisoning, which had taken hundreds of lives in poor tenements, was finally eliminated with the mandatory replacement of obsolete gas refrigerators and water heaters. Monitoring systems for the measurement of air pollution were set up by laboratory experts in the health department. Major support for air-pollution control came only with the establishment of a new department in 1949.

Accidental poisonings took lives every year, particularly of children.

A Poison Control Center to serve thousands of doctors and patients was set up in 1955. Its information service still works day and night. The center's roster of the composition of antidotes for thousands of compounds is used by New Yorkers and non-New Yorkers.

Realization of the hazards of ionizing radiation grew out of the development of the atom bomb. A radiation-control unit was set up in 1950, but it had insufficient help. In March 1958 the Board of Health, with the help of the nation's chief experts in medicine and industrial radiation, adopted legislation designed to protect the public from unnecessary exposure to radiation. Under the leadership of an expert from the Atomic Energy Commission, the first comprehensive program aimed at protecting the public against radioactive hazards in the country was established. It was soon found that improper installation and use of x-ray equipment in doctors' and dentists' offices offered the greatest dangers. Elimination of these hazards and protection against radiation accidents were the first points of emphasis. The unit was informed about the movement of all radioactive materials through the city.

Old Problems Continued

The Sanitary Code or, as it was renamed in 1958, the Health Code, is the basic body of law through which health protection for New Yorkers is regulated. Unrevised for 45 years, it had become an indigestible mass of obsolete, conflicting, and modern regulations covering many aspects of health and business affairs. It was not only recodified, but substantively rewritten with the help of the Columbia University legislation-drafting service. After three years of study and negotiation, the new code was adopted in 1958 and has become a model for modern health laws. Many picturesque laws were abandoned, including one that required the commissioner to police the streets at night in search of horses that had died in harness and had been abandoned, "causing a light to be placed at the head and tail" so that accidents could be avoided!

The story of fluoridating the city's water supply was full of ups and downs. The procedure was first recommended after careful studies in 1952; report after report followed. The issue became a political one, even as chlorination had been a half century before. In 1965 the fluorides were in the water. Thirty-five years of dental care provided to the poorest children by the department's large dental service had protected some, but the treated water would do much more.

Family planning—or birth control, as it was called in earlier days—was another controversial subject. In the 1930's the department had an unwritten agreement with the Catholic Church that women referred to clinics would not be pressured or coerced, and that employees would not be required to participate in any activity that would offend their consciences. Some municipal hospitals gave contraceptive service in the late 1950's. In the 1960's the climate changed and more direct action was taken. Soon national leadership and funds came to the rescue and service in family planning was made widely available.

Research and Evaluation

Research in the laboratory had been important since the days of Herman M. Biggs, William H. Parks, and Anna Williams. Several departmental units had published important studies in epidemiology, pediatrics, disease control, statistics, and so on. Basic laboratory research was intensified in 1941 by the establishment of the Public Health Research Institute, a semi-independent unit whose staff was free from routine diagnostic work and could concentrate on basic problems in viral, infectious, and metabolic diseases. It was probably the first municipal research institute devoted exclusively to public health but its scope remained limited. Its record has been an enviable one.

Changes in the health and medical scene demanded other approaches in research. The leading causes of death and disability were changing. Man's ever-increasing ability to control and change his physical environment created new risks. New scientific knowledge and technologies were awaiting wider application. It was felt that even as large an organization as the Department of Health, which had more than 5,000 employees and a budget that was nearing 50 million dollars, should examine its own operations and its future development more carefully. Two approaches were chosen: one via the so-called Health Research Council, to focus on problems the department was ill-equipped to handle; the other, through an internal group more closely related to the department's efforts, intended to work on problems the department could handle.

The establishment of the Health Research Council (HRC), begun in 1954 and formalized in 1958, established a unique approach—another first in the history of the department. A survey indicated that New York City was unusual in the multiplicity of its resources and the magnitude and diversity of its health problems. Its medical-care services were scattered, undermanned, and were failing to keep up with the health problems of the time. Its medical schools and teaching hospitals had difficulty in keeping teachers, high-caliber technicians, and research scientists. Space for needed facilities was inadequate. Yet there was talent here and an enormous medical establishment that was not being used to find answers to the growing problems. A municipally financed effort focusing on some of the most acute problems seemed appropriate. Careful planning went into the development of the new Health Research Council, which was patterned somewhat after the British Medical Research Council but whose scope was widened to include the social sciences, engineering, and any discipline that could possibly throw light on health problems. It does not duplicate other research efforts. Experts from the Medical Research Council in Great Britain, from the National Institutes of Health, from the Rockeller Institute and the Rockefeller Foundation, from medical schools, and prominent citizens helped design the new council. Its professional activities are placed largely in the hands of a group of scientists and laymen; the government maintains budget allocations and certain veto power over contracts, but it does not assume responsibility for approval of specific research proposals. The council supports research in universities, colleges, medical schools, and city agencies. A goal of one dollar per person per year was established as an initial rough rule-of-thumb guide for financing. From the beginning, the emphasis has been put on assisting the careers of young research scientists, studying the medical and health problems of particular relevance to the city, and aiding scientific education and training. It is already clear that the support given the career-scientist program has strengthened local hospital and teaching institutions by enabling them to maintain stable positions for highly qualified staff members and creating openings for able scientists who are thus attracted to the city. About $10 million for career scientist awards have been committed by the city. One of three applications has been refused. At the end of 1965, 172 scientists were being supported and at work in many of the city's municipal and voluntary hospitals where their presence has meant better care for patients.

There are also institutional project grants focusing on problems that particularly concern New Yorkers, such as alcoholism and narcotics addiction, the large number of infant deaths, chronic diseases of the aged, delivery and management of medical care, mental illness, more specific knowledge about the flow of sewage-polluted waters into New York harbors, and the sources of air pollution.

One success achieved by the council has been in the control of narcotics addiction. After World War II addiction to heroin grew alarmingly. The degradation, the crime, and the lack of effective control were scandalous. The council found that there was almost no knowledge about how the drug worked, even in single-celled animals; it sought persons who might be interested. Finally one brilliant investigator, at work on another problem at The Rockefeller University, undertook the task. With the help of a colleague (his wife), the usefulness of methadone was discovered. By the use of this substance hundreds of young persons are staying away from heroin, are back at work, and are no longer a burden to themselves, to society, or to their families.

Federal, private, and city funds are often employed jointly in a project of the Research Council. Obsolete and half-forgotten storage space has been converted into laboratory space, and more than 100 new laboratories are being developed without building a single new structure. These laboratories are scattered from Coney Island to Washington Heights. They have cost the city only 3 million dollars, a paltry sum compared to the cost of housing them in new buildings.

The municipal funds have acted to a considerable extent as "seed" money. For every dollar of tax money the city has put into the HRC nearly five dollars in additional federal or private funds has been received.

The benefits obtained from research come in unexpected ways; their value does not become apparent for many years, but the HRC has already justified its expenditures. Achievements have ranged from a speed-up in immunization against measles to the treatment of many psychotics at day hospitals so that they can continue to live at home with their families.

With the realization that any large organization needed its own office of research, program planning, and development, the department, as stated above, was reorganized in 1955 to include such an entity. The unit receives municipal, federal, and private funds. It has evaluated a variety of departmental programs, including the management of school children with heart disease and of satellite clinics for maternal and child care. It has helped to plan follow-up services for men who were rejected by the selective service, whereby these New Yorkers could be returned to their community with their health problems under control. It works for and with other city departments. It promotes research on emerging health problems. Little is known about the cost of chronic-disease programs or about the total expenditures of New Yorkers for medical care, but the economic studies underway are obtaining the facts. An entire new chapter in health economics has been opened. This pattern of having internal research and development units has been copied. Clearly research must move out of the biomedical laboratory into the community, particularly into the area of the delivery of health services, if a major problem of our times is to be solved. This demands a new and different commitment on the part of official departments, universities, and research institutions. Government — federal, state, and local—will need to finance these efforts generously, not only to use the nation's resources more effectively but possibly to hold down mounting costs of health care, and above all to improve the health of everyone.

The Need for Reappraisal

Is the present structure of governmental organization in New York City adequate for meeting today's problems? Obviously the delivery of personal health services is badly in need of reorganization. Other city units have not been sufficiently used. For example, the wealth of information in the Medical Examiner's Office has not been subjected to epidemiological scrutiny. Nor have many health problems. Within the decade separate departments of air pollution and mental health have been established, and much of the regulation of health hazards in housing has been transferred to other departments. These regroupings of functions come and go. What is important is that their functions be carried out better under the new plan, where they are often better financed.

One important factor in health affairs for more than half a century has been the development and maintenance of a delicate balance between the powers of state and city governments. When the Metropolitan Board of Health was established 100 years ago, it was perhaps dimly seen that health problems in the already overcrowded urban areas could probably best be solved locally. Wide powers have been vested in the city's Board of Health and its decisions with hardly any exceptions have been upheld by the courts. One exception concerned the amount of water allowed in that favored New York food, corned beef. The board fought for more meat and less water, but federal standards, the court ruled, took precedence. The board's work seldom makes the news, but its tradition of excellence is unbroken. For many years mayors have appointed to the board only persons eminently well qualified as scientists, doctors, lawyers, health experts, and administrators who have represented no interest other than the welfare of citizens. Similarly, its counterpart, the Public Health Council of the State of New York, has been largely free of vested interests. It has respected the opinion of and stood behind the activities of the city's Board of Health when necessary. The relations between officials in the two departments have usually kept the same delicate balance of mutual respect regardless of the relation between governors and mayors. The positions have been held, particularly after 1913, when Herman M. Biggs left New York City and became the first commissioner of health in the state, by professionally competent persons who keep each other informed of problems and have members of their staffs solve them. New York City, because of its richer facilities and more specialized personnel, could and often did set higher standards than could be set for the rest of the state. This was true even for medical care until the advent of Medicare and Medicaid in 1966. In other words, health has not been a field on which politicians fought their battles. As Mayor LaGuardia said years ago, there is no difference between the tubercle bacillus that attacks a Republican or a Democrat, hence the wise politician has kept partisan politics out of the field of health. The politician has learned that good health services are good politics. This does not mean that the health worker does not have to win wide public support for programs and work effectively with the political leaders in power. The trick is not to become embroiled in the petty partisan political battles but to win wide political support. And that too is a matter of delicate balance.

Another delicate balance is maintained between the department and the board. In 1927 an amendment to the *Charter of the City of New York* (section 1167 of the 1901 charter) provided that the commissioner become head of the department. However, most of the administrative powers remained with the board because of a failure to amend other sections of the charter which specifically authorized the Board of Health to act in an administrative capacity. The new charter of 1938 defined the powers and duties of the commissioner so as to give him all of the powers and duties except those specifically conferred by law on the Board of Health.

The board has wide powers over all matters affecting the health of citizens. It has used its broad powers sparingly and wisely. Since the 1930's the department has brought to the board only matters of major importance and has relied on the board to enact legislation. The power of the Board of Hospitals has changed the situation to a certain extent, so far with no unhappy results. The citizen can call on the Board of Health for review of what he considers arbitrary action by the department. He can, of course, also go to the courts.

The relations of the board and the department with organized groups are likewise worthy of note. The board, in carrying out its chief function of writing the basic health laws and regulations for the city, necessarily consults with a wide variety of commercial, union, charitable, and professional interests. The views of all concerned are sought, chiefly by letter and in hearings before the board. The department, concerned with enforcing regulations and administering a large program of health activities, also crosses the conflicting interests of many people. It has made wide use of professional advisory committees, recognized experts in special fields, and voluntary health groups. There are several standing committees and many ad hoc committees. Representatives of the department choose members of these committees usually in consultation with the groups concerned. In contrast to the Department of Hospitals, it works with many more outside groups and is concerned with many health activities other than its own operations. Relations with the county medical societies have been carried on mainly through the attendance of the commissioner at the department's five-county coordinating council. Care is taken to inform medical, dental, and nursing societies of proposed activities before they are publicly announced, but recommendations made by these groups have not necessarily been adopted. The guiding principle has been to choose the health of the majority of New Yorkers, not the special interests of the professionals. There are also a variety of interdepartmental boards to consider subjects of mutual concern.

Today's health problems are changing, just as they have in the past century. A revolution is under way. Some of its manifestations are conspicuous, such as air and water pollution, pesticides, the ever-rising costs of medical care, the burden of caring for the mentally retarded and the emotionally handicapped, and the problem of where to go for what when one is ill. Some problems are hard to understand and deal with, particularly those caused by the archaic organization of the total system of delivering personal health services. New approaches are being made through regionalization in water, air pollution, and for the care of cancer, heart, and stroke patients; through payment of bills for the elderly through Medicare and for others through Medicaid; through wider use of ancillary personnel; through health planning at state and community levels; through direct attacks on poverty and through changes in techniques of operational research, to name but a few. More money is now available, largely through the federal government, to support the new activities. Community-wide planning is on its way. Were more assistance through the great foundations also available, as in the past, sounder programs difficult to accomplish with public funds alone might well evolve. But it is clear that with 1966 another wave of change has begun.

In Retrospect

What of the results of these efforts? The simplest answer is probably that in the 100 years covered, life expectancy had risen from 45 to 70 years. The death rate had fallen by two thirds. Major epidemics have disappeared. Despite the unattractiveness of much of modern living, the stench and extreme filth of even the poor areas is largely gone. Health problems have not all been solved; new ones have come and will continue to come. Today a major reevaluation in medical care is facing the city. In solving this current problem, as in solving problems of earlier years, the answers lie not only with the politicians and the health professionals but with the climate of the time.

What lessons are to be learned from the past? Seven stand out.

First, success has been achieved whenever the health affairs of the city have had strong scientific and professional leadership, and when there have been citizens, various professional groups, and political leaders sincerely interested in the common good.

Second, the social and economic climate of the times has a marked influence on what can be and is done. Health education, mental health, and family planning are examples of programs that died out and re-flowered later.

Third, the larger battles seem to have been won when efforts have centered on what can best be done at a particular time to reach a larger goal, when there is readiness to shift tactics as new techniques and new obstacles are found. Progress has seemed to come in spurts, but even then it has usually gone one step at a time. When that step is based on solid scientific evidence, the desired goal can usually be attained more readily. Closing schools and swimming pools did not control poliomyelitis, but vaccine did.

Fourth, a certain amount of patience is essential. Fluoridation of water supplies came after 10 years of continuous effort. More effective delivery of personal health services to all will take its decade or more, also.

Fifth, the importance of a sound administrative structure in city government staffed by highly-skilled professionals able to move from one health problem to another has been amply demonstrated in these past 100 years. The ability of such a structure to circumvent bureaucratic controls and political interference has also been shown, though such a process wastes a great deal of time and effort and does not always succeed.

Sixth, the strong tradition of the integrity, professional, and scientific expertise of the Board of Health and of the Department of Health and their ability to mobilize private resources, maintained over many years, has been of major importance in the protection of the health of New Yorkers.

Seventh, a strong research component is essential to good administration.

May New Yorkers be wise enough to remember these lessons in the coming days of the increasingly noisy revolution in health affairs that is taking place. And may New Yorkers salute that hard core of devoted health workers in the city service who have made possible the achievements I have briefly and inadequately recounted.

THE DEVELOPMENT OF PSYCHIATRY IN NEW YORK CITY: AN OVERVIEW

George Mora, M.D.

Medical Director
The Astor Home for Children
Rhinebeck, N. Y.

Introduction

A historical presentation of the development of psychiatry in New York City can hardly avoid being incomplete and, perhaps, somewhat unilateral. No matter what philosophical school of psychiatry one adheres to, what chronological period one focuses on, or what relations and boundaries one establishes for the field of psychiatry, it is probable that others may disagree and that their rationale may be justifiable. As in any other historical presentation the events which have occurred are factual data which cannot be disputed, but their interpretation in the context of the political, social, economic, and cultural scene can differ according to the viewpoint of the observer.

Moreover, it is not improbable that the interpretation of relatively recent events in psychiatry may be vitiated by several factors: 1) psychiatry is still at a "preparadigmatic" level (Kuhn)[1] and, therefore, its methodology and conceptualization into a definite area of knowledge in terms of core and boundaries remains somewhat vague even in our time; 2) it has become increasingly evident in recent years that much writing on the history of medicine and science is influenced by "inductivistic" or "presentistic" bias (Agassi, Stocking):[2, 3] i.e., events of the past are emphasized or minimized in terms of their relevance to the present instead of being placed in their historical context; 3) somewhat related to the latter point is the difficulty of writing of contemporary events that involve many people who are still active in the field and many concepts and practices which are still not clearly defined; 4) finally, the social scene in the city of New York has changed to an extent unmatched in any other larger conglomerate in the United States and perhaps in the world; we may note, for example, the influx of the Puerto Rican population and the movement of the middle class toward suburbia.

Bearing these limitations in mind I propose to describe in the following paragraphs the developments in the field of psychiatry since the beginning of the century, placing my main emphasis on the last few decades. The fact that I have followed these developments from a distance without being closely involved in them may perhaps represent an advantage in terms of objectivity.

Important Aspects

Four main factors can be isolated with a certain degree of accuracy: 1) the hospital tradition; 2) the European psychoanalytic influence; 3) the organicistic trend; 4) the role played by social phenomena.

1) The importance of institutional medical settings, such as state hospitals and general hospitals, in the development of psychiatry has been well recognized. It probably had its origin in the strong influence exercised on psychiatry by the New York State hospital system and by the general hospitals of New York City. It is worth noting that John Gray of the Utica State Hospital was editor of the *American Journal of Insanity* from 1855 to 1886. The New York State Care Act, which divided the state into hospital districts, was passed in 1890. Bellevue Hospital opened an "Insane Pavillion" in 1879. The New York State Psychiatric Institute was founded in 1896 under the name of "Pathological Institute" of the New York State Hospital service.[4]

In 1907-1909, shortly after his arrival in New York City, Adolf Meyer introduced clinical notes at Manhattan State Hospital. Many of the early psychoanalysts in New York City held positions in hospitals, especially at the Manhattan State Hospital where, in fact, psychoanalysis was introduced about 1908. Later, in 1926, the New York Psychoanalytic Society could not be licensed as a clinic because it was not affiliated with a hospital.

In the 1940's the first attempts to introduce psychoanalytic training in the context of a university setting were initiated in New York City. This took place at the New York Medical College Psychoanalytic Institute in 1944 and at Columbia University Psychoanalytic Clinic in 1945. By that time some general hospitals had initiated psychiatric services. The most outstanding among them is the Payne Whitney Psychiatric Clinic, inaugurated at the New York Hospital in 1932.[5]

2) Psychiatry in New York City has had the constant characteristic of being first influenced by trends developed in Europe. The profes-

sional interplay between New York City and Europe is a unique feature in the development of American psychiatry. This factor is particularly evident in relation to the development of psychoanalysis, both in terms of the unitary aspect of the early psychoanalytic movement—from the beginning of our century to the 1940's—and of the fragmentation of psychoanalytic schools—from the 1940's to the present.

Although Freud lectured in Worcester, Mass., and not in New York City in 1909, New York City for a number of years had almost a monopoly of psychoanalysis. The New York Psychoanalytic Society was founded by Abraham A. Brill in 1911. Brill, Freud's translator, remained active in New York City for many years and Freud's translations were published in New York City. In the 1920's a number of New York City psychiatrists such as C. P. Oberndorf, A. Kardiner, I. Hendrick, L. S. Kubie, B. D. Lewin, W. V. Silverberg, C. Thompson, and G. Zilboorg, went to Europe to be analyzed by Freud and his pupils. Conversely, during the same years a number of psychoanalysts such as O. Rank, S. Lorand, S. Ferenczi, P. Schilder, F. Wittels, followed in the 1930's by A. Adler, H. Nunberg, G. O. Roheim, and S. Rado, came to New York City to lecture or to settle.

As late as 1929, the New York Psychoanalytic Society had 50 members, more than the American Psychoanalytic Association, which had only 46. In the same year didactic analysis became a requisite for admission to the New York society. In 1931 psychoanalytic training was introduced at the newly founded New York Psychoanalytic Institute. In 1932 the *Psychoanalytic Quarterly* was founded by a group of psychoanalysts in New York City.[6]

3) The fact that for many years the psychoanalytic movement presented itself in a rather compact way may have tended to overshadow the importance of the "organicistic" trend, which was also characterized by strong ties between Europe and New York City. Opposition to psychoanalysis always ran very high in New York City, as is evidenced by the attacks of some neurologists, notably Foster Kennedy and Bernard Sachs.

Interestingly enough, in the decades between the late 19th and the early 20th century, neurology—notably through George Beard's "neurasthenia" and S. Weir Mitchell's "rest cure," in New York City and Philadelphia respectively—had fostered the practice of long-term doctor-patient relations, which in time would become the conscious aim of psychoanalysis and of Meyer's psychobiology. More important than this, however, are the developments in the field of pathologic anatomy, histology, heredity, mental deficiency, and others.

In 1913 the *Spirocheta pallida* was isolated in paretic brains by Noguchi and Moore at the Rockefeller Institute in New York City. In the 1920's the New York Psychiatric Institute, which acquired its present name in 1929, took upon itself, under the direction of George H. Kirby, the task of carefully testing some new methods for the biological treatment of mental illness, in particular the malaria treatment of general paresis, which had been introduced by von Jauregg in Vienna in 1918, and some new pathogenetic theories of mental disorders, such as that of focal infections, advanced by Henry Cotton at the State Hospital in Trenton, N. J.[7]

In the late 1930's treatment of psychosis by means of insulin shock was introduced in New York City by M. Sakel in association with Bernard Wortis at Bellevue Hospital. This was soon followed by L. Bini and U. Cerletti's electric shock treatment, introduced in New York City by R. J. Almansi, D. J. Impastato, and a few others. Study of the insulin-shock treatment was continued by others, such as A. M., M. D., and R. R. Sackler, and the whole area of shock treatment was presented in a comprehensive work by L. B. Kalinowski and P. H. Hoch. At the same time a number of studies on the effects of various "drugs of the mind" were made by New York City psychiatrists. The first study on marijuana intoxication was made by W. Bromberg at Bellevue in 1934. Finally, at the New York Psychiatric Institute, its new director, L. Kolb, in the late 1940's did some basic research on the effect of lobotomy which had been introduced by W. Freeman and F. W. Watts in Washington, D.C. a few years previously.

Other important studies are those on hereditary factors in schizophrenia, conducted by F. J. Kallman and J. D. Rainer, also at the New York Psychiatric Institute, and on mental deficiency by G. A. Jervis at Letchworth Village, and by J. Wortis at Bellevue Hospital-New York University. This organicistic trend, which received impetus from the introduction of chemotherapy in the early 1950's, eventually led to the foundation of the Society for Biological Psychiatry, which has always maintained its stronghold in New York City.

4) The impact of social factors on psychopathology is common to all large urban conglomerates. Poverty, lack of housing, urbanization,

industrialization, deficient education, social mobility, ethnic conflicts, all lead to psychiatric disorders. In New York City these problems have been magnified by the continuous wave of immigrants who, consequently, have created great cultural conflicts. Individuals, schools, agencies, and organizations have traditionally been aware of these factors and have attempted to deal with them in different ways.

The New York Children's Aid Society began to place children in foster homes and institutions in 1853. It was followed by the Child Study Association of New York, founded in 1881. The first meeting of the National Conference of Charities and Correction, which in 1917 became the National Conference of Social Work, took place in New York City in 1874. The Henry Street Settlement was opened in New York City in 1896. In 1898, the New York School of Philanthropy organized summer sessions, which were continued for several years. As soon as Adolf Meyer began to work at the Manhattan State Hospital in 1907, he recognized the importance of studying the social backgrounds of his patients. Mrs. Meyer helped him in this endeavor, earning recognition as the "first American social worker." A year before, in 1906, the New York State Charities Aid Association had inaugurated an assistance plan for after-care of patients discharged from mental hospitals.[8] Following the establishment of the Connecticut Society for Mental Hygiene in 1908 by Clifford Beers, a National Committee on Mental Hygiene was founded in New York in 1909, and Thomas V. Salmon was appointed as medical director in 1912.[9] The Child Welfare League of America was founded in New York City in 1920. In 1929 the New York School of Social Work began to operate. It was followed a few years later by the New School of Social Research, which has played an important role up to the present time.

Large voluntary agencies, such as the Federation of Protestant Welfare Agencies, the Catholic Charities, and the Jewish Board of Guardians, which later became an agency of the Federation of Jewish Philanthropies, were also organized in the 1920's. Some important foundations located in New York City, such as the Commonwealth Fund, the Rockefeller Foundation, and the Milbank Memorial Fund, contributed actively to the psychiatric movement by granting funds for research, training, and service. As a part of this, the child guidance movement gained impetus in the 1920's.[10] In 1921 the Bureau of Children's Guidance was established under B. Glueck and M. Kenworthy for five years as a part of the Commonwealth Fund Program for the Prevention of Delinquency. It was followed by the Institute for Child Guidance, under L. Lowrey, which was located in New York City and provided training in child psychiatry and in social work from 1927 to 1933.[11] Also, as an expression of this concern for social issues, the New York City Court of General Sessions from 1931 on began to have all offenders examined; this was done under the direction of Karl Bowman and, later, of Walter Bromberg.

Even psychoanalysis, in spite of its exclusive early emphasis on the doctor-patient relation was affected by the social situation of New York City. Early in the 1930's a number of analysts, such as B. Glueck, W. A. White, A. A. Brill, and M. Kenworthy, taught at the New York School for Social Work. In response to the political distress caused by Nazi persecution of Jews, an Emergency Committee on Relief and Immigration was formed in New York City by the American Psychoanalytic Association under L. S. Kubie and B. D. Lewin. As a result of the work of persons attached to this committee, as well as others, a number of "illustrious immigrants" (or about to be illustrious) arrived in this country in the late thirties and early forties: this group included W. Reich, T. Reik, O. Fenichel, E. Simmel, S. Bernfeld, E. Kris, A. Waelder, E. Fromm, and F. Redlich. In spite of the encouraging attitude of some other centers, notably the Menninger Foundation in Topeka, Kans., most of the newcomers considered the Midwest too "American" and preferred to settle in New York City so as to be able to maintain contact with Europe. Some even founded their own group, such as the T. Reik's Society for Psychoanalytic Psychology (1941), which later became the National Association for Psychoanalysis. In the same year (1941), were founded the Association for Advancement of Psychoanalysis, which later (1942-1943) became the William A. White Institute, and the American Institute for Psychoanalysis, established by Karen Horney. Previous to that, in 1939, the American Association for the Advancement of Psychotherapy, which has had as its forum the *American Journal of Psychotherapy*, was founded in New York City. In 1945 the Post-graduate Center for Psychotherapy was opened. Up to the present time it has been directed by L. Wolberg. Recently its name has been changed to Postgraduate Center for Mental Health.

A common characteristic of these various groups has been involvement with social issues, whether the social situation in New York City fostered such an involvement or, conversely—as in the case of Karen Horney, who moved to New York City from Chicago—whether social conditions represented a more receptive environment for ideas already developed elsewhere. Be this as it may, the fact remains that some of the most outstanding representatives of the so-called "neo-Freudian movement," such as Geza Roheim, Ruth Benedict, Margaret Mead, Abraham Kardiner, Karen Horney, Erich Fromm, and Rollo May, found New York City the most suitable place for the development of their ideas. Even in the case of H. S. Sullivan his original ideas on the psychoanalytic treatment of psychosis were developed at the Sheppard Pratt Hospital in Maryland, but found fertile ground only at the White Institute in New York City. It was also in New York City that J. L. Moreno made his early attempts in psychodrama in the 1930's and S. R. Slavson initiated his group work with children at the Jewish Board of Guardians.

By the late 1940's a conceptual definition of social psychiatry had been offered by T.A.C. Rennie at New York Hospital; attempts at family therapy had been initiated by N. Ackermann; the School of Applied Psychoanalysis, which aimed to integrate psychoanalytic and anthropological research, had been founded; and the Treatment Center for psychoanalytic treatment of poor patients had been operating, first as a Veterans Administration mental hygiene clinic and then in the New York Psychoanalytic Institute.[12]

In summary: four main trends have been identified in the development of psychiatry approximately from the beginning of the century to the end of World War II:

1) The hospital tradition, stemming both from the strong state-hospital and general hospital systems.

2) The psychodynamic tradition, due to the strong relation between New York City and Europe and fostered by the immigration to this country of many European psychoanalysts.

3) The organicistic tradition, which was also influenced by the strong relation between Europe and New York City.

4) The impact of social factors on psychopathology, a pervasive and almost unique feature of psychiatry in New York City.

Recent Trends

At this point some general considerations and comments related to the recent developments of psychiatry in New York City are in order.

Obviously it is very difficult for anyone to comprehend and to present objectively a situation as complex as that of psychiatry in New York City. The fact that no institute for the history of medicine was ever founded in New York City does not explain this state of affairs, since traditionally medical historians have shied away from psychiatric themes. Interestingly enough, three recent publications on the development of psychiatry were prepared almost exclusively by psychiatrists not working in New York City.[13-15] Iago Galdston, editor of one of these volumes, as former executive secretary of the committee on Medical Information of the New York Academy of Medicine, was instrumental in the preparation of several collaborative works on various aspects of psychiatry. Also, a number of psychiatrists and historians interested in the history of psychiatry, e.g., G. Zilboorg, A. Deutsch, G. Rosen, N. D. C. Lewis, B. Nelson, O. Diethelm, J. Ehrenwald, P. Cranefield, E. T. Carlson, and J. Schneck have been active or are still active in New York City. But no comprehensive study on the development of psychiatry in New York City has ever been attempted. In regard to psychoanalysis, much useful material can be found in the two studies on psychoanalysis in the United States published, respectively, by the New York City psychoanalysts C. P. Oberndorf[6] and J. Millet.[16]

The reasons for this lack of a special study of New York developments may be difficult to ascertain. It would be an oversimplication to attribute this fact to a strict adherence of each member of the psychiatric profession to a particular school of thought, with a consequent inability to comprehend the contributions of other schools of thought. Indeed, both all-encompassing presentations of modern psychiatry—S. Arieti's *American Handbook of Psychiatry* and A. D. Freedman and H. I. Kaplan's *Comprehensive Textbook of Psychiatry*—originated in New York City.

Rather, a certain degree of electicism has been a pervasive feature of psychiatry in New York City. No matter how vehement the controversy between the organicistic and the dynamic schools has been, a certain dialogue between neurology and psychiatry has always been carried on there. The first two psychoanalysts in New York City, A. A. Brill and C. P. Oberndorf, were initially introduced to Freud's work at the beginning of the century by two neurologists, Frederick Peterson and Louis Casamajor, respectively. The American Psychopathological Association, founded in 1911 and closely identified with New York City—

where its annual meeting takes place—has traditionally represented a common ground for discussion of neurological and psychiatric matters, as recently brought forth in a comprehensive review by F. Freyhan.[17]

Later, from the 1930's and 1940's up to the present time, the New York Psychiatric Institute of Columbia University has served as a crossroads between persons of various psychiatric orientations. It was there that, in the 1930's, Flanders Dunbar composed her encyclopedic work on psychosomatic medicine, establishing a bridge between medicine and psychodynamics. Likewise, at the Columbia Psychoanalytic Institute, David Levy established a tie between psychodynamics and child development with his very important studies on the mother-child relationship. In the same setting, Sandor Rado developed his so-called "adaptional psychodynamics," which opened the way toward brief and realistic psychotherapy. Before then, however, at Bellevue Hospital, Paul Schilder—whose impact on New York City psychiatry has been outstanding, as is evidenced by the establishment of the Schilder Society—had opened more than one avenue toward neurology with his basic studies on muscle tone, body image, and sensory perception—which anticipated today's gestalt psychiatry—and toward interpersonal and social theory with his early attempts at group psychotherapy. This latter was anticipated in New York City by Triggant Burrow's "philoanalysis," by Cody Marsh's lectures to mental patients, and by Moreno's "theatre of spontaneity."

In New York City psychoanalysis itself, though originally organized by Freud into a compact society responsible for therapy, training, research, and publication, broke down into a number of independent organizations. In 1956 some members of the American Psychoanalytic Association and of other New York City organizations founded the American Academy of Psychoanalysis as a forum for a broader discussion of psychodynamics in the contex of social issues. Unquestionably the representatives of the neo-Freudian movement, who for some years attempted to integrate psychodynamics with social and anthropological findings, were influential in the formation of this academy. True, the main development in the field of orthodox psychoanalysis is constituted by the studies on ego psychology carried on by H. Hartmann, E. Kris, and R. M. Loewenstein in New York City, and was influenced by many trends, from child development to the social sciences. Likewise, child analysis in New York City had some of its most well-known representatives, such as D. Levy, R. Spitz, M. Fried, M. Ribble, H. Bruch, followed in time by the emphasis on child psychoses and autism (represented by L. Bender, L. Despert, W. Goldfarb, M. Mahler), and later by the importance of longitudinal studies such as those conducted by S. Chess and A. Thomas at the New York Medical College and later at Bellevue-New York University.

According to the best European tradition, some of the early child analysts, such as B. Bornstein, as well as adult analysts in New York City, have been laymen. The controversy in regard to lay analysis has been especially lively in New York City. Opposing it are the attempts to establish psychoanalysis in the realm of medical schools, at Columbia University, at the New York Medical College and, more recently, in 1961, at the State of New York University Downstate Medical Center of Brooklyn. In defense have arisen the voices of some, such as K. R. Eissler, with his ponderous *Medical Orthodoxy and the Future of Psychoanalysis*. Aside from orthodox psychoanalysis, a number of laymen are also involved in continuing the tradition of Alfred Adler and Carl G. Jung almost exclusively in New York City on the American continent. Jung, however, has had very few followers in this country because of the esoterism of his formulations and because of the lack of immigrants to join his adherents.

Actually, the issue of orthodoxy of psychoanalysis risks becoming purely academic, at least in New York City. A few facts are sufficient to support this statement: the radical departure from psychoanalysis initiated by N. Ackerman with his family therapy, leading to the creation of the Family Institute in 1960; the combined use of psychoanalysis and drug therapy advocated by some, such as M. Ostow and others; the existential emphasis of some types of psychotherapy (T. Hora, H. Kelman, I. Progoff); the interest in psychodynamics on the part of the main religious denominations, as evidenced by the work of S. Blanton, N. V. Peale, and by the courses offered at the New York Theological Seminary. Of particular significance is the relation between psychology and psychiatry. Although this is a national issue involving all kinds of aspects and problems, such as licensing and insurance, it is particularly outstanding in New York City: here psychologists have contributed effectively to the development of mental health in general while, conversely, psychiatrists have contributed to the development of psychology. For example, E. Oberholzer introduced the Rorschach test in New York City in the early 1920's.

From a broader perspective, psychiatric practice in New York City has been affected, until very recently at least, by the economic situation of its residents; namely, by the presence of a substantial number of sophisticated upper-class residents able to afford private psychotherapeutic treatment. The statistics recently published by I. Rogow show that New York City has almost one quarter of the analysts in the United States and that, of 4,000 psychiatrists in New York State, 3,000 work in New York City.[18] That psychiatry is perceived very differently by various groups in New York City has been shown recently in the survey *Public Health Image of Mental Services* (1967), edited by J. Elinson, E. Padilla, and M. E. Perkins under the sponsorship of the New York City Community Mental Health Board.

The fact that psychiatry and psychoanalysis have traditionally tended to develop in urban middle and upper class communities started to cause concern in the early 1950's, when local, state, and federal agencies began to realize the value of psychiatric treatment and prevention. In 1955 the Mental Health Study Act provided for establishment of a Joint Commission on Mental Illness and Health, to which New York City psychiatrists substantially contributed. By the time *Action for Mental Health* was ready (1961), the *Midtown Manhattan Study*, published in 1962 and 1963 as *Mental Health in the Metropolis*, showing the extent and vastity of the psychiatric problems in New York City, was in an advanced stage.

Since then a "fourth revolution" has occurred in psychiatry with the advent of community psychiatry.[19] It is unquestionable that many ideas and projects related to community psychiatry have originated in New York City, as evidenced by two very important books, the *Handbook of Community Psychiatry*, edited by L. Bellak, and *Mental Health for the Poor*, edited by F. Riessman; both were published in 1964. Vigorous leadership in the field of community psychiatry was exercised by the late Commissioner of Mental Hygiene, Paul Hoch,[20] followed by the present Commissioner, A. Miller. The Community Mental Health Board, under the chairmanship of H. Tompkins and the directorship of M. Perkins, initiated a variety of new therapeutic programs, designed especially for disadvantaged and minority groups. Study of the mental health of these groups produced some clinical advances. It is enough to mention the description of the so-called "Puerto Rican syndrome," by no means accepted by everyone, and of the so-called "social breakdown syndrome" presented by E. Gruenberg, as well as the advance brought about by E. Auerswald and S. Minuchin at the Wiltwyck School for Boys in the understanding of the dynamics of multiproblem families.

In line with this new philosophy, psychiatry came close again to everyday medical practice and, indeed, showed a return to the philosophy of the beginning of the century. A number of voluntary general hospitals established psychiatric wards for acute mental disorders: The Mount Sinai Hospital, St. Luke's Hospital, Roosevelt Hospital, and St. Vincent's Hospital. Likewise, as J. Cotton stated in a synthetic review a few years ago,[21] psychiatry has increasingly acquired importance in the six medical schools located in New York City. Although each department has developed its own approach, especially evident in its research and training program, all have been affected by the psychodynamic school as well as by the social situation. Under L. Kolb, the Department of Psychiatry of the College of Physicians and Surgeons, located mainly in the New York State Psychiatric Institute, has established close liaison with adjacent state hospitals. It has become known for its Division of Community Psychiatry which, until recently, was directed by V. Bernard and has provided training for professionals qualified to work in the field of community mental health, as well as for fostering the research on epidemiology of psychiatry carried on by E. Gruenberg. Cornell University's Department of Psychiatry, directed by W. Lhamon, which includes both the Payne Whitney Clinic of the New York Hospital and the Westchester Division of the New York Hospital in White Plains (known as Bloomingdale), has been involved especially in research on neurophysiology and metabolism and has developed a very active Department of Social Psychiatry of the New York University School of Medicine, directed by A. Leighton and, recently, by A. Kiev. The Department of Psychiatry of New York University School of Medicine, under B. Wortis, has had an illustrious tradition in child psychiatry; for many years this group was led by L. Bender. The same school has also had an important division of forensic psychiatry and an association with the Institute of Physical Medicine and Rehabilitation. The New York Medical College, which will soon expand in Westchester County, has an important Department of Psychiatry, directed by A. Freedman and known especially for its divisions of child psychiatry and of community psychiatry, as well as for its research and service programs for drug addicts. The Downstate Medical

College of the University of the State of New York has a newly built Department of Psychiatry directed by C. Kaufman, whose research focuses on the life and development of primates and on a combined neurophysiological and psychoanalytic study of dreams; this work is conducted by C. Fisher. Finally, the Albert Einstein School of Medicine, established about 15 years ago, has had from its beginning a good Department of Psychiatry, which for several years was led by M. Rosenbaum and has had a strong psychoanalytic orientation and an important division of social and community psychiatry.

Aside from programs solidly built into the academic medical structure, an important feature of psychiatry in New York City is constituted by the proliferation of special programs designed for particular kinds of patients in terms of age, psychopathology, and other dimensions. In just one field, that of child psychiatry, it is enough to think of the services provided for New York City children by the Hawthorne Cedar Knoll School, sponsored by the Jewish Board of Guardians, the Astor Home for Children and the Kennedy Child Study Center, both sponsored by Catholic Charities, the Ittleson Center for Research, the Wiltwyck School for Boys, the Children's Day Treatment Center and School, the League School, the Manhattan School for Seriously Disturbed Children, the Child Development Center, the Northside Development Center, and the University-Affiliated Mental Retardation Center of New York Medical College—each providing a highly specialized type of program.

While all these programs, like others in various fields of psychiatry, have received their support from well-established voluntary organizations, others have been developed in recent years, mainly with local and state support, to face critical problems, such as drug addiction. For instance, the program for drug addicts developed at the Riverside Hospital, followed by the Methadone Maintenance Treatment Program at the Beth Israel Medical Center, represent two of the most important endeavors made by New York City in this area. But increasingly, professionals and mental health supporters by and large have become aware of the limitations of official psychiatry in the handling of this problem. Consequently, a considerable number of groups, sponsored by a variety of organizations and staffed by so-called "paraprofessionals" or by former patients, have become involved in a variety of programs related in one way or another to emotional disturbances. As early as 1948, the

Fountain House was opened in New York City by ex-mental patients aiming at individual and social rehabilitation. More recently, in 1964, in relation to the increasing emphasis on drug addiction, Daytop Lodge was opened in Staten Island as a pilot project for the rehabilitation of drug addicts and eventually was expanded to other counties. It is too early to judge the effect of programs of this sort on the problem of drug addiction and of mental illness in general, but their importance cannot be minimized. In some psychiatric centers, notably at the Lincoln-Morrisania in the Bronx, the influence of the paraprofessionals has altered the over-all program. In a way, the participation of laymen from minority groups, which in New York City is particularly important, is beneficial but stressful as well, at least at the present moment, for the success of the community mental health movement. In particular, it has been pointed out that the problems presented by the Puerto Rican community may remain chronic because of its persistent ties with Puerto Rico, in contrast with the European immigrants of the past who had to break entirely with their countries of origin, thus facilitating their absorption into the American culture.

It would appear that the special social situation in New York City has influenced the development of psychiatry and of the mental health movement in two opposite directions. On the one hand, it has facilitated the development of new ideas, especially by fostering interdisciplinary exchanges. This is exemplified by the influence of sociological theory on psychiatry as shown in the work of R. Merton and, vice versa, by the influence of psychoanalysis on anthropology which is associated with the names of Ruth Benedict and Margaret Mead. Also, New York City has represented a crossroads for all kinds of movements. For instance, three of the most important psychiatric lectures annually delivered by outstanding men in this country are given in New York City: The Freud Anniversary Lecture Series, the Samuel W. Hamilton Memorial Lecture, and the Thomas William Salmon Memorial Lectures, sponsored respectively by the New York Psychoanalytic Institute, the American Psychopathological Association, and the New York Academy of Medicine. In addition, for many years New York has been the headquarters for nationwide interdisciplinary organizations, such as the National Committee for Mental Hygiene, under G. Stevenson, the American Orthopsychiatric Association, the Academy of Religion and Mental Health and, up to a few years ago, the central office of the American

Psychiatric Association, led by A. Davies. Likewise, New York City has been traditonally the most important center in this country for the dissemination of information on mental health and psychiatry: among the most important sources of information are the reports of the Group for the Advancement of Psychiatry, published in New York City, and the publications of the Research Center for Mental Health of New York University. Very valuable also is the *Bulletin of the New York State District Branches of the American Psychiatric Association*, to which psychiatrists of the district branch of New York City, known as the New York Society for Clinical Psychiatry, often contribute. Also, the city houses a number of firms which publish books in the field of psychiatry, notably, Basic Books, Free Press-Macmillan, and Pergamon. Each firm specializes in certain special areas, such as the history of psychiatry, i.e., Stechert-Hafner, in collaboration with the New York Academy of Medicine. The field of psychoanalysis is mainly represented by the International Universities Press, which is known especially for the three series: *The Psychoanalytic Study of the Child*, *Psychological Issues*, and *The Annual Survey of Psychoanalysis*. Among the yearly publications devoted to a psychiatric topic are the *Proceedings of the American Psychopathological Association*, edited by J. Zubin and, up to his death, by P. Hoch, and the *Proceedings of the American Academy of Psychoanalysis*, edited by J. Masserman; both are published by Grune & Stratton. Finally, a number of psychiatric journals are published in New York City. Especially noteworthy are *Mental Hygiene*, *Psychosomatic Medicine*, *Comprehensive Psychiatry*, *The Psychoanalytic Review*, *The American Journal of Psychotherapy*, *The Journal of the American Psychoanalytic Association*, *The Journal of Religion and Health*, the *Journal of the American Academy of Child Psychiatry*, and *Psychiatric Quarterly*. While the latter is primarily conceived of as an expression of the New York State hospital system, a number of these journals are the official publications of associations located in the City.

On the other hand, it would appear that many ideas have developed in New York City but have been implemented elsewhere because of New York's especially complex urban problems. For instance, in the first decade of this century, Meyer's ideas on psychiatric prevention and the mental hygiene movement had their origin in New York City, but the leadership of the child psychiatric movement was soon taken over by Chicago, Boston, and other cities, in which the demonstration child guidance clinics were founded in the 1920's. The same applies to the community mental health movement. New York City contributed a great deal to the origins of this movement but in implementation it lags behind many other cities. To be sure, the city has always taken psychiatry very seriously, as is evidenced by the work of the New York City Department of Mental Health and Mental Retardation Services established some years ago. Yet a simple survey of the existing facilities, inclusive of federal, state, city, and voluntary programs in the field of mental health—heavily concentrated in certain areas of the city and almost nonexistent in others—proves to be almost impossible. This may explain the attitude of caution and dissatisfaction which has been expressed by some, including Laurence Kolb, toward the community mental health movement, which has been viewed as a panacea for all kinds of psychiatric problems.

Despite this, the trend toward community mental health continues to increase in New York City without interruption. A short while ago the Community Service Society, the city's oldest private social agency—originally founded in 1848 under the name of the Association for Improving the Condition of the Poor—decided to change its approach from family casework and individual counseling to direct work with existing neighborhood groups. The same change of emphasis has recently become the policy of the Family Service Association of America, the country's largest federation of counseling services,whose headquarters is located in the city. In the last few years a number of New York City psychiatrists and psychiatric agencies have contributed to the formulation of the report of the Joint Commission on Mental Health for Children, recently published under the title *Crisis in Child Mental Health: Challenge for the 1970's*. As a concrete step toward the implementation of the recommendations included in the report, Senator Jacob K. Javits of New York on December 10, 1970 introduced a bill called the Comprehensive Community Child Development Act of 1971, which aimed to establish child development programs at a community, state, and federal level in the context of the new concept of "child advocacy," which provides for an increasing role of parents in the organization of programs for children.

The development of psychiatry in New York City is very difficult to assess; only certain trends can be identified with a fair degree of certainty. However, no matter how difficult an assessment may be, it is likely that the situation of psychiatry in New York City will remain unusually challenging and complex for future decades, and that it will continue to stimulate new ideas and to lead to new programs in psychiatry.

REFERENCES

1. Kuhn, T. S.: *The Structure of Scientific Revolutions.* Chicago, Univ. Chicago Press, 1961.
2. Agassi, J.: *Towards an Historiography of Science.* Gravenhage, Mouton, 1963. *History and Theory,* Beiheft 2.
3. Stocking, G. W.: On the limits of "presentism" and "historicism" in the historiography of the behavioral sciences. *J. Hist. Behav. Sci. 3:* 211-18, 1965.
4. Deutsch, A.: *The Mentally Ill in America. A History of Their Care and Treatment from Colonial Times.* Garden City, Doubleday, 1937, passim.
5. Russell, W. L.: *The New York Hospital. A History of the Psychiatric Service, 1771-1936.* New York, Columbia Univ. Press, 1945.
6. Oberndorf, C. P.: A *History of Psychoanalysis in America.* New York, Grune & Stratton, 1953.
7. Hall, J. K., ed.: *One Hundred Years of American Psychiatry.* New York, Columbia Univ. Press, 1944.
8. *American Journal of Psychiatry.* Centennial Anniversary Issue, 1844-1944.
9. Bond, E. D.: *Thomas W. Salmon, Psychiatrist.* New York, Norton, 1950.
10. Stevenson, G. S. and Smith, G.: *Child Guidance Clinics: A Quarter Century of Development.* New York, Commonwealth Fund, 1937.
11. Lowrey, L. G., ed.: *Orthopsychiatry. 1923-1948. Retrospect and Prospect.* New York, American Orthopsychiatric Association, 1948.
12. Wangh, M., ed.: *Fruition of an Idea: Fifty Years of Psychoanalysis in New York.* New York, Int. Univ. Press, 1962.
13. Stokes, A. B., ed.: *Psychiatry in Transition, 1966-1967.* Toronto, Univ. Toronto Press, 1967.
14. Talkington, P. C. and Bloss, C. L., eds.: *Evolving Concepts in Psychiatry.* New York, Grune & Stratton, 1969.
15. Galdston, I., ed.: *Psychoanalysis in Present-Day Psychiatry.* New York, Brunner-Mazel, 1969.
16. Millet, J. A. P.: Psychoanalysis in the United States: In: *Psychoanalytic Pioneers.* Alexander, F., Eisenstein, S. and Grotjahn, M., eds. New York, Basic Books, 1966.
17. Freyhan, F. A.: The psychopathologist—What man of science? *Compr. Psychiat. 5*:391-402, 1970.
18. Rogow, A. A.: *The Psychiatrists.* New York, Putnam's, 1970.
19. Linn, L. The Fourth Psychiatric Revolution. *Amer. J. Psychiat. 124*:1043-048, 1968.
20. Lewis, N. D. C. and Strahl, M. O., eds.: *The Complete Psychiatrist. The Achievements of Paul H. Hoch, M.D.* Albany State Univ. New York Press, 1968.
21. Cotton, J. M.: Psychiatry in New York City. *Amer. J. Psychiat. 121*:1007-010, 1965.

NONUNION OF FRACTURES IN ANTIQUITY, WITH DESCRIPTIONS OF FIVE CASES FROM THE NEW WORLD INVOLVING THE FOREARM

T. D. Stewart, M.D.

National Museum of Natural History
Smithsonian Institution
Washington, D.C.

Extensive search of the literature of paleopathology reveals that many of the references to fracture of the long bones concern malpositioned union whereas only an occasional reference mentions nonunion (pseudoarthrosis). This finding, particularly the scanty mention of any cases of nonunion, is reflected in four of the most recent general books on the subject: Two do not mention nonunion at all;[1, 2] the third simply says of ancient Egyptian remains that "cases of malunion and nonunion have been found";[3] and the fourth cites only two early cases, both of the ulna and both presumably from France.[4]

This hint at the situation existing in ancient times contrasts sharply with reports on the outcome of modern treatment of fractures. For instance, the records of a single clinic in Tennessee have yielded a total of 964 cases of nonunion of the long bones requiring renewed efforts to obtain healing.[5] Although the length of time required to accumulate all of these cases is not stated, the last 122 were recorded between 1959

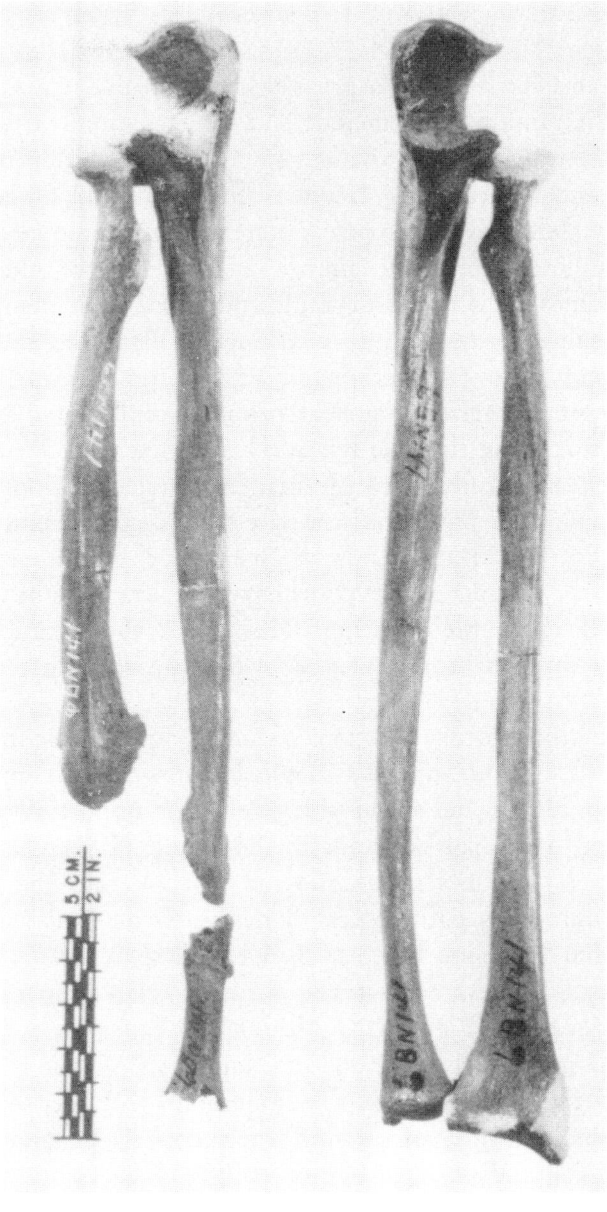

Fig. 1. Anterior aspect of the right forearm bones of skeleton No. 6BN141 (Frank H. McClung Museum) from the Eva site in northwestern Tennessee. Fractures of both bones had resulted in nonunion. Only a portion of one of the distal fragments was recovered. Photograph courtesy of the Smithsonian Institution, Washington, D.C.

and 1965. Nearly a third of the latter series involved bones of the forearm.

If, as seems likely, such a great disparity really exists between the frequency of nonunion in ancient and modern times, it is, of course, mainly caused by modern man's newly acquired dependence upon machinery and the resulting frequent comminution of his bones. The degrees of violence to which man's bones are now frequently subjected when human and mechanical failures lead to accidents seldom occurred in ancient times. It is understandable, therefore, that many of today's fractures challenge—and a few continue to defy—the most ingenious reparative techniques that orthopedic science has devised.[6]

In view of the serious medical problem represented by nonunion today, it is surprising that the relatively new science of paleopathology has shown so little interest in the matter. Further, as indicated above, what little evidence from the past is cited in the general literature is from the Old World and tends to give undue prominence to Egypt, where factors favoring preservation have encouraged study. These circumstances lead to the question: How does the situation regarding nonunion in the prehistoric New World compare with that in ancient Egypt?

Before taking up this question, I should explain that my interest in this matter dates from my visit to the University of Tennessee in the fall of 1973. Having taken advantage of that opportunity to look at the collection of Indian skeletons in the Frank H. McClung Museum, I had the good fortune to be allowed to look into the storage area containing numerous pathological bones, each carefully wrapped and labeled, which Madeline Kneberg Lewis had segregated from the Eva site skeletons.[7] There I came across a case of nonunion of both bones of a right forearm (Figure 1). Although I had seen a few cases of nonunion of individual bones in the National Collection in Washington, this was the first case of double nonunion I had ever seen. Intrigued by the unusual character of the find, I immediately arranged to borrow the skeleton for study.[8]

Geographical Comparisons

Observations on fractures occur occasionally in reports on American archeological sites, but their reliability often depends upon whether or not the lesions had been diagnosed by medical authorities. Rather than spend time assembling data from these dubious and widely scattered sources, I decided to settle for the indications in three major reports (see accompanying table) which together yield a larger number of long-bone fractures than is given in the classic study on ancient Egyptian cemeteries.[9] Three conclusions stand out from the data: 1) In America, as in Egypt, the forearm bones were fractured most frequently. 2) In Egypt, because of the need to use the left arm to parry blows from the *naboot* (a stout staff), the ulna was fractured more often than the radius, whereas in America, for some unknown reason, the radius seems to have been fractured more often than the ulna. 3) Nonunion was about equally rare in the ancient Old and New Worlds.

It is noteworthy, too, that both the Egyptian and American samples represent peoples from diverse cultures and periods. The Egyptian cemeteries range from pre-Dynastic times (before 3000 B.C.) to the end of the Roman Period (642 A.D.) and probably beyond.[14] In contrast, Indian Knoll is a shell-midden site in northwestern Kentucky dating back to Archaic times, roughly 5,000 years ago;[15] Pecos is a New Mexico Pueblo site of the "apartment-house" type which was more-or-less continuously occupied from about 800 to 1840 A.D.[16] And to round out these two single-site samples, "Midwest" is a summation of data from at least nine sites, all but one in Illinois, ranging in age from Late Archaic to near the end of pre-Columbian times.[17]

In general, numbers in the American sample populations vary with the robusticity of the bones—slender bones such as the fibula being recovered less often than stouter bones such as the femur. For this reason the numbers in the American skeletal populations examined (Indian Knoll, 521;[18] Pecos, 503;[19] Midwest 976+[20]) do not constitute satisfactory bases for comparison. This limitation may not apply to the Egyptian cemeteries (4,403 individuals.)[21]

Although the variations in the numbers of bones comprising the American samples make for unreliable comparisons, the differences in frequencies of fractures between sites cannot be ignored. Why should Pecos have so few fractures? Why should Indian Knoll have so many more fractures of radii than of other long bones? Why should more fractures occur on the left side at Indian Knoll, whereas more occur on the right side at Pecos and Midwest? To what extent do these differences reflect the different training of the observers rather than the different ways of life of the aboriginal American populations? Since

INDICATIONS FROM ANTIQUITY OF THE RELATIVE VULNERABILITY OF THE LONG BONES TO FRACTURE

Long bone	Old World: Egypt[10] No.	Old World: Egypt[10] %	New World: Indian Knoll[11] No.	New World: Pecos[12] No.	New World: Midwest[13] No.	New World: Combined No.	New World: Combined %
Clavicle	21	17.8*	6	0	3	9	7.1
Humerus	9	7.6	6†	10	9	25	19.8
Radius	20 }	44.9	26	0	5	31 }	36.5
Ulna	33 }		7†	1	7‡	15 }	
Femur	16	13.6	4	6	8	18	14.3
Tibia	10	8.5	5	2	11	18	14.3
Fibula	9	7.6	3	0	7	10	7.9
Total	118	100.0	57 {19 rt. 38 lt.	19 {12 rt. 7 lt.	50 {33 rt. 17 lt.	126	99.9

* Includes two cases of nonunion.
† One humerus and two ulnas are said to be "unhealed."
‡ Includes one case of nonunion.
rt. = right; lt. = left.

answers to these questions are not yet forthcoming, the distribution of fractures in ancient times deserves much more study—including, of course, their relation to age, sex, and area of the bone involved. So much for fractures in general.

What about the evidence of nonunion in ancient times? The Egyptian sample includes two cases of nonunion of the clavicle and the Midwest sample includes one case of nonunion of the ulna (see footnote to table). In the Indian Knoll sample the term "unhealed" is used by Snow in connection with fractures of a humerus and two ulnas; it could mean that one or more of these fractures was in an early stage of healing, or that one or more had failed to unite. Assuming the latter interpretation to be correct, the combined American samples still include only four cases of nonunion, all involving long bones of the upper extremity, whereas the Egyptian sample includes only two cases, both involving the clavicle. In all of these ancient samples the bone most often failing to unite is the ulna—three cases, followed by the clavicle—two cases, and the humerus—one case.

Probably the most remarkable case of nonunion included (see table) is the one in the Midwest sample involving the ulna. It is one of six·

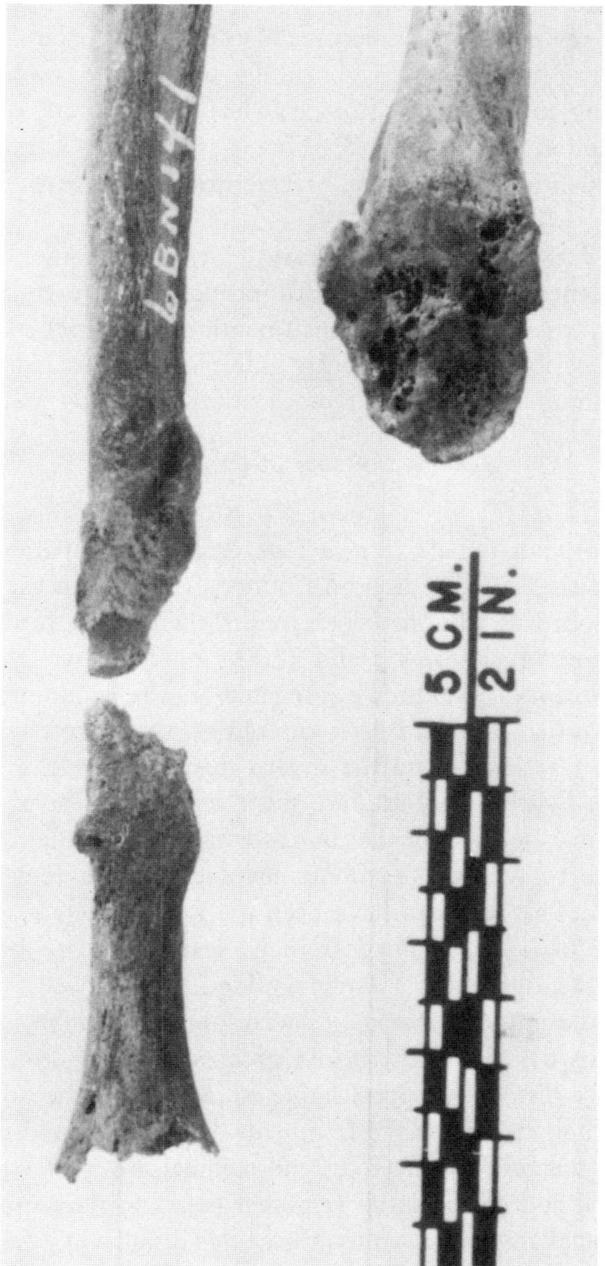

Fig. 2. Enlarged posterior view of the pseudoarthrosis shown in Figure 1. Note the large false articular surface of the proximal radial fragment. Photograph courtesy of the Smithsonian Institution, Washington, D.C.

fractures sustained by one male(?) Indian found in the late-prehistoric Vandeventer site in Illinois. Fractures of the right maxilla, left clavicle, right femur, right tibia, and right fibula had healed (with only the femur showing much malpositioning), but the fracture of the right ulna had resulted in nonunion.[22] This is a striking example of the notorious tendency, noted above, of fractures of the forearm bones to fail to unite.

In view of the rarity of prehistoric cases of nonunion in general, with the tendency for these rare cases to occur in forearm bones more often than in other long bones, I shall continue this brief survey of the subject by describing five previously unreported cases from the New World, beginning with the one from Tennessee already mentioned.

Descriptions of New Cases

1) *Frank H. McClung Museum No. 6BN141*—a badly fragmented skeleton of an adult female from a Late Archaic occupation level (ca. 3000 B.C.) in the Eva site, Benton County, Tenn. Both the radius and ulna on the right side had been fractured in their distal thirds and show no signs of uniting (Figures 1 and 2). As noted above, the proximal parts of these bones had been segregated in the museum collections circa 1961. No diagnosis had been entered on the wrappings, and both the published reference[23] and the record made in the field in 1940 by the excavator, Charles H. Nash, are silent on the subject of pathology. Usually, when a bone lesion is not recognized in the field, no special effort is made to recover the bones involved or the remaining fragments thereof. This seems to have been the case here.

The piece of bone, assumed from its scarred end to be the distal fragment of the right ulna (shown in Figures 1 and 2), was located elsewhere in the museum storage, as were numerous bones of the right hand (not shown). Since the styloid process is absent, the orientation of this putative distal fragment relative to the rest of the bone is problematical. Although both ulnar fragments have roughened and grossly pointed ends where they meet, when attempts are made to articulate them the distal end of the distal fragment seems to flare too soon.

The proximal fragment of the radius ends distally in a false articular surface which is fairly large, rough, and faces more anteriorly than distally—suggesting thereby that the distal radial fragment had a corresponding surface facing more posteriorly than proximally. Thus, the

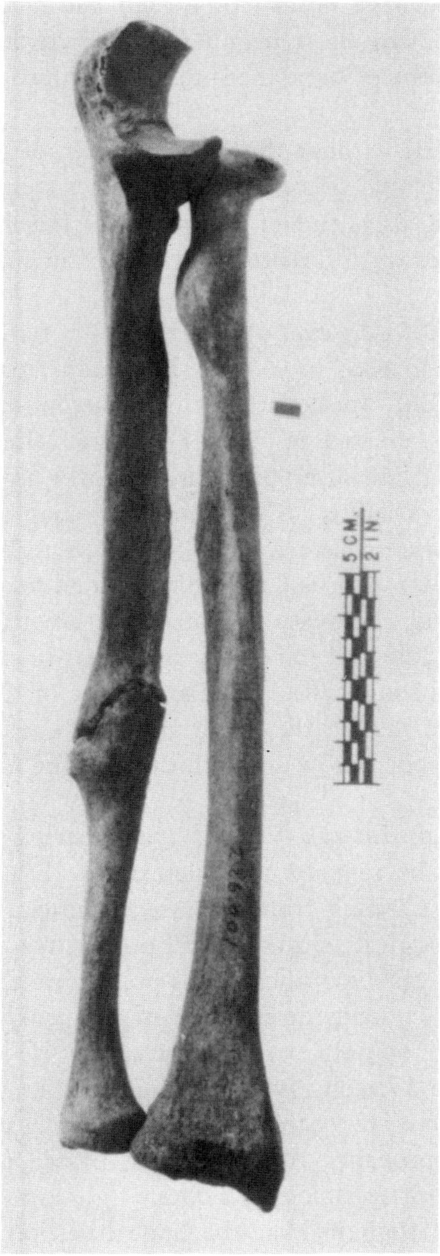

Fig. 3. Anterior aspect of the left forearm bones of skeleton No. 226,001 (U.S. National Museum) from a mound near Palo Alto, Calif. The fracture of the ulna had resulted in nonunion. Photograph courtesy of the Smithsonian Institution, Washington, D.C.

two fragments may have fitted closely and had a fibrous union. Unfortunately, a search of the remainder of the skeleton did not reveal the rather sizable piece of bone that must have constituted the ununited distal fragment.

Incidentally, even without the putative piece of ulna and the hand bones, amputation would be ruled out by the existence of a false articular surface on the distal end of the proximal radial fragment. I shall deal with the matter of differential diagnosis after presenting the other cases.

2) *U.S. National Museum No. 226,001*—a fairly complete male skeleton recovered in 1897 by Arthur L. Bolton from an earth mound near Palo Alto, Calif. In donating this skeleton to the Smithsonian Institution, Bolton referred to it as a "Digger" Indian, a term then widely used in the West, often opprobriously, for any group of Indians that dug for roots. There is no way now of telling whether the burial dates from prehistoric or historic times. Bolton noted in his accompanying letter that the left ulna had an "unknit" fracture.

As Figures 3 and 4 show, a diagonal fracture had occurred at the junction of the middle and lower thirds so that in the pseudoarthrosis the fairly large and rough false articular surface of the upper fragment faces anteriorly and that of the lower fragment faces posteriorly. The fit of the two surfaces is now so close that a tight fibrous union seems certain.

3) *U.S. National Museum No. 239,370*—a partial skeleton of uncertain sex recovered in 1887 by the Hemenway Expedition under the direction of Frank Cushing from an unrecorded site in the Gila River Valley, Ariz. Although its chronological provenance is unknown, there is no reason to doubt its identification as prehistoric Pueblo Indian. The expedition report[24] contains no mention of the proximal fragment of a fractured left ulna, the only part now remaining (Figure 5, left). Apparently, after the Hemenway Collection was transferred from the Army Medical Museum to the U.S. National Museum early in this century someone, probably Aleš Hrdlička, placed this fragment in a general assemblage of pathological bones.

The illustration suggests that the bone had been fractured in the middle third long enough before death to result in a false end, which is flattened from side to side and sharply pointed. In the absence of the other parts of the forearm, amputation cannot be absolutely ruled out—

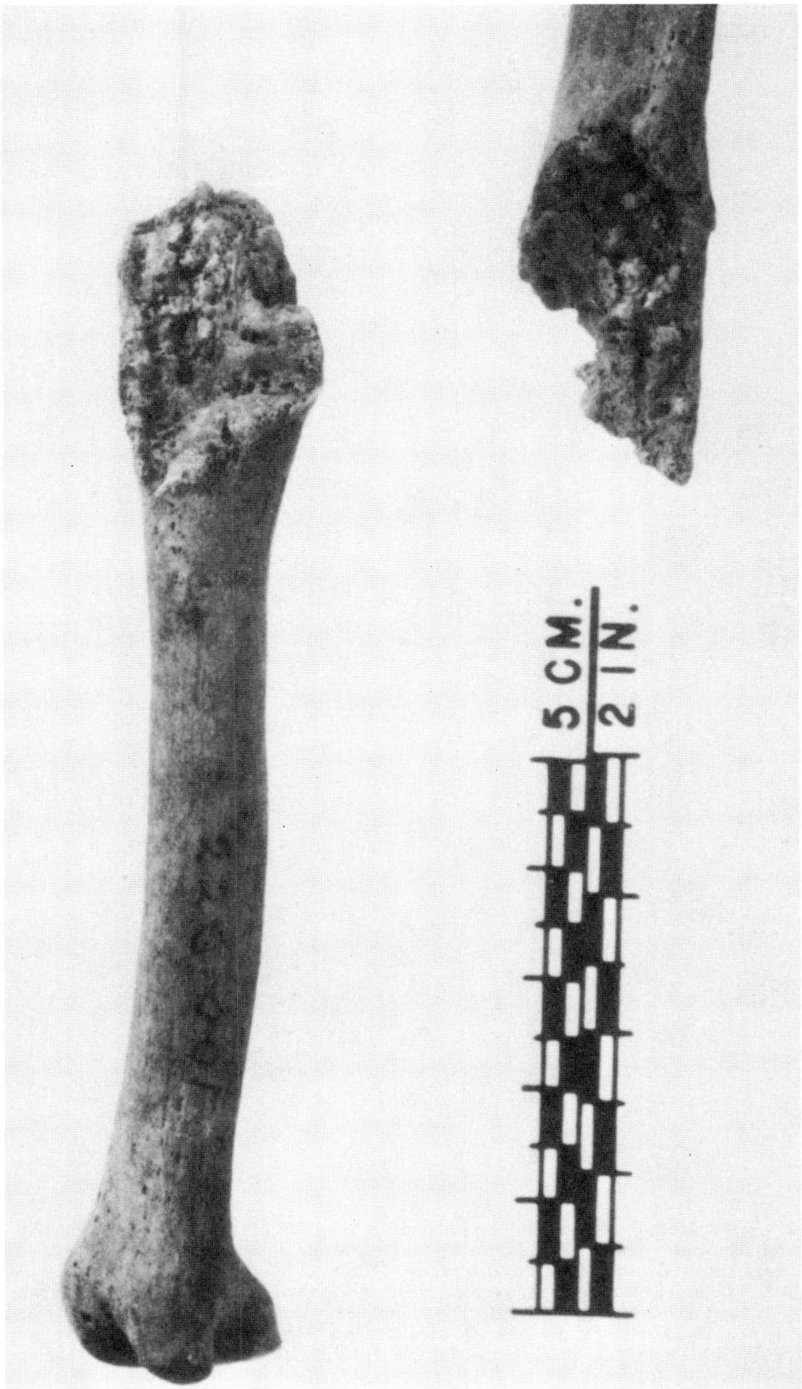

Fig. 4. Enlarged view of the pseudoarthrosis shown in Figure 3 as separated to expose the false articular surfaces. Photograph courtesy of the Smithsonian Institution, Washington, D.C.

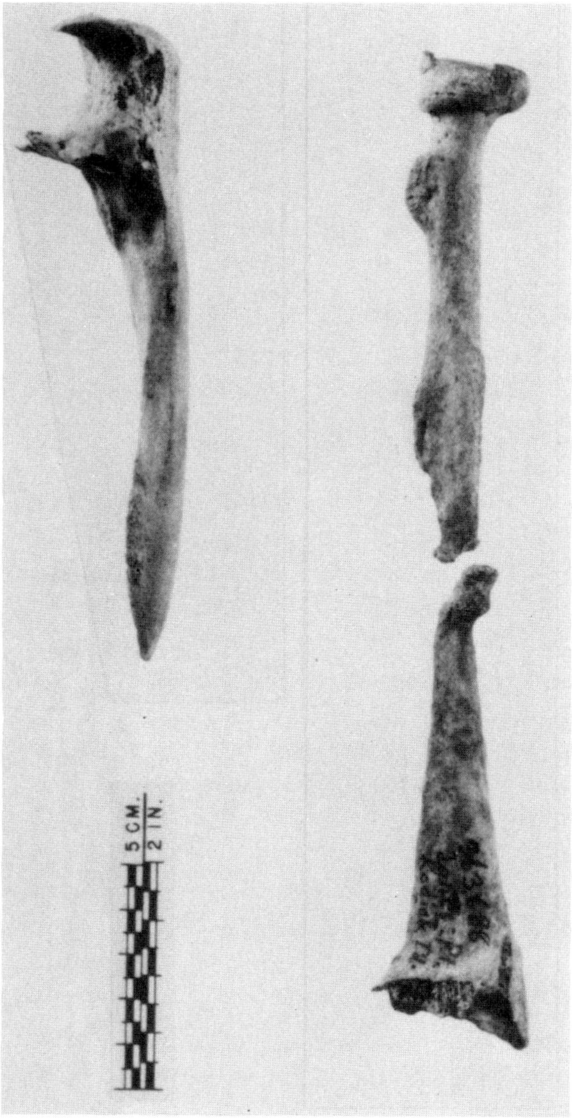

Fig. 5. *Left:* Medial aspect of the left ulna of partial skeleton No. 239,370 (U.S. National Museum) from the Gila River Valley, Ariz. This is assumed to be a fracture which had resulted in nonunion and atrophy of the distal end of the proximal fragment. The distal fragment was not recovered. Note the arthritic lipping of the superior joint. *Right:* Anterior aspect of left radius No. 363,688 (U.S. National Museum) found isolated in the Uyak site on Kodiak Island, Alaska. Fracture had resulted in nonunion and considerable atrophy on each side of the fracture line. Note the arthritic lipping of the superior and inferior joints. Photographs courtesy of the Smithsonian Institution, Washington, D.C.

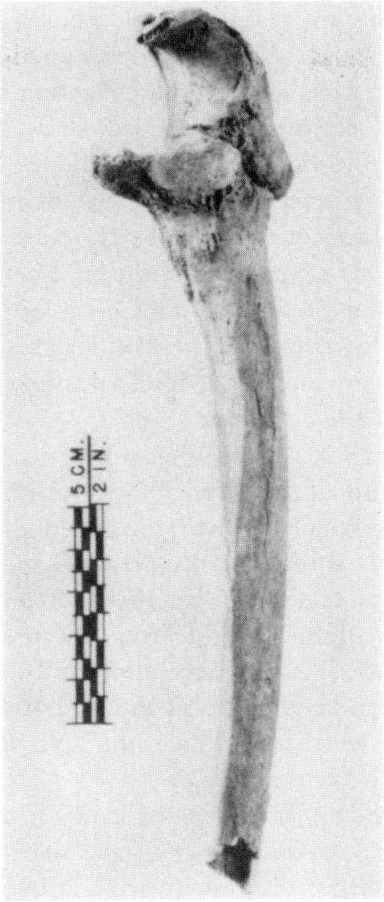

Fig. 6. Medical aspect of a left ulna from Feature No. 9, a secondary burial, at the Anllulla site in Guayas Province, Ecuador. Fracture through the superior joint has resulted in nonunion. Photograph courtesy of the Smithsonian Institution, Washington, D.C.

but it seems unlikely, as the next case will demonstrate. Whatever the situation was, the margins of the semilunar notch show fairly marked arthritic lipping.

4) *U.S. National Museum No. 363,688*—a number of isolated radii of uncertain sex recovered by Aleš Hrdlička in 1931 from the Jones Point site (also called Our Point site) on Kodiak Island, Alaska, near the confluence of Larson and Uyak Bays. Since depth records do not seem to have been kept for these isolated bones, the fractured left

radius in question (Figure 5, right) could be either Aleut or pre-Aleut, in either case prehistoric. Although I recorded the presence of this fractured bone when I catalogued the collection in 1931, Hrdlička did not mention it in his site report.[25] Records show that the specimen was already in the assemblage of pathological bones before Hrdlička died in 1943. I may have placed it there in 1931 or he may have done this when he studied the collection in the early 1940s.

The two fragments taper toward the midshaft, where they end in irregular but rather pointed ends. This gives no clue as to what happened to the ulna. However, like the pseudoarthrosis, the lipping of the joint margins at the proximal and distal ends bears witness to the considerable duration of the condition.

5) *Anllulla Feature 9.* While this study was in progress, Douglas Ubelaker of the National Museum of Natural History began studying the skeletal remains which he had recovered during the summer of 1973 from urn burials at the Anllulla site in Guayas Province, Ecuador. By coincidence, he came across a fractured left ulna (Figures 6 and 7) among the contents of one of the urns (Feature 9) and generously allowed me to include it here. Since almost all of the skeletons in the urns are incomplete and represent secondary burials, the accompanying radius has not been identified and may not have been included. Judging from size, the bone is from a male.

Unlike the preceding fractures, this one is through the proximal joint rather than through some part of the shaft. As can be seen, the fracture line passed diagonally downward and backward from the midpart of the joint so that the plane of the pseudoarthrosis is visible when the proximal fragment is viewed in the anterior aspect and when the distal fragment is viewed in the posterior aspect. The fit of the two surfaces is now as close as that in No. 2, thus again suggesting a tight, fibrous union. However, the pseudoarthrosis may have been responsible for the marked arthritic lipping around the semilunar notch.

Discussion

Since four of the five new cases of ununited fracture of forearm bones presented here are from the National Collection, the reader may have gained the impression that this condition is more common than the figures in the table indicate. However, the National Collection includes a far larger representation of New World aboriginal populations

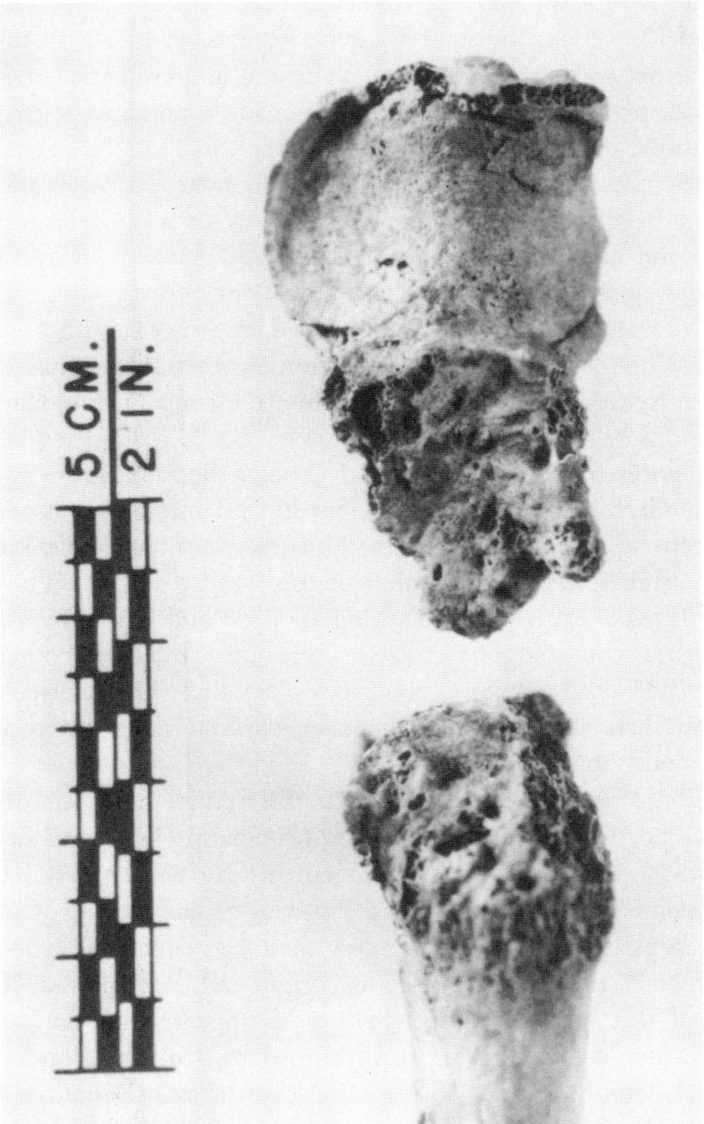

Fig. 7. Enlarged views of the pseudoarthrosis shown in Figure 6 as separated to show the false articular surfaces. Note the arthritic lipping of the margins of the proximal part of the semilunar notch. Photograph courtesy of the Smithsonian Institution, Washington, D.C.

than do the three samples in the table combined; an estimate of possibly 10 times as many individuals would not be an exaggeration. Also, Hrdlička, who was medically trained, studied a large part of the collection, and I have seen most of what he never saw. It is probable, therefore, that between us we detected all of the ununited fractures of forearm bones present, especially since we made a point of segregating all such unusual cases.

As for ununited fractures of other long bones in the National Collection, I have seen only three or four—one of a clavicle and two or three of the neck of the femur. The latter finding is in keeping with the tendency for fractures of the femoral neck to be more common in old age—a category not well represented in American aboriginal populations. The scarcity, then, of nonunion in other long bones reinforces the claim that the bones of the forearm are especially vulnerable in this respect.

It is noteworthy that F. Wood Jones called attention to the fact that in modern man, unlike the ancient Egyptians, at least as many fractures occur in the leg bones as in the forearm bones.[26] We know now that the same applies to nonunion of the fractures of these two sets of bones.[27] This is explained, according to F. Wood Jones, by the Egyptians' custom of going barefoot or wearing sandals: in other words, avoiding heels. Be that as it may, it is clear that the American aborigines, who had the same custom, also suffered rarely from leg-bone fractures and nonunion thereof.

Finally, I return to the matter of differential diagnosis of isolated proximal portions of forearm bones terminating in blunt or pointed false ends, especially when such specimens are poorly documented. A case in point in the literature is the partial right forearm of a IX Dynasty Egyptian from Sedment described by Brothwell and Møller-Christensen.[28] Aside from place of origin, all information about the history of this specimen seems to have disappeared by the time of its transfer after World War II from University College, London, to the British Museum (Natural History). Nevertheless, the authors declare that "The distal halves of these two bones, together with the hand, had *certainly* been missing for some time before death" (italics mine). A picture and x ray show that the radius and ulna are fused in partial pronation by a bony bridge just above the false ends. In this position the lateral surfaces of the ends are seen to taper medially. It was this appearance of the ends, rather than any documentation, apparently, that led the authors to conclude that the distal part of the arm had been lost in life through deliberate amputation. There is a single word of qualification in the title of their publication and this is not repeated in the text. They never mention the possibility of nonunion, and they support the diagnosis of amputation solely with historical records from Egypt relating to the severing of the *hands* of war prisoners.

As for the bony bridge connecting the two proximal fragments just above the false ends, the authors simply call attention to its presence and make no effort to explain how it relates to the process of amputation. Presumably, they were unaware that F. Wood Jones illustrated two healed fractures of Egyptian forearm bones in which similar bridges had developed.[29] He characterized the union in these cases as "by development of callus-formation." In view of the combined evidence from Jones' study and the new cases presented above, I am led to conclude that a diagnosis of amputation in the case from Sedment needs far more qualification than one word confined to the title of the publication.

I would like to drop the matter at this point, but unfortunately it extends further. Already Brothwell's and Møller-Christensen's doubtful diagnosis has led one American anthropologist astray in the field of paleopathology. Among the badly preserved and incompletely recovered skeletal remains from the ancient Mayan site of Altar de Sacrificios in the Peten region of Guatemala described by Saul[30] are portions of two fused bones judged to be a radius and an ulna. As in the Egyptian "amputation," the fusion is by a bony bar. Although neither of these putative forearm bones shows evidence of a false end, Saul cites the case of the Egyptian "amputation" as a possible explanation of what happened to this ancient American. Why is it that a bizarre explanation is often so much more attractive than a simpler one?

NOTES AND REFERENCES

1. Wells, C.: *Bones, Bodies and Disease.* New York, Praeger, 1964.
2. Jarcho, S., editor: *Human Palaeopathology.* New Haven, Yale University Press, 1966.
3. Brothwell, D. and Sandison, A. T., editors: *Diseases in Antiquity.* Springfield, Ill., Thomas, 1967. See especially page 603 in chapter 47 on Trauma and Disease of the Postcranial Skeleton in Ancient Egypt by Philip Salib.
4. Janssens, P. A.: *Palaeopathology: Diseases and Injuries of Prehistoric Man.* London, Baker, 1970. See p. 33.
5. Boyd, H. B., Anderson, L. D., and Johnston, D. S.: Changing concepts in

the treatment of nonunion. *Clin. Orthop. 43*:37-54, 1965.
6. Marmor, L., editor: Management of nonunion. *Clin. Orthop. 43*:5-167, 1965.
7. Lewis, T. M. N. and Lewis, M. K.: *Eva: An Archaic Site.* Knoxville, University of Tennessee Press, 1961.
8. I am indebted to Dr. Alfred K. Guthe, Director of the Frank H. McClung Museum, for the loan of skeleton 6BN141 and for answers to questions relating thereto.
9. Smith, G. E. and Jones, F. W.: *The Archaeological Survey of Nubia. Report for 1907-1908. II. Report on the Human Remains.* Cairo, Nat. Print. Dept., 1910.
10. Ibid., pp. 337-40.
11. Snow, C. E.: Indian Knoll skeletons of site Oh 2, Ohio County, Ky. *Univ. Kentucky Rep. Anthrop. 4*:454-84, 1948.
12. Hooton, E. A.: *The Indians of Pecos Pueblo: A Study of Their Skeletal Remains.* New Haven, Yale University Press, 1930. See pp. 312-30.
13. Morse, D.: Ancient Disease in the Midwest. *Ill. State Mus. Rep. Invest.* No. 15, 1969. See Table 1.
14. Smith and Jones, op. cit., pp. 337-40.
15. Snow, op. cit., p. 381. In 1948 Snow knew only that the specimens were from Archaic times. Their chronological age was not established until the carbon-14 test came into use.
16. Hooton, op. cit., pp. 10-12.
17. Morse, loc. cit.
18. Snow, op. cit., p. 384.
19. Hooton, op. cit., p. 312.
20. Morse, loc. sit.
21. Smith and Jones, op. cit., pp. 337-40.
22. Morse, op. cit., Plate 4.
23. Lewis and Lewis, op. cit., p. 137.
24. Matthews, W., Wortman, J. L., and Billings, J. S.: The human bones of the Hemenway collection in the United States Army Medical Museum at Washington. *Mem. Nat. Acad. Sci. 6*:1-286, 1891.
25. Hrdlička, A.: *The Anthropology of Kodiak Island.* Philadelphia, Press of the Wistar Institute of Anatomy and Biology, 1944.
26. Smith and Jones, op. cit., pp. 294-98.
27. Boyd, Anderson, and Johnston, loc. cit.
28. Brothwell, D. R. and Møller-Christensen, V.: A possible case of amputation, dated to c. 2000 B.C. *Man 63*:192-94, 1963.
29. Smith and Jones, op. cit., p. 314.
30. Saul, F. P.: The human skeletal remains of Altar de Sacrificios: An osteobiographic analysis. *Harvard Univ. Peabody Mus. Archaeol. Ethnol. Papers 63*:1-123, 1972.

PREHISTORIC MULTIPLE MYELOMA

DAN MORSE, M.D.
Research Associate

R. C. DAILEY, Ph.D.
Associate Professor and Chairman

JENNINGS BUNN
Department of Anthropology
Florida State University
Tallahassee, Fla.

MULTIPLE myeloma is a malignant tumor originating in the bone marrow. It is a fatal disease and is usually generalized and extensive. It can involve all the bones of the skeleton but has predilection for the vertebrae, ribs, skull, and pelvis.[2, 3] According to Dahlin,[2] multiple myeloma is the commonest primary malignant tumor of bone. In the Mayo Clinic series, myeloma accounted for 1,286, or 43%, of all malignant primary bone tumors and 32% of all primary bone tumors, both benign and malignant. It occurs more often in males and in the older groups, being most common in those over 50 and rare in those under 40. Solitary lesions occur, but most authorities believe this is a precursor to generalized distribution.[2, 3]

The tumor arises in the marrow spaces and invades the bone, leaving discrete rounded holes of various sizes. These holes have sharply demarcated borders which show little or no condensation of bone. Gross specimens and x-ray reproductions are described as being "punched out," as if the lesions might have been made by a paper-punch. In the long bones, the tumor invades the cortex and eventually reaches the outer surface. In the skull, it starts in the diploic space and progresses into and through the inner table, outer table, or both. The x ray is invaluable for the study of archaeological specimens, since it visualizes defects that have not yet reached the surface of the bone.

Clinically the diagnosis is confirmed by biopsy of the tumor. Archaeologically a differential diagnosis would include first an osteolytic carcinomatous metastasis. Discreteness of the individual lesions and extensive distribution favor myeloma. This is even more characteristic in other conditions of the skeleton, such as osteitis fibrosa cystica, histiocytosis X, leukemia, and possibly fibrous dysplasia.

In 1932 William Ritchie and Stafford Warren[6] reported a case of possible multiple myeloma in a prehistoric American Indian. This specimen was derived from a "senile male" and was one of 43 skeletons excavated in 1930 from an Indian site near Binghamton, N.Y. According to Ritchie and Warren,[6] the date of occupation of this "Clark" site was about 800 A.D. Gross and x-ray appearance demonstrated the presence of discrete destructive lesions throughout the entire skeleton. In 1941 Williams, Ritchie, and Titterington[7] reported similar lesions in a child, about 10 years of age, who probably dated from around 1200 A.D.

Sheilagh Brooks and Jerome Melbye[1] in 1967 described a female skeleton, with an estimated age at time of death of 40 years or more. This individual was excavated from the Kane Mound near St. Louis, Mo., and belonged to the Mississippian culture; the probable occupation date was about 1200 A.D. All the skeletal elements contained bone perforations ranging in size from 2 to 17 mm.

While examining skeletal material in the R. H. Lowie Museum of Anthropology, University of California, Berkeley, Don Brothwell called attention to multiple myeloma in a prehistoric California Indian. This was reported by me[5] in 1969. According to information supplied by Dr. Albert B. Elsasser, the skeleton, that of a female aged 45, was excavated by Ronald L. Olson in 1930. The occupation site was known as "site 100," Santa Cruz Island; the estimated date was between 300 A.D. and 1450 A.D. (Late Horizon). The specimen was riddled with osteolytic lesions of various sizes.

In the past few months the staff of the Department of Anthropology at Florida State University has become aware of four additional cases of possible multiple myeloma in prehistoric Americans. The reports follow.

Sowell Mound

In the summers of 1967 and 1968 the Department of Anthropology at Florida State University conducted salvage excavations of the Sowell Mound, located in Bay County, Fla., near Panama City. More than 20,000 bones and bone fragments were collected. These are believed to be the discards of at least five different archaeological parties, begin-

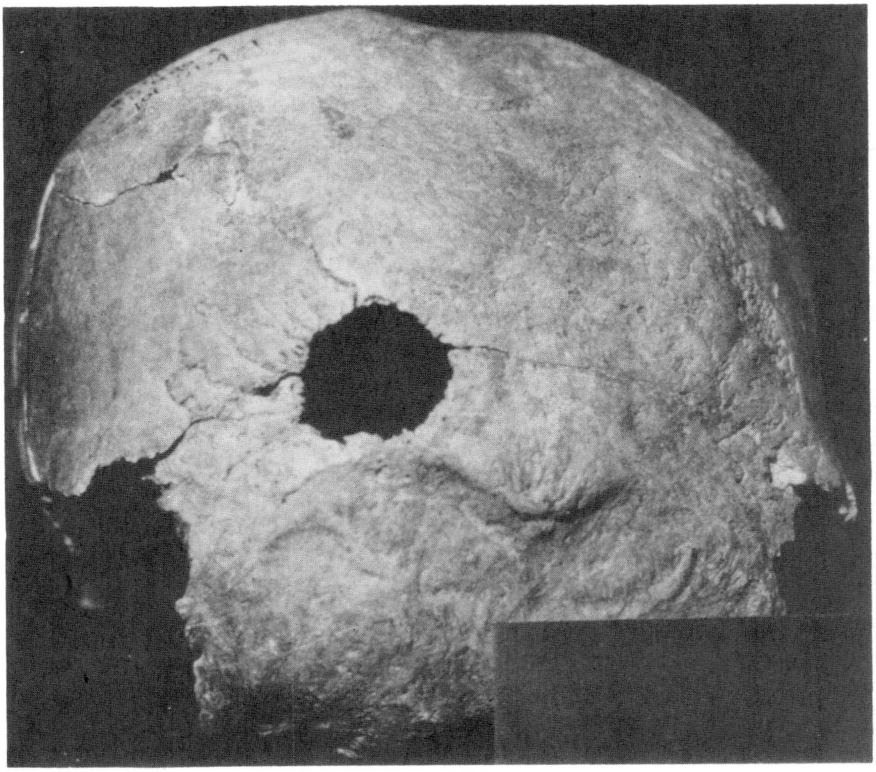

Fig. 1. Sowell Mound skull. Posterior view, showing large myelomatous lesion in occipital bone.

ning with that of Clarence Moore, who apparently investigated and excavated more than 40 Indian sites in the northwest Florida coast for a four-month period during the summer of 1902, including the Sowell excavation.[4] The Indian culture represented is most probably Weeden Island; the approximate dates could range between 500 A.D. and 1200 A.D. One carbon dating of the site was submitted by Lamar Gammon. This was derived from oyster shells; the result was: 610 A.D. ± 125 years.

Among the bone fragments found, it was possible to piece together some 26 cranial vaults. One of these (shown in Figure 1) is Specimen Number 1; it is a cranium without a lower jaw or face. From the orbits

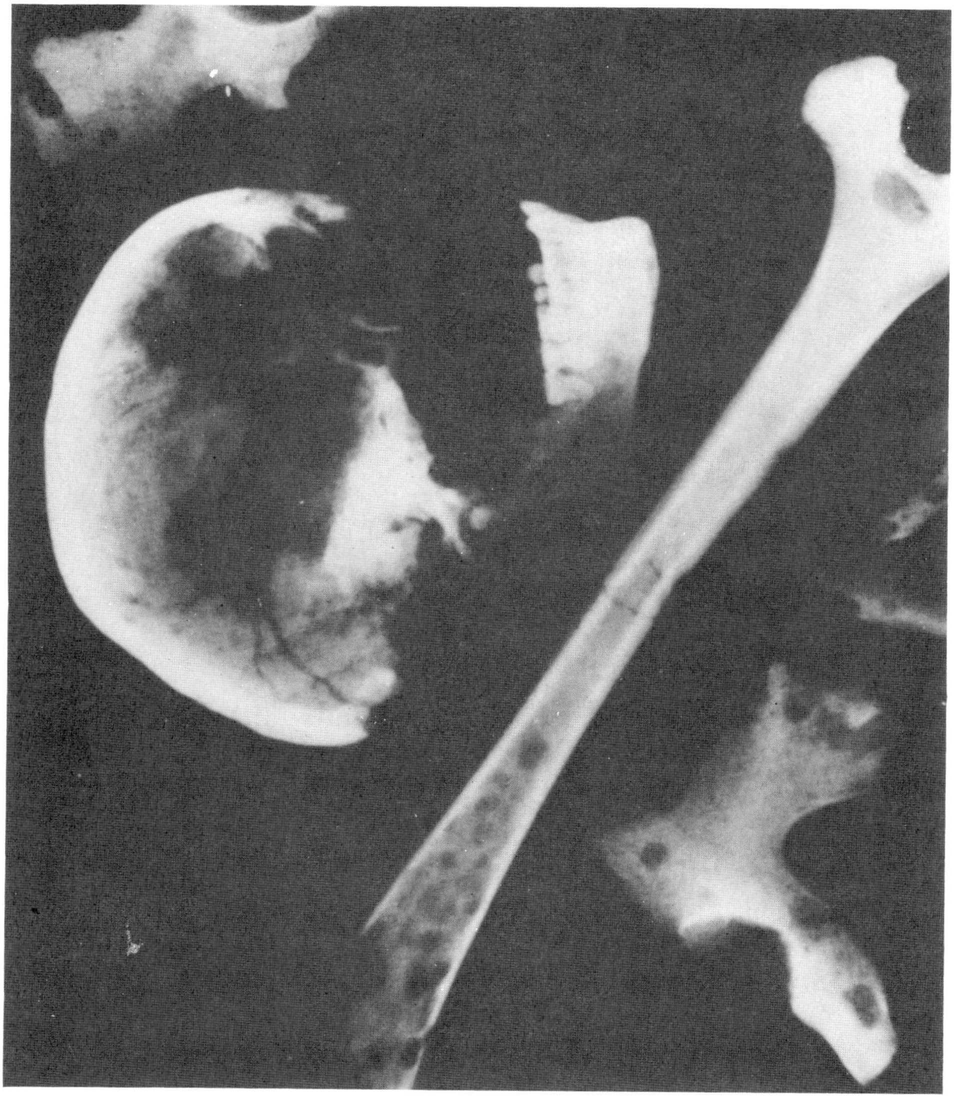

Fig. 2. Calico Hills Burial Number One. X ray showing "punched-out" lesions in all the bones.

and the closure of sutures, it is estimated that the individual was a male aged 45. There is a large circular opening on the left side of the occipital bone, measuring 24 mm. in diameter. The hole penetrates both tables; there is no evidence of reaction in adjacent bone. In the right frontal bone there is a circular lesion 8 mm. in diameter. There is a hole measuring 2 mm. in the posterior portion of the right parietal. Both of these penetrate only the outer table of the skull. On the inside of the cranium there are eight openings which range in size from 1 to 10 mm. in diameter and which penetrate the inner table only. X-ray examinations confirm these findings and reveal in addition many indefinite smaller osteolytic areas, representing tumors that had not yet reached the surface.

In the long-bone fragments there were five specimens showing evidence of cystic lesions which could be myeloma, but there is no way in which these bones could be matched with the pathological cranium. The cranium is definitely osteosclerotic. This is true of many of the other cranial vaults and quite a few long bones. In addition, in more than 1,000 teeth recovered there are no cavities. This suggests that the drinking water may have contained an excess of fluorine. The mound is located in an area occupied by the Naval Coastal Systems Laboratory and has been so altered by recent developments that the source of water used by the aboriginal populations cannot be ascertained.

Calico Hills, Burials One and Two

One of the authors (J.B.), undertook salvage excavations in one of the three Calico Hills mounds which is in Jefferson County, Fla., on the west bank of the Wacissa River. It had been destroyed almost totally by a series of previous excavators. Mr. Bunn recovered the remains of eight burials, one of which was a cremation. All the skeletons were incomplete and had been damaged postmortem. They had to be sprayed many times with Krylon in order to prevent complete disintegration. Two of the eight showed evidence of myeloma.

From pottery previously excavated it could be determined that the culture was probably assignable to Late Swift Creek and Early Weeden Island. An uncertain estimate of occupation date for the mound would be between 200 A.D. and 900 A.D.

Calico Hills Burial Number One (Figure 2) is an incomplete, fragmented female skeleton consisting of a cranial vault, some fragments of

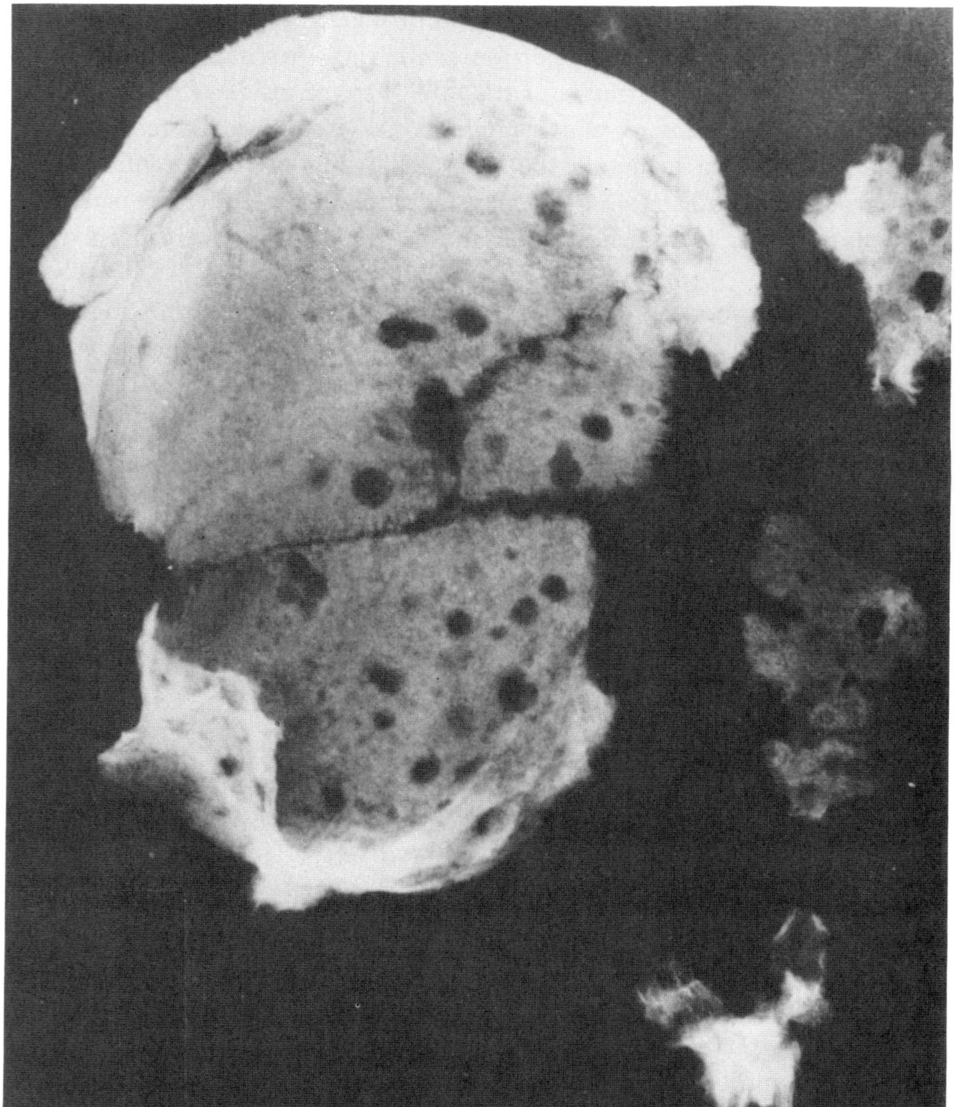

Fig. 3. Calico Hills Burial Number Two. X ray of portion of skull.

skull and face, lower jaw, a few long bones, and some pieces of ribs, vertebrae, scapulae, and pelvis. This skeletal age is about 25 years. Gross and roentgenological examination reveal involvement of all available skeletal elements, with numerous punched-out areas varying in size from 1 to 13 mm. Taking into consideration changes due to postmortem degeneration, the density of the bones appears to be within normal limits.

Calico Hills Burial Number Two (Figures 3 and 4) consists of the top of a skull with part of an occipital bone and one orbit, plus several fragments of skull and facial bones. On the basis of the appearance, this is a female and appears to be young. The age at death might be guessed at 25 years or less. The lesions are numerous. They are discrete, unaccompanied by osseous reaction, and are identical to those seen in Burial Number One.

Mangum Mound

In 1963 the Mangum Mound (Site No. MCL 9) in Claiborne County, Miss., on the Natchez Trace Parkway, was excavated by Charles F. Bohannon for the National Park Service. Approximately 62 skeletons were recovered, boxed, and stored. Anticipating publication of the data, the National Park Service contracted with the Department of Anthropology of Florida State University to do a complete skeletal analysis. When the material was prepared for examination, one specimen was found to be extensively diseased. The site has not been dated accurately; apparently it belongs to the Late Mississippian Period, circa 1300 A.D.

The burial in question, consisting of nearly all the postcranial bones, was in a separate box and was labeled Burial No. 4. Analysis of these bones suggests that this is a female with an approximate age of 35. The field notes said that Burial No. 4 was a group burial representing four separate individuals. In separate bags were portions of four skulls, each labeled Burial No. 4. All four of the portions of the skull were x rayed; only one was definitely female. It was designated Burial No. 4B. Lesions were revealed by the x ray, and resembled those discovered in the postcranial bones. A description of this skeleton and of "B" skull follows:

The postcranial skeleton consists of 21 vertebrae, 34 rib fragments, the pelvis, scapulae, all the long bones, and most of the bones of the hands and feet. The greatest pathological involvement is in the body of

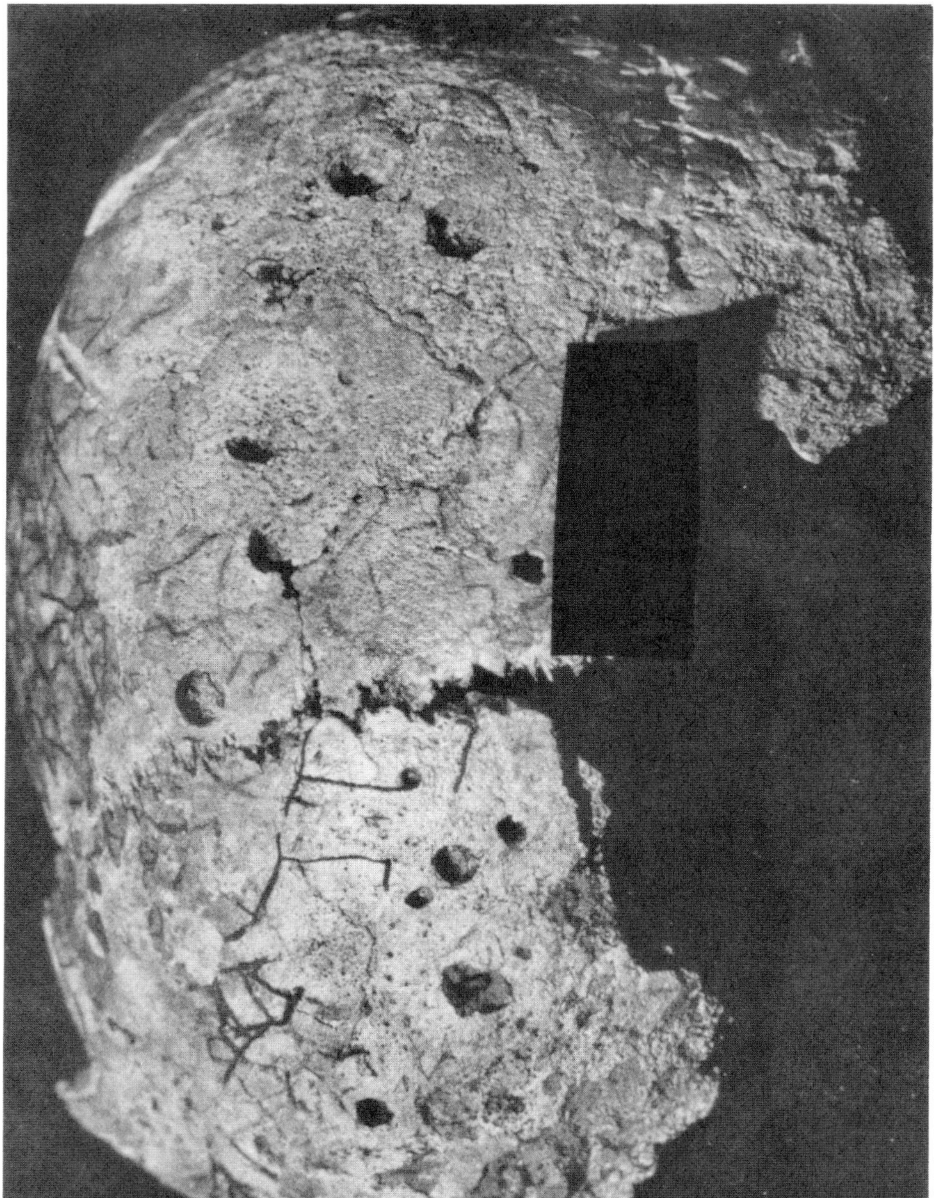

Fig. 4. Calico Hills Burial Number Two. Outer surface of portion of cranium, showing multiple “punched-out” holes penetrating outer table.

the seventh cervical vertebra. This vertebra reveals the presence of seven distinct punched-out areas, whose borders show no bony reaction. The areas vary in size from 2 to 7 mm. X-ray examination demonstrates two additional radiolucent areas not seen on the gross specimen, indicating nonpenetration of bone surface. Other vertebrae showing involvement, detected either by inspection or by roentgen examination, are the cervical 1, 2, and 3; the thoracic 1, 2, 3, 4, 6, 7, 8, 9, 11, and 12; and the lumbar 2, 3, and 5. Other bones affected include 11 of the 34 rib fragments, the pelvis, and the right scapula.

Skull B (Figure 6) is that of a female about 35 years old. The x ray shows many areas of rarefaction of varied size; these appear to be the same as those seen in multiple myeloma. These are confined mostly to the left parietal bone. These punched-out areas are not detected by simple inspection. The surface of the outer table seems normal. On the inside there is a large circular region of roughened superficial erosion. The lesion appears as if the inner table has been almost completely destroyed. The diploic space is exposed, but there is no extension through the outer table. The area of involvement includes the entire left parietal and the posterior portion of the left side of the frontal; there is some extension past the squamous suture onto the left temporal bone. The borders of this erosion are demarcated by a ridge of what appears to be roughened nodular periosteal proliferation. If this is a large myelomatous area, the tumor could have originated in the diploic space and destroyed the inner table completely. One would expect that it would erode the outer table also, but it did not. Another feature not typical of myeloma is the build-up of osseous nodules on the borders. In addition, this skeleton demonstrates marked generalized osteoporosis. The long bones are feather-light.

Comment

Four cases of possible prehistoric multiple myeloma are presented. Two of these, Calico Hills Burial One and Two, are so typical in appearance that the diagnosis of multiple myeloma is fully justified. In the cranial vault from the Sowell Mound the disease is not as extensive as one would expect and the bone shows marked osteosclerosis, but myeloma is still the best possibility. The Mangum Mound Case (Figure 6) is also most likely one of multiple myeloma, but the atypical lesion on the inside of the skull reduces confidence in the diagnosis.

A word should be said about the age. Statistics indicate great rarity

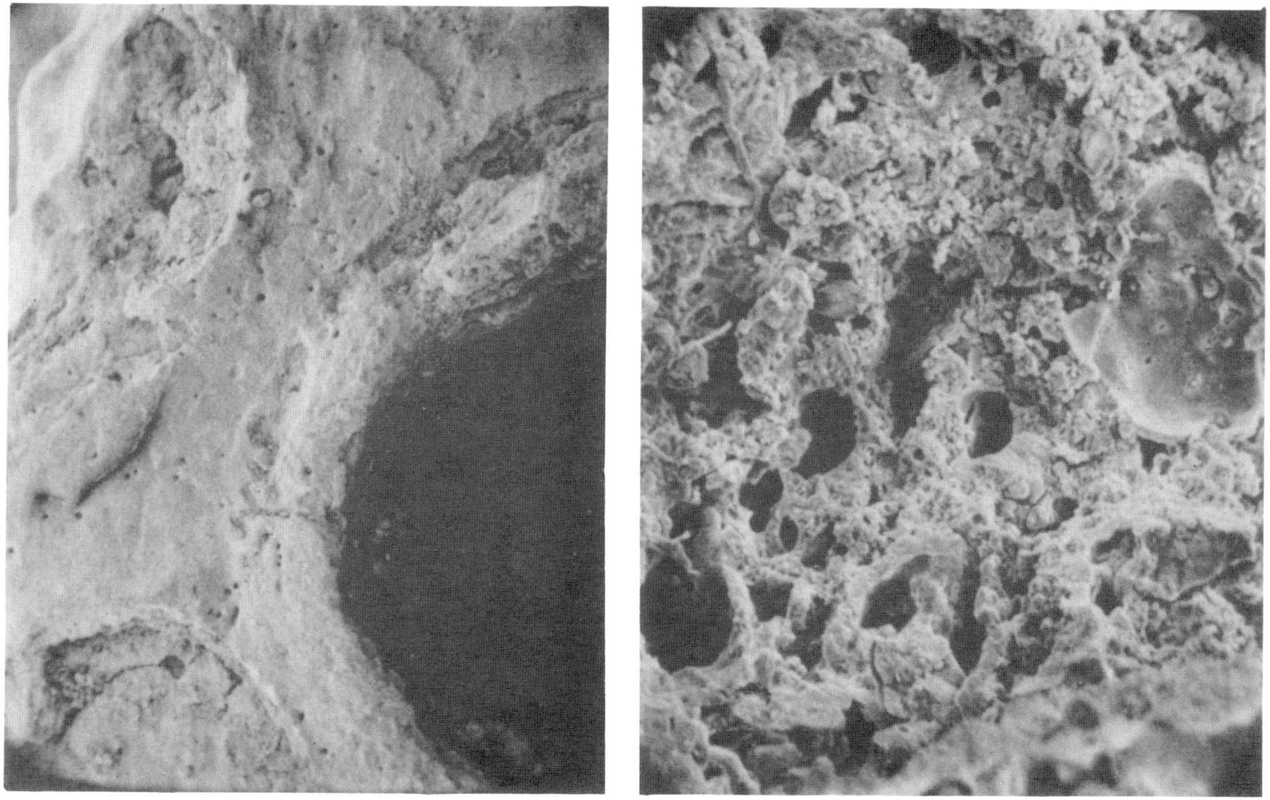

Fig. 5. Calico Hills Burial Number Two. Scanning electron micrographs of bone lesions in skull fragment, demonstrating possible mild osseous condensation at edge of bone lesion. A × 22 and B × 1050. These photographs were made with the scanning electron microscope in the Department of Psycho-Biology, Florida State University; Ron Parker, operator.

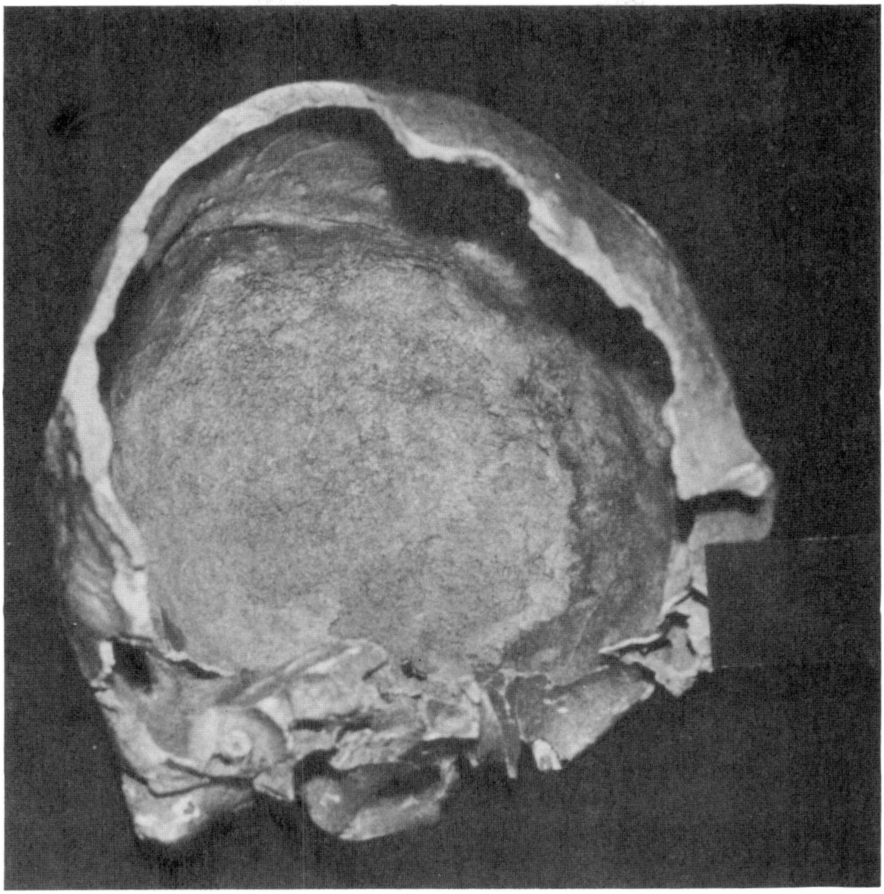

Fig. 6. Mangum Mound Burial. Inside of skull, showing atypical destruction of large portion of inner table.

of myeloma in persons under 40. Three of our four cases were below the age of 40, but one should remember that quoted incidence rates are frequently based on American and European cases and may not necessarily apply to other population groups.

A preliminary report of this paper was read at the annual meeting of the American Association of Physical Anthropology held at Dallas, Tex., in May 1973. After the presentation several physical anthropologists stated that they had seen many similar cases (unreported) in their prehistoric Indian collections. This leads one to the opinion that multiple myeloma in the prehistoric American Indian was not a great rarity.

REFERENCES

1. Brooks, S. T. and Melbye, J.: Skeletal Lesions Suggestive of Pre-Columbian Multiple Myeloma. Technical Series No. 7. In: *Paleopathology* 1, Wade, W. D., editor. Museum of Northern Arizona, Flagstaff, Ariz., 1967, pp. 23-29.
2. Dahlin, D. C.: *Bone Tumors.* Springfield, Ill., Thomas, 1967, pp. 11, 124, 127.
3. Luck, J. V.: *Bone and Joint Diseases.* Springfield, Ill., Thomas, 1950, p. 538.
4. Moore, C. B.: Certain aboriginal remains of the northwest Florida coast. *J. Acad. Nat. Sci. 12:*167-74, 1902.
5. Morse, D.: *Ancient Disease in the Midwest.* Reports of Investigations, No. 1. Springfield, Ill., Illinois State Museum, 1969, p. 144.
6. Ritchie, W. A. and Warren, S. L.: The occurrence of multiple bony lesions suggesting myeloma in the skeleton of a pre-Columbian Indian. *Amer. J. Roentgen. 28:*622-28, 1932.
7. Williams, G. D., Ritchie, W. A., and Titterington, P. F.: Multiple bony lesions suggesting myeloma in a pre-Columbian Indian aged ten years. *Amer. J. Roentgen. 46:*351-55, 1941.

MEDICAL NUMISMATICS: A DENARIUS COMMEMORATING ROME'S FIRST DOCTOR, ARCAGATHUS (219 B.C.)*

ADRIAN W. ZORGNIOTTI

Clinical Associate Professor of Medicine
Principal Lecturer, History of Medicine
New York University School of Medicine, New York, N. Y.

PLINY, in his *Natural History*,[4] quotes Cassius Hemina as saying that the first doctor (*medicus*) to come to Rome was Arcagathus, who arrived from the Greek Peloponnese in 219 B.C. and was treated with extraordinary kindness. Arcagathus was accorded the rights of citizenship (*ius Quiritium*). With public monies a medical shop (*taberna*) was purchased for his use at the Acilia Cross Roads. Prior to this, Rome had no physicians and home remedies were used.

Because he was an expert wound surgeon (*vulnerarius*), he immediately became popular. This happy state did not last. Arcagathus' vigorous use of the knife and cautery soon led to his being called executioner (*carnifex*). The cause of medicine appears to have been set back by public revulsion to his methods. In fact, about 100 years elapsed before we hear that another Greek physician (Asclepiades of Bithynia, ca. 100 B.C.) had taken up residence in Rome.

The coin we are examining, a denarius of the Acilia gens (family), was struck in Rome in 54 B.C. (see figure). The obverse shows the goddess Salus wearing a laurel crown, earrings, and a *torque* (necklace). Varro[5] tells us that Salus was of Sabine origin. Transplanted to Rome, she was associated with the general well-being (*salus publica*). In 302 B.C. a temple in her honor was erected near the Quirinal Hill by C. Junius Bubulcus.[6] During the late Republic, Salus became identified with her Greek counterpart Hygeia. With this came a change in meaning to the well-being of the emperor (*salus Augusta*), for whom annual prayers and vows (*vota*) were offered. Behind the head of the goddess appears the inscription SALUTIS.[1]

The reverse of the coin represents a statue of Salus which can, with

*Three notes on medical numismatics by the editor in chief of the *Bulletin* have appeared in previous issues: Medical numismatic notes I. *Bull. N.Y. Acad. Med. 45*:512-14, 1969; Medical numismatic notes II. The Montrose lunatic hospital. *Bull. N.Y. Acad. Med. 45*:637-39, 1969; and Medical numismatic notes III. The filtering-stone warehouse. *Bull. N.Y. Acad. Med. 45*:1124-25, 1969.

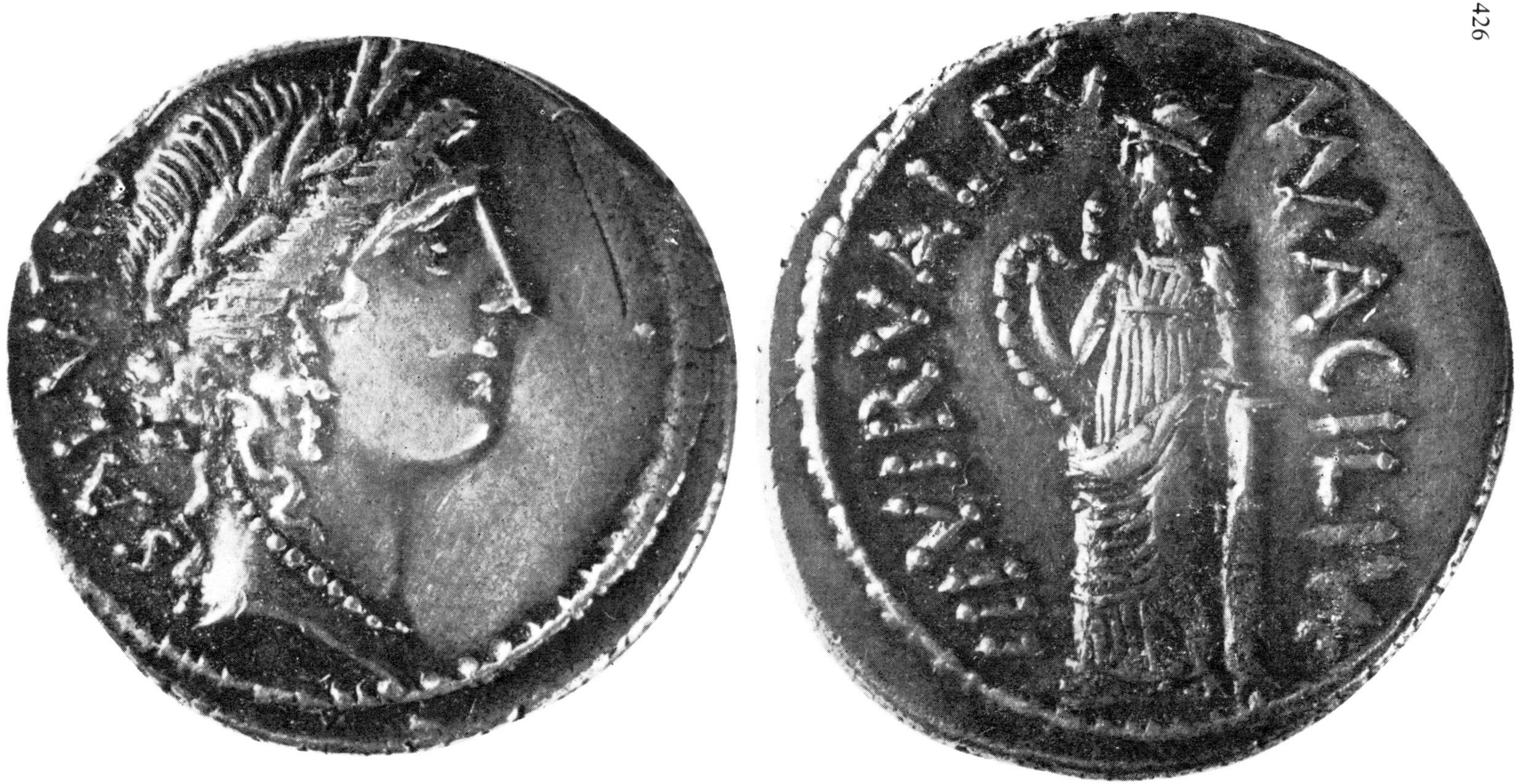

Roman denarius struck in 54 B.C. by a member of the Acilia family. Both sides depict the goddess Salus and commemorate the first doctor to come to Rome in 219 B.C. Obverse; reverse.

reasonable certainty, be identified according to Pliny[8] as the work of the Greek sculptor Niceratus; the statue stood in the Temple of Concord. Salus is depicted leaning on a column and holding a serpent in her right hand. The inscription is of considerable interest and reads M·ACILIUS III·VIR VALETV. It refers to the moneyer, Manius Acilius Glabrio, who became proconsul to Africa under Augustus. The abbreviation III·VIR refers to the board of three directors of the mint (*tresviri*) of which he was a member. It was usual for young men beginning their public careers to be given these posts. The tresviri were permitted considerable latitude in selecting the subject matter of the money they issued.[2] Hence it was usual to recall events associated with the family name—in this case, a contribution to the health and welfare of Rome.[3] VALETV appears to be an abbreviation for *valetudo* and is the word which most means health in the sense of freedom from disease. However, in certain contexts it can also mean ill health, in fact, military hospitals were called *valetudinaria*.

As Roman coins go, this one is unusually well documented. Although no direct reference exists in ancient writings to a connection between this coin and the ill-fated Arcagathus (did he go back to Greece?), there is enough information to support this supposition.

The coin is included in the numismatic collection of the New York Academy of Medicine, in the collection of the Numismatic Society, New York, N.Y., and in my private collection.

NOTES AND REFERENCES

1. Stevenson[7] lists various personifications: *Salus, Salus Augusta, Salus Exerciti, Salus Generis Humani, Salus Provinciarum,* etc. From this and other evidence we can surmise that Salus personified the broader connotation of welfare rather than "health" as we know it. The use of the word SALUTIS in the inscription is almost entirely restricted to coins of the *Acilia Gens*. On other coins (mainly of the empire) where Salus is depicted, the inscription reads SALUS.
2. The Romans were, perhaps, the most expert in understanding and utilizing the propaganda value of coins. Augustus has been shown by recent scholarship to have been unusually skillful at manipulating opinion, after the Battle of Actium and throughout his reign, by means of coins which had a vast circulation.
3. Babelon,[9] the outstanding expert on Roman republican coinage, confirms the prevalent opinion that the Acilia claimed to have introduced medicine to Rome and that they derived their name from the Greek ἀχέομαι, to heal.

4. Pliny: *Natural History,* XXIX, 6.
5. Varro: *On the Latin Language,* V, 74.
6. Livy: Book IX, 34.
7. Stevenson, S.M.: *Dictionary of Roman Coins*. London, 1889, pp. 713-16.
8. Pliny: *Natural History,* XXV, 4.
9. Babelon, E.: *Description Historique et Chronologique des Monnaies de la République Romaine,* vol. 1, pp. 100-07. Paris, 1885-1886. Reissued. Bologna, Forni, 1963.

MEDICAL NUMISMATIC NOTES, XV: SOME MEDICAL ASPECTS OF GREEK AND ROMAN COINS*

WILLIAM K. BEATTY

Librarian and Professor of Medical Bibliography
Northwestern University Medical School
Chicago, Ill.

SINCE any discussion of Greek and Roman medicine should open with a bow to Hippocrates or Galen it would be fitting to begin this essay with the statement that Galen was the first to describe coin lesions of the lungs. Unfortunately, because of the medium required for the demonstration of such lesions, not even the remarkable extensibility of lung tissue would cover such an anachronism.

Greek and Roman coins demonstrate a great variety of medical and medically related subjects. Hippocrates, strange as it may seem, is not a popular subject. He appears on few coins, one of the more fitting examples being a Coan coin of 55 B.C.[8-24†] Much better off is the god of medicine, Aesculapius, who is represented in many forms on a large number of coins from a broad variety of cities, states, and regions.

Before becoming a divinity Aesculapius achieved great fame as a practicing physician. Ultimately he suffered an attack of *hubris*, a condition not unknown among medical men down through the centuries, and was led into the great error of raising one of his patients from the dead. Retaliation was quick and Olympian. Pluto, god of the underworld, who was the immediate loser in this negative population growth, protested at once to his superior brother, Zeus. Zeus responded by hurling a low and inside thunderbolt at Aesculapius who, as a result, suffered for the rest of his life from a shortened leg. This condition is shown on a bronze coin from Hadrianapolis minted during the reign of Alexander Severus (222-235 A.D.).[2-4]

The prescription for raising a patient from the dead at that time consisted of a potion which had Gorgonian blood as its main compo-

*Presented at a meeting of the Israel Numismatic Society of Illinois, held in Skokie, Ill., March 28, 1973.

†Reference superscripts are composed in most cases of the number of the reference joined by a hyphen to the number of the figure in that reference work.

nent. The face of Medusa, the most famous of the three sisters, is depicted as almost overflowing a striking coin.[8-10] Unhappily the useful fluid involved is no longer obtainable either generically or under the original label.

Aesculapius usually appears in the traditional form of a distinguished middle-aged or elderly individual. A few examples of him as a young man exist, a good one being on a tetradrachm from Zakynthos.[2-6] The god of medicine achieved his greatest popularity on coins during the reigns of Commodus (180-192 A.D.) and Caracalla (211-217 A.D.). If Aesculapius had had his choice of emperors he probably would have disapproved of both.

Although most of the members of Aesculapius' family are less famous than he, several appear on coins. His wife, Epione, is shown on an early coin,[8-13] on which she is presumably pouring medicine from a vial into a mixing bowl. An alternative suggestion, which takes into account her husband's many travels and great involvement in cultic activities, is that she is mixing herself a good strong drink.

The best known younger member of the family is a daughter, Hygeia. She usually appears with her father (e.g., a bronze coin[2-17] from Hadrianapolis at the time of Antoninus Pius, 138-161 A.D.). The Romans had a happy knack for bringing their gods down to earth by combining representations of deities and earthly rulers. A bronze coin[2-31] from Pergamon (165 A.D.) shows Marcus Aurelius as Aesculapius and his wife Faustina as not Epione, but Hygeia.

A lesser-known but intriguing member of the family is Telesphoros, who started out as a local divinity around Pergamon and later became assimilated as a son of Aesculapius. The Greek word, telesphoreo, has the basic meaning of bringing to a head, completing; hence it easily came to include the concept of convalescence. Telesphoros, therefore, was the divinity of convalescence, the son who completed the work of his father, the god of medicine. Telesphoros (Figure 1) is easily identified by his pointed mantle and generally hooded demeanor. He appears on Pergamene coins from the time of Hadrian (117-138 A.D.), and his circulation was substantially increased in the third century when he received credit for ending an outbreak of pestilence in Athens. A charming brother-and-sister combination, Hygeia and Telesphoros, appear on a bronze coin[2-20] from Hierapolis. Other groupings of members of the family are also extant.

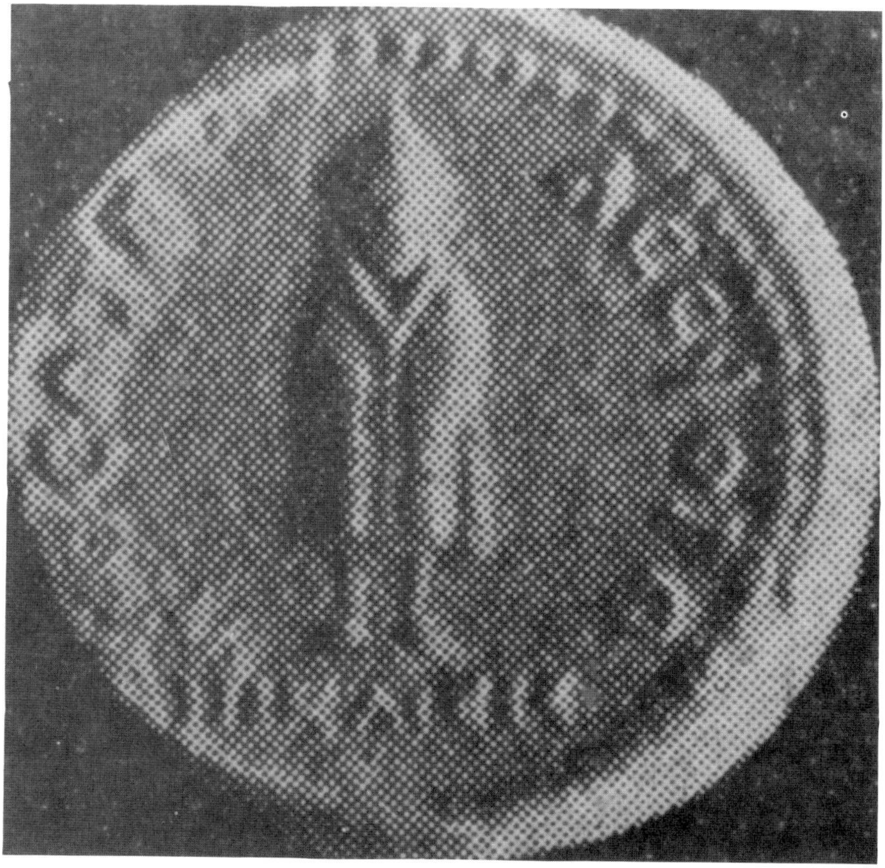

Fig. 1. Telesphoros, an assimilated son of Aesculapius, who served as the divinity of convalescence. Reproduced by permission from Bernhard, O.: Ueber Heilgötter auf Griechischen und Römischen Münzen. *Schweiz. Med. Wschr.* *55*:258-64, 1925, Figure 18 (a bronze coin from Nicaea).

In 214 A.D. Caracalla made a state visit to Pergamon, and a coin[8-25] of that time shows the emperor saluting the serpent of Aesculapius with Telesphoros looking on, mantled in appropriate dignity. State visits are usually processions of solemn character. However, Caracalla's trip to Pergamon loses a little of this atmosphere according to one commentator who stated that the emperor's real motive was a last-ditch effort to free himself from one of the venereal diseases.

Greek and Roman divinities are brought together on a Roman gold coin (200 A.D.) that portrays both Aesculapius and Salus.[14-2] Salus, as an indigenous Roman goddess of health, plays an interesting role in the assimilation of medical aspects of the two civilizations. A silver denarius[3-1] of the Roman Republic has Salus on the obverse and Valetudo on the reverse. Valetudo was the Roman counterpart of Hygeia, but she gradually declined as Salus increased her scope and eventually took over related attributes, including care of the Aesculapian serpent.

Salus was a popular divinity for many years. Livia, the wife of Augustus, appeared on a bronze coin[2-30] as Salus. One of the more fascinating numismatic appearances she made was in the bisexual form of a gynecomastic Aesculapius on a coin[7-9] minted about 260 A.D.

Occasionally one coin will include several medical aspects. Such a coin[8-38] from Berytus in Phoenicia shows Eshmun-Aesculapius, a transitional compound of the Phoenician and Greek divinities. Not only are these two strands woven together, but Aesculapius is shown wearing the Phrygian cap, which calls to mind the deformity of the gallbladder that has been given this name.

Many divine attributes appear on coins. The Aesculapian staff is depicted in a wide variety of shapes and situations; the first known Aesculapian coin,[8-14] minted at Larissa between 450 and 400 B.C., shows the staff. The city of Cos eventually took over the Aesculapian staff as its municipal device. Serpents are not always creeping creatures; a copper coin[2-9] from Nicaea demonstrates a flying staff, perhaps the symbol of an early disaster relief team. Another serpent in a hurry is shown on horseback on a coin[1-161] of the time of Caracalla from Lydian Philadelphia (Figure 2).

The Aesculapian serpent was a powerful symbol of medical success, and at least one con man took advantage of this symbolism. Alexandros of Abonuteichos had domesticated a large serpent, for which he designed a cloth head with movable jaws.[22] The serpent, professionally known as Glycon, was supposedly a reincarnation of Aesculapius himself. Upon receipt of fitting sums of acceptable coins Glycon would make oracular statements in response to his questioners. A Nicomedian copper coin (217 A.D.) depicts this human-headed Aesculapian serpent.[1-82]

The Roman Senate was usually a practical body, and when Rome suffered from a severe plague in 291 B.C. the Senate sent a band of

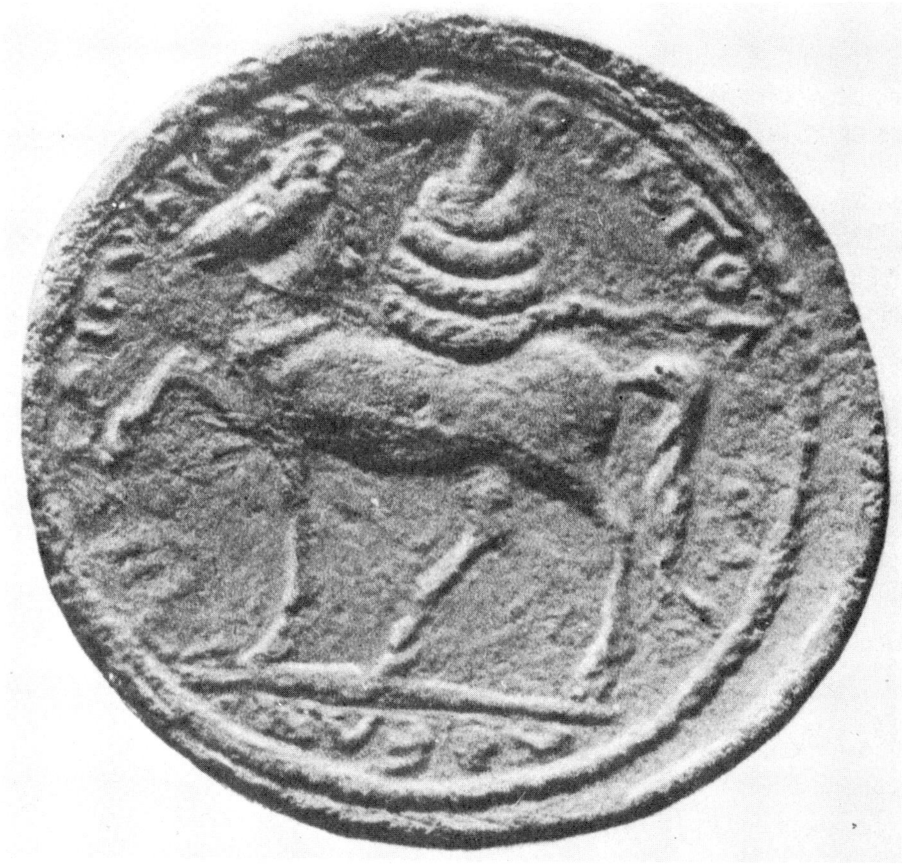

Fig. 2. An Aesculapian serpent moving a little more quickly than usual. Reproduced by permission from Bernhard, O.: *Griechische und Römische Münzbilder in ihren Beziehungen zur Geschichte der Medizin*. Zürich, Füssli, 1926, Figure 161.

nine men to Epidaurus to request aid from one of the most powerful sources of the Aesculapian cult. The temple priests assigned one of the Aesculapian serpents to the Roman group, and all made the long trip back on shipboard. As the ship was moving up the Tiber the serpent snaked overboard, swam to a nearby island, and moved ashore. A temple was built on the spot, and the remains can still be seen.[11, 7] A coin[20-54] from the time of Antoninus Pius shows this historic scene in some detail (Figure 3). The galley is seen approaching two arches of the Pons

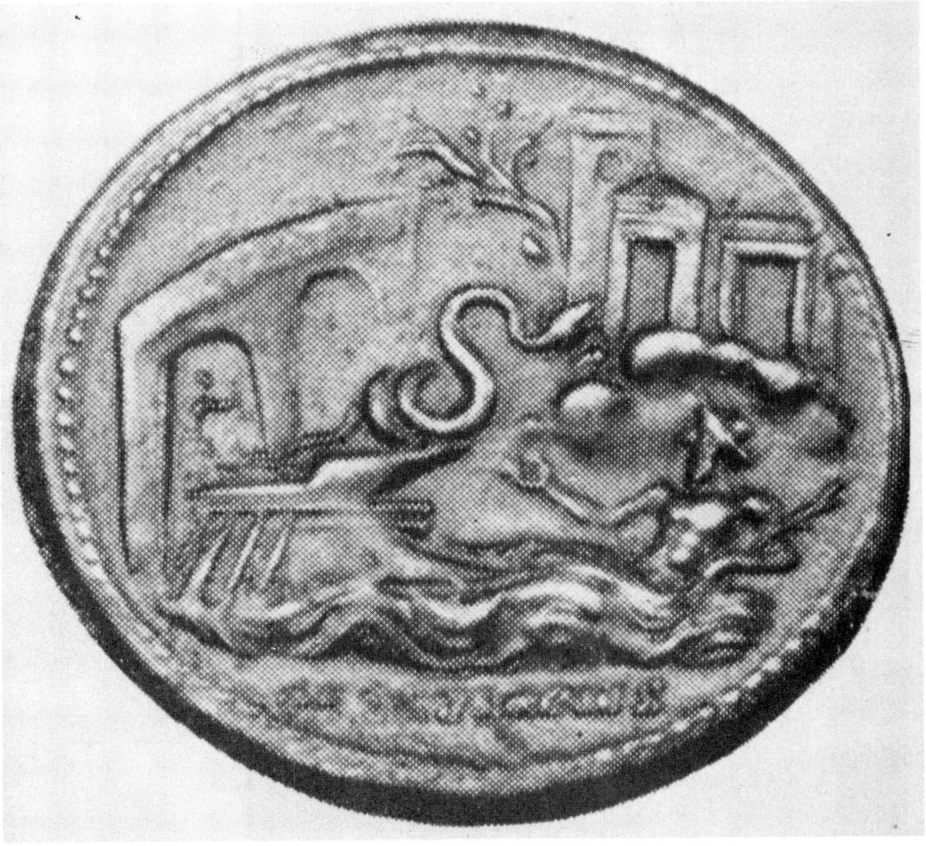

Fig. 3. An Aesculapian serpent arriving at Rome during the plague of 291 B.C. This is one of the most attractive ancient coins with medical interest. Reproduced by permission from Sutherland, C. H. V.: *Art in Coinage: The Aesthetics of Money from Greece to the Present Day*. New York, Philosophical Library, 1956, Figure 54.

Fabricius (now the Ponte Quattro Capi); the erect serpent is on the prow, the god of the Tiber is comfortably reclining and making welcoming gestures, and the Aventine Hill looms in the background. This is a beautiful example of the coin-designer's art.

When Aesculapius and his agents were not traveling they usually dwelt in substantial and often impressive buildings. A bronze coin[2-24] of Nikopolis (c. 230 A.D.) exhibits one of these temples, and a Pergamene coin[8-17] shows three different varieties (Figure 4). These Aesculapian temples often served as rudimentary medical schools. It is ironic in this time of staggering cuts in federal funds for medical educa-

Fig. 4. Three Aesculapian temples on a coin from Pergamon. Reproduced by permission from Hart, G.: Ancient coins and medicine. *Canad. Med. Ass. J.* *94*:77-89, 1966, Figure 17(c).

tion to see a medical school depicted on a coin. It would be far better to have the coins in the schools rather than the schools on the coins.

The temples had their secret rooms and areas, which were usually kept locked. Symbolic keys were exhibited in processions honoring Aesculapius, and at least one of these keys was pictured on a coin.[8-18]

As the religious and political tides of the Roman Empire ebbed and flowed the Aesculapian staff accordingly rose and fell. It reached its nadir at the time of Constantine the Great on a coin[8-28] from Constantinople that pictures a Christian cross above a Roman standard; both rest on a low-lying serpent.

On a Pergamene coin [8-26] the staff and snake share the scene with a mouse. This is not as odd as it might seem on first glance when it is recalled that the Greeks and Romans relied heavily on imported grain for their food supply. Mice ate grain, dearth of grain often led to famine, and famines were frequently accompanied by diseases. The mouse thus became associated with Apollo Smintheus, as readers of the Iliad will recall. A fifth century B.C. coin[17-9] from Selinus in Sicily shows Apollo and Diana in a chariot; Apollo is aiming his bow and arrow at the spirit of the plague. The other side of this coin shows the god of the river Selinus bearing a thank offering to Aesculapius. This coin commemorates the project sponored by Empedocles to drain a large swamp by combining two rivers (one of which was the Selinus) and to strike a blow against the endemic malaria.

Coins were used not only to memorialize great acts by rulers but also to commemorate familial productivity. Marcus Aurelius had a silver denarius struck depicting his wife, Faustina, on one side,[21-50] and their two children on the other.[21-49] Faustina was a productive empress and Marcus Aurelius was a bit of a denarius-pincher, and this combination later produced a reminting of the same obverse with its striking portrait of Faustina but with a new reverse,[21-50] which now showed four children in charge of a suitably medical demigoddess, Fecunditas.

In addition to divine and human creatures, Greek and Roman coins also show medical equipment. Cupping glasses appear on several coins,[2-14] usually with either Aesculapius or Telesphoros.

Diseases were occasionally commemorated, and several examples date from the brief reign of Valerian (250-254 A.D.). There is some doubt about the real disease which the Romans then called the Cyprianic pest, but the best guess seems to be typhus.[15] The coins show Apollo holding a laurel branch in his right hand.

Many medical plants are depicted on ancient coins. Probably the most mysterious of these is silphium, a plant that was the numismatic trademark of Cyrene for three and a half centuries. Theophrastus wrote that silphium popped up de novo after a heavy thunderstorm, but there is good evidence that it was known before his time. Some authorities believe that silphium either was, or was closely related to, *Ferula tingitana*, in which case it still crops up in North Africa.

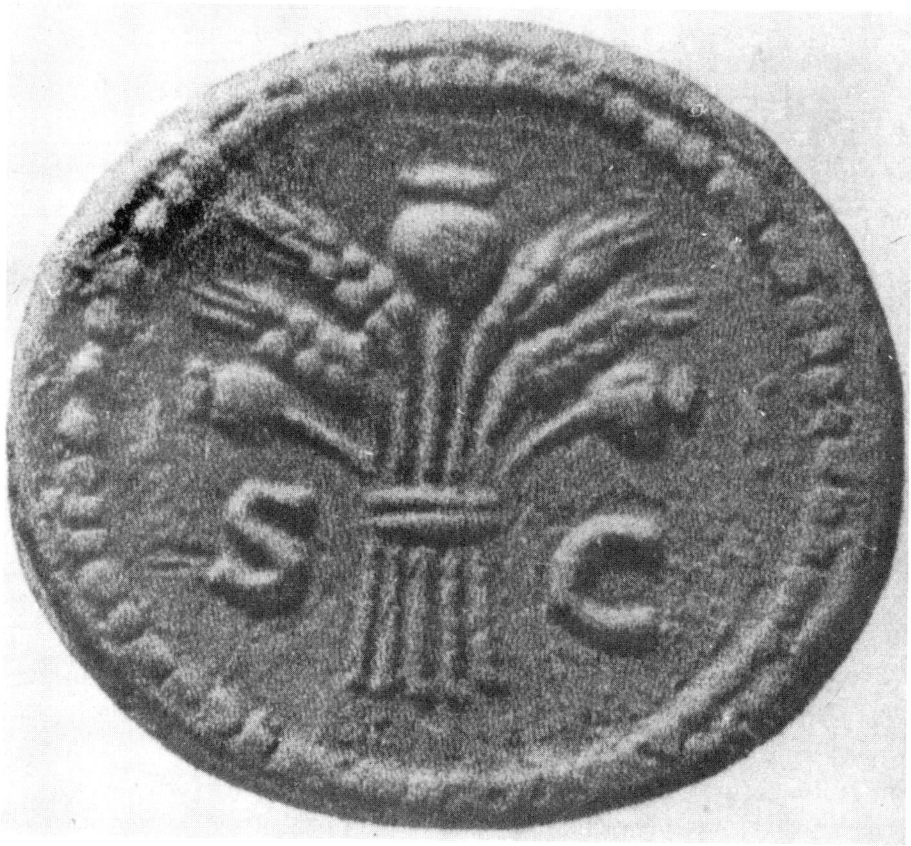

Fig. 5. Poppies had many medicinal uses. This combination of poppy heads and wheat ears is a charming mixture. Reproduced by permission from Bernhard, O.: *Griechische und Römische Münzbilder in ihren Beziehungen zur Geschichte der medizin.* Zurich, Füssli, 1926, Figure 225.

Cyrene used large quantities of silphium for both medicinal and condiment purposes. Gemmill has written informatively and enjoyably on the subject[5, 6] The plant first appeared on a Cyrenean coin about 600 B.C., and by the middle of the sixth century it had become solidly established on the country's coins.[8-30] In fact, the Cyreneans may have gone overboard on their promotion of silphium. A visitor to the area, Antiphanes, wrote (after he had left): "I want to say good-bye to Cyrene, to all horses, silphium, chariots, silphium stalks, steeple-chasers, silphium leaves, fevers, and silphium juice."

Hellebore is shown on a coin[8-33] from Pherae, and a pomegranate appears on a silver stater[1-227] from Side in Pamphylia. The pomegranate was used as a vermifuge and to assuage a variety of female pains. In addition to the medicinal appeal of this plant there is a typically Hellenic twist in that the Greek word for pomegranate was "sida."

The lily, useful to counteract burns, snake bites, and menstrual pains, is shown on a copper coin[1-228] from Syria. The poppy shows up several times, and may have created a problem in determining which side of the coin was "heads." An attractive design combining three poppy heads and four ears of wheat is depicted on a bronze coin[1-225] from the reign of Domitian (Figure 5).

In addition to official coins, a variety of unofficial coin-shaped items are pertinent to this subject. These tesserae were often worn around the neck to ward off diseases or, if put on too late, to cure them. An interesting example[16-1] from Ephesos (first century A.D.) shows the deer of Artemis in her role as guardian of health. The fact that so few tesserae still exist may be assigned to the same cause that makes our western pioneers' household "remedy books" so rare—they were used to the point of disintegration.

As a final example of this brief survey of the medical aspects of Greek and Roman coins may be cited a fascinating series discovered and described by Dr. Gerald D. Hart.[9] Parthia fought with Greeks and Romans for so many years that she can legitimately be included in a discussion of those two civilizations. For several centuries the kings of Parthia suffered from a small hereditary tumor which Dr. Hart suggests was probably a trichoepithelioma. Dr. Hart illustrated several examples of this tumor from current case histories, and compared the appearances of the tumor on the coins with those in current photographs. The results are striking. One of the monarchs, Volagases II (77-147 A.D.), was apparently vainer than the others. The first coins issued with his portrait show the usual tumor, but later issues have the tumor obscured by a conveniently handsome curl. If medicine concerns itself with both the abnormal and the normal here is a splendid numismatic example of a delightfully normal condition.

The references appended to this review have been selected both for their information and to provide material for those who would like to go further into this fascinating field.

REFERENCES

1. Bernhard, O.: *Griechische und Römische Münzbilder in ihren Beziehungen zur Geschichte der Medizin.* Zürich, Füssli, 1926.
2. Bernhard, O.: Ueber Heilgötter auf Griechischen und Römischen Münzen. *Schweiz. Med. Wschr. 55*:258-64, 1925.
3. Boyce, A. A.: Salus and Valetudo. *J. Hist. Med. 14*:79-81, 1959.
4. Foy-Vaillant, J.: *Numismata Imperatorum Romanorum.* Paris, Jombert, 1692.
5. Gemmill, C. L.: Medical numismatic notes, VIII: Coins of Cyrene. *Bull. N.Y. Acad. Med. 49*:81-84, 1973.
6. Gemmill, C. L.: Silphium. *Bull. Hist. Med. 40*:295-313, 1966.
7. Gluckman, L.: The physician and numismatist. *New Zeal. Med. J. 64*:156-61, 1965.
8. Hart, G. D.: Ancient coins and medicine. *Canad. Med. Assoc. J. 94*:77-89, 1966.
9. Hart, G. D.: Trichoepithelioma and the Kings of ancient Parthia. *Canad. Med. Assoc. J. 94*:547-49, 1966.
10. Jarcho, S.: Medical numismatic notes, VII: Mithridates IV. *Bull. N.Y. Acad. Med. 48*:1059-64, 1972.
11. Kerenyi, K.: *Asklepios: Archetypal Image of the Physician's Existence.* New York, Pantheon, 1959.
12. Klawans, Z. H.: *An Outline of Ancient Greek Coins.* Racine, Wis., Whitman, 1959.
13. Laing, L. R.: *Coins and Archaeology.* New York, Schocken, 1970.
14. McNaught, J. B.: Physicians on coins. *Stanford Med. Bull. 2*:78-85, 1944-1945.
15. Mallory, W. J.: Coins and medals in medicine. *Med. Rec. 90*:495-98, 1916.
16. Obermajer, J.: The tesserae of Ephesos in the history of medicine. *Med. Hist. 12*:292-94, 1968.
17. Reich, J.: Medizinische Münzen und Medaillen. *Deutsch. Med. Wschr. 50*: 1657-59, 1924.
18. Schouten, J.: *The Rod and Serpent of Asklepios, Symbol of Medicine.* Amsterdam, Elsevier, 1967.
19. Storer, H. R.: *Medicina in Nummis,* Storer, M., editor. Boston, Wright & Potter, 1931.
20. Sutherland, C. H. V.: *Art in Coinage: The Aesthetics of Money from Greece to the Present Day.* New York, Philosophical Library, 1956.
21. Wear, T. G.: *Ancient Coins.* Garden City, N.Y., Doubleday, 1965.
22. Zorgniotti, A. W.: Alexander of Abonoteichus: False priest of Asclepius. *J.A.M.A. 224*:87-89, 1973.
23. Zorgniotti, A. W.: Medical numismatics: A denarius commemorating Rome's first doctor, Arcagathus (219 B.C.). *Bull. N.Y. Acad. Med. 46*:448-50, 1970.

INDEX